SURGICAL RECALL
Ninth Edition

SURGICAL RECALL
Ninth Edition

Recall Series Editor and Senior Editor

Lorne H. Blackbourne, MD, FACS
Trauma, Surgical Critical Care
Houston, Texas

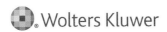
. Wolters Kluwer

Philadelphia • Baltimore • New York • London
Buenos Aires • Hong Kong • Sydney • Tokyo

Not authorised for sale in United States, Canada, Australia, New Zealand, Puerto Rico, and U.S. Virgin Islands.

Acquisitions Editor: Matt Hauber
Development Editors: Andrea Vosburgh, Kelly Horvath
Editorial Coordinator: Tim Rinehart
Marketing Manager: Phyllis Hitner
Production Project Manager: Barton Dudlick
Design Coordinator: Stephen Druding
Art Director, Illustration: Jennifer Clements
Manufacturing Coordinator: Margie Orzech
Prepress Vendor: Aptara, Inc.

Ninth Edition

9 8 7 6 5 4 3 2

Printed in Singapore

Library of Congress Cataloging-in-Publication Data

Names: Blackbourne, Lorne H., editor.
Title: Surgical recall / Recall series editor and senior editor, Lorne H.
  Blackbourne.
Other titles: Recall series.
Description: 9th edition. | Philadelphia, PA : Wolters Kluwer, [2022] |
  Series: Recall series | Includes bibliographical references and index.
Identifiers: LCCN 2020041909 | ISBN 9781975152949 (paperback)
Subjects: MESH: Surgical Procedures, Operative | Examination Questions
Classification: LCC RD37.2 | NLM WO 18.2 | DDC 617.0076–dc23
LC record available at https://lccn.loc.gov/2020041909

shop.lww.com

MKO322

Dedication

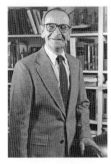

This book is dedicated to the memory of Leslie E. Rudolf, Professor of Surgery and Vice-Chairman of the Department of Surgery at the University of Virginia. Dr. Rudolf was born on November 12, 1927, in New Rochelle, New York. He served in the U.S. Army Counter Intelligence Corps in Europe after World War II.

He graduated from Union College in 1951 and attended Cornell Medical College, where he graduated in 1955. He then entered his surgical residency at Peter Brigham Hospital in Boston, Massachusetts, and completed his residency there, serving as Chief Resident Surgeon in 1961.

Dr. Rudolf came to Charlottesville, Virginia as an Assistant Professor of Surgery in 1963. He rapidly rose through the ranks, becoming Professor of Surgery and Vice-Chairman of the Department in 1974 and a Markle Scholar in Academic Medicine from 1966 until 1971. His research interests included organ and tissue transplantation and preservation. Dr. Rudolf was instrumental in initiating the Kidney Transplant Program at the University of Virginia Health Sciences Center. His active involvement in service to the Charlottesville community is particularly exemplified by his early work with the Charlottesville/Albemarle Rescue Squad, and he received the Governor's Citation for the Commonwealth of Virginia Emergency Medical Services in 1980.

His colleagues at the University of Virginia Health Sciences Center, including faculty and residents, recognized his keen interests in teaching medical students, evaluating and teaching residents, and helping the young surgical faculty. He took a serious interest in medical student education, and he would have strongly approved of this teaching manual, affectionately known as the "Rudolf" guide, as an extension of ward rounds and textbook reading.

In addition to his distinguished academic accomplishments, Dr. Rudolf was a talented person with many diverse scholarly pursuits and hobbies. His advice and counsel on topics ranging from Chinese cooking to orchid raising were sought by a wide spectrum of friends and admirers.

This book is a logical extension of Dr. Rudolf's interests in teaching. No one book, operation, or set of rounds can begin to answer all questions of surgical disease processes; however, in a constellation of learning endeavors, this effort would certainly have pleased him.

John B. Hanks, MD
Professor of Surgery
University of Virginia
Charlottesville, Virginia

Editors

SENIOR EDITOR
Lorne H. Blackbourne, MD, FACS
Trauma, Surgical Critical Care
Houston, Texas

EDITORS
Roland Paquette, PA-C
Assistant Professor/Clinical Associate
Academic Coordinator
Department of Physician
    Assistant Studies
UT Health San Antonio
San Antonio, Texas

M. Azfar, MD, FRCSEd, FACS
Consultant Surgeon, HOD General
    Surgery and Acting Chief of
    Service, Al Rahba Hospital
President, ACS UAE Chapter
Abu Dhabi, UAE

Paul B. Allen Sr., DSc, MPAS, PA-C
Associate Professor, Program Director
    and Chair
Department of Physician Assistant
    Studies
School of Health Professions
University of Texas Health Science
    Center
San Antonio, Texas

Seeyuen J. Lee, MD, MPH, FACS
Associate Program Director
Advanced GI/Minimally Invasive
    Surgery Fellowship
Houston, Texas

Shiree A. Berry, MD, FACS
Trauma and Acute Care Surgeon
Regional Trauma Medical Director
Envision Surgical Services
Houston, Texas

Joshua Slaven, CRNA
Chief CRNA
Houston Northwest Medical Center
Houston, Texas

Samer ElFallal, DO
Chief of Neurosurgery
HCA Houston Healthcare Northwest
Houston, Texas

Matt Carrick, MD, FACS
Trauma Medical Director
Medical City Plano
CMO and Senior Vice President
Envision Surgical Services
Plano, Texas

Dennis Metaxas, MD
Chief Department of Anesthesiology
HCA Houston Healthcare Northwest
Houston, Texas

Preface

This edition of *Surgical Recall* has been distilled even further to allow optimal performance on BOTH the shelf exam and the wards. Rapid-Fire "microvignettes" throughout the text are once again provided so you can test your knowledge and also get familiar with finding the words in every vignette that are the key to unraveling the puzzle they hold.

The formula for success on the shelf exam is simple:

Disease Information (raw data facts) ×
Disease Recognition in a Vignette = SUCCESS on the SHELF Exam.

The formula for success on the wards is also straightforward:

Clinical Care Knowledge × Performance = Optimal WARD SUCCESS.

This text is unique in that it holds the knowledge in a very concise manner—in a self-study, right- and left-column format—to excel on both the Wards and the Shelf exam.

Once again, our Pre-Book and Post-Book Tests allow you to self-assess vignette subject knowledge and reveal what areas to restudy until the material is mastered.

Furthermore, we are excited to introduce you to our new feature, "Three-Dimensional Surgical Vignette Chess." This testing opportunity is broken up into information nuggets followed by questions and immediate answers. These new vignettes are in a three-column format instead of the two-column format the rest of the book uses. Since this is a new format, we would love your feedback!

Lorne H. Blackbourne, MD, FACS
Trauma, Surgical Critical Care
Round Rock, Texas

Figure Credits

Chapter 9 (carotid endarterectomy)
Lawrence PF, Bell RM, Dayton MT. *Essentials of General Surgery.* 5th ed. Philadelphia, PA: Wolters Kluwer; 2012:545.

Chapter 13 (Puestow procedure)
Jarrell BE. *NMS Surgery.* 6th ed. Baltimore, MD: Wolters Kluwer; 2016; Fig. 14-2.

Chapter 13 (Nissen)
Jarrell BE. *NMS Surgery.* 6th ed. Baltimore, MD: Wolters Kluwer; 2016; Fig. 20-5.

Chapter 13 (Heineke-Mikulicz pyloroplasty)
Mulholland MW. *Greenfield's Surgery.* 6th ed. Baltimore, MD: Wolters Kluwer; 2016; Fig. 43-14.

Chapter 13 (Pringle maneuver)
Blackbourne LH. *Advanced Surgical Recall.* 4th ed. Baltimore, MD: Wolters Kluwer; 2015:86.

Chapter 13 (percutaneous endoscopic gastrostomy)
Blackbourne LH. *Advanced Surgical Recall.* 4th ed. Baltimore, MD: Wolters Kluwer; 2015:101.

Chapter 15 (suprapubic catheter)
Carter P. *Lippincott Textbook for Nursing Assistants.* Philadelphia, PA: Wolters Kluwer; 2015; Fig. 24-6C.

Chapter 17 (causes of hypercalcemia mnemonic)
Blackbourne LH. *Advanced Surgical Recall.* 4th ed. Baltimore, MD: Wolters Kluwer; 2015:17.

Chapter 37 (cricothyroidotomy)
Britt LD, Peitzman A, Barie P. *Acute Care Surgery.* Baltimore, MD: Wolters Kluwer; 2012; Fig. 64-5A.

Chapter 37 (pneumothorax)
Daffner RH. *Clinical Radiology.* 4th ed. Baltimore, MD: Wolters Kluwer; 2013; Fig. 4-95B.

Chapter 37 (anterior hip dislocation)
Blackbourne LH. *Advanced Surgical Recall.* 4th ed. Baltimore, MD: Wolters Kluwer; 2015:672.

Chapter 37 (brown recluse spider bite)
Blackbourne LH. *Advanced Surgical Recall.* 4th ed. Baltimore, MD: Wolters Kluwer; 2015:179.

Chapter 41 (sleeve gastrectomy)
Jarrell BE. *NMS Surgery.* 6th ed. Baltimore, MD: Wolters Kluwer; 2015; Fig. 19-2.

Chapter 41 (gastric bypass)
Lawrence PF, Bell RM, Dayton MT, et al. *Essentials of General Surgery.* 5th ed. Baltimore, MD: Wolters Kluwer; 2012; Fig. 13-14.

Chapter 41 (lap-band)
Daffner RH, Hartman M. *Clinical Radiology.* 4th ed. Baltimore, MD: Wolters Kluwer; 2013; Fig. 8-45A.

Chapter 42 (loop colostomy)
Albo D. *Operative Techniques in Colon and Rectal Surgery.* Baltimore, MD: Wolters Kluwer; 2015; Fig. 44-1B.

Chapter 47 (sigmoid volvulus)
Moore KL, Agur AMR, Dalley AF. *Clinically Oriented Anatomy.* 7th ed. Baltimore, MD: Wolters Kluwer; 2013; Fig. 2-18 (box image).

Chapter 48 (anal fissure triad)
Mulholland MW. *Greenfield's Surgery.* 6th ed. Baltimore, MD: Wolters Kluwer; 2016; Fig. 37-2.

Chapter 51 (French system)
Blackbourne LH. *Advanced Surgical Recall.* 4th ed. Baltimore, MD: Wolters Kluwer; 2014:129.

Chapter 51 (liver segments)
Blackbourne LH. *Advanced Surgical Recall.* 4th ed. Baltimore, MD: Wolters Kluwer; 2014:130.

Chapter 55 (spiculated mass)
Daffner RH, Hartman M. *Clinical Radiology.* 4th ed. Baltimore, MD: Wolters Kluwer Health; 2013; Fig. 6-10.

Chapter 55 (rectus abdominis flap reconstruction)
Mulholland MW. *Greenfield's Surgery.* 6th ed. Philadelphia, PA: Wolters Kluwer;
2016; Fig. 19-4.

Chapter 56 (gastrinoma triangle)
Mulholland MW. *Greenfield's Surgery.* 6th ed. Philadelphia, PA: Wolters Kluwer
Health; 2016; Fig. 56-8.

Chapter 65 (endovascular repair)
Zelenock GB, Huber TS, Messina LM, et al. *Mastery of Vascular and
Endovascular Surgery.* Philadelphia, PA: Lippincott Williams & Wilkins; 2005;
Fig. 22-3.

Chapter 68 (paronychia)
Henretig FM, King C, eds. *Textbook of Pediatric Emergency Procedures.*
Philadelphia, PA: Wolters Kluwer; 1997; Fig. 71-1.

Chapter 68 (Jersey finger)
Miller MD, Chhabra AB, Konin J, et al. *Sports Medicine Conditions: Return to
Play: Recognition, Treatment, Planning.* Philadelphia, PA: Wolters Kluwer; 2013;
Fig. 3-10.

Chapter 73 (Colles' fracture)
McKenney MG, Mangonon PC, Moylan JA. *Understanding Surgical Disease:
The Miami Manual of Surgery.* Philadelphia, PA: Lippincott-Raven; 1998.

Chapter 73 (Lachman test)
Redrawn from Spindler KP, Wright RW. Clinical practice. Anterior cruciate
ligament tear. *N Engl J Med.* 2008;359:2135–2142.

Chapter 74 (Kocher's point)
Spector SA. *Clinical Companion in Surgery.* Philadelphia, PA: Lippincott
Williams & Wilkins; 1999.

Chapter 74 (bitemporal hemianopsia)
Blackbourne LH. *Advanced Surgical Recall.* 4th ed. Baltimore, MD: Wolters
Kluwer; 2015;706.

Contents

SECTION IV
SUBSPECIALTY SURGERY

Pre- and Post-Book Study Test for the Shelf Exam

HOW TO USE THIS CHAPTER

First cover the right-hand side of the page (i.e., cover the answers). Then answer all the microvignettes on the left-hand side. Record the number answered correctly at the bottom of the page before reading the book (Pre-test) and then after finishing the book (Post-test). This will facilitate self-assessment of vignette subject knowledge and reveal what areas to restudy until the material is mastered.

TOP 100 CLINICAL SURGICAL MICROVIGNETTES

1.	Elderly female, SBO, and air in biliary tract	Gallstone ileus
2.	Elderly female with pain down inner aspect of thigh	Obturator hernia (Howship–Romberg sign)
3.	Abdominal pain, hypotension, and abdominal pulsatile mass	Ruptured abdominal aortic aneurysm (AAA)
4.	Abdominal pain "out of proportion" to abdominal exam	Mesenteric ischemia
5.	Arm pain and syncope with arm movement	Subclavian steal syndrome
6.	Increasing creatinine on ACE inhibitor	Renal artery stenosis
7.	Child with MIDLINE neck mass	Thyroglossal duct cyst
8.	Child with LATERAL neck mass	Branchial cleft cyst
9.	Crush injury and dark urine	Myoglobinuria
10.	Emesis, chest pain radiating to back, and mediastinal air	Boerhaave's

SCORE YOUR ANSWERS: Pre- and Post-Book Self-Assessment of Surgical Knowledge

Pre-test: _____/10

Cumulative: Pre-test: _____/10

Post-test: _____/10

Cumulative: Post-test: _____/10

11.	**Lower GI bleed + technetium pertechnetate scan**	Meckel's diverticulum
12.	**Flushing, diarrhea, and right-sided heart failure**	Carcinoid
13.	**Pneumaturia and LLQ pain**	Colovesical fistula
14.	**Desmoid tumor, osteoma, and colon cancer**	Gardner's syndrome
15.	**Epigastric pain radiating to back and flank ecchymosis**	Hemorrhagic pancreatitis
16.	**Pancreatitis and palpable epigastric mass**	Pancreatic pseudocyst
17.	**Liver abscess with "anchovy paste"**	Amebic abscess
18.	**RUQ pain, travel, and exposure to sheep**	Hydatid cyst
19.	**Caput medusae**	Portal hypertension
20.	**45-year-old female with RUQ pain for 12 hours, fever, and leukocytosis**	Acute cholecystitis
21.	**Elderly male with large nontender palpable gallbladder**	Pancreatic cancer (Courvoisier's sign)
22.	**Female taking birth control pills with liver mass**	Hepatic adenoma
23.	**Liver tumor with "central scar"**	Focal nodular hyperplasia
24.	**Pancreatic mass, gallstones, diabetes, and diarrhea**	Somatostatinoma
25.	**RUQ bruit and CHF in young adult**	Liver hemangioma
26.	**Excruciating pain with bowel movement**	Anal fissure
27.	**Abdominal pain, diarrhea, and anal fistulae**	Crohn's disease
28.	**EKG with "peaked" T waves**	Hyperkalemia
29.	**Buccal mucosa with pigmentation**	Peutz–Jeghers syndrome

SCORE YOUR ANSWERS: Pre- and Post-Book Self-Assessment of Surgical Knowledge

Pre-test: _____/19   Post-test: _____/19

Cumulative: Pre-test: _____/29   Cumulative: Post-test: _____/29

30.	LLQ pain, fever, and change in bowel habits	Diverticulitis
31.	Elevated urine 5-HIAA	Carcinoid
32.	Institutionalized, abdominal pain, vomiting, and distention, with proximal colonic dilation	Sigmoid volvulus
33.	Infant with projectile vomiting	Pyloric stenosis
34.	Newborn with failure to pass meconium in first 24 hours	Hirschsprung's disease
35.	Infant with bilious vomiting	Malrotation
36.	Newborn with abdominal defect and umbilical cord on sac	Omphalocele
37.	Teenager with knee pain and "onion skinning" on x-ray	Ewing's sarcoma
38.	Pulmonary capillary wedge pressure <18, CXR with bilateral pulmonary infiltrates, and PaO_2:FiO_2 ratio <300	Acute respiratory distress syndrome (ARDS)
39.	Increased peak airway pressure, low urine output, and urinary bladder >25 mm Hg	Abdominal compartment syndrome
40.	Newborn with inability to "pass an NGT"	Esophageal atresia
41.	Traumatic blinding in one eye followed by blindness in the contralateral eye 2 weeks later	Sympathetic ophthalmia
42.	Miotic pupil, ptosis, and anhidrosis	Horner's syndrome
43.	Traumatic head injury, conscious in ER followed by unconsciousness	Epidural hematoma ("lucid interval")
44.	"Worst headache of my life"	Subarachnoid hemorrhage
45.	Hematuria, flank pain, and abdominal mass (palpable)	Renal cell carcinoma

SCORE YOUR ANSWERS: Pre- and Post-Book Self-Assessment of Surgical Knowledge

Pre-test: _____/16

Cumulative: Pre-test: _____/45

Post-test: _____/16

Cumulative: Post-test: _____/45

46.	60-year-old white male with painless hematuria	Bladder cancer
47.	RUQ pain, jaundice, and fever	Cholangitis
48.	Epigastric pain radiating to back, with nausea and vomiting	Pancreatitis
49.	Chest pain radiating to back and described as a "tearing" pain	Aortic dissection
50.	40-year-old male with tachycardia/hypertension and confusion on postoperative day #2	Alcohol withdrawal
51.	Marfanoid body habitus and mucosal neuromas	MEN II-b
52.	Psammoma bodies	Papillary thyroid cancer
53.	Sulfur granules	*Actinomyces* infection
54.	Thyroid tumor with AMYLOID tissue	Thyroid medullary cancer
55.	PALPABLE neck tumor and hypercalcemia	Parathyroid cancer
56.	Hypertension, diaphoresis (episodic), and palpitations	Pheochromocytoma
57.	Jejunal ulcers	Zollinger–Ellison syndrome
58.	Pituitary tumor, pancreatic tumor, and parathyroid tumor	MEN-I
59.	Necrotizing migratory erythema	Glucagonoma
60.	Medullary thyroid cancer, pheochromocytoma, and hyperparathyroidism	MEN-IIa
61.	Hypokalemia refractory to IV potassium supplementation	Hypomagnesemia
62.	Newborn with pneumatosis	Necrotizing enterocolitis (NEC)

SCORE YOUR ANSWERS: Pre- and Post-Book Self-Assessment of Surgical Knowledge

Pre-test: _____/17

Cumulative: Pre-test: _____/62

Post-test: _____/17

Cumulative: Post-test: _____/62

63.	Child with abdominal mass that crosses midline	Neuroblastoma
64.	Child <4 years with abdominal tumor that does NOT cross midline	Wilms' tumor
65.	"Currant jelly" stools and abdominal colic	Intussusception
66.	Femur fracture, respiratory failure, petechiae, and mental status changes	Fat embolism
67.	Hearing loss, tinnitus, and vertigo	Ménière's disease
68.	Adolescent boy with nasal obstruction and recurrent epistaxis	Juvenile nasopharyngeal angiofibroma
69.	Child <5 years sitting upright and drooling, with "hot-potato" voice	Epiglottitis
70.	Angina, syncope, and CHF	Aortic stenosis
71.	Tobacco use, asbestos exposure, and pleuritic chest pain	Mesothelioma
72.	Supracondylar fracture and contracture of forearm flexors	Volkmann's contracture
73.	Tibia fracture, "pain out of proportion," pain on passive foot movement, and palpable pulses	Compartment syndrome
74.	25-year-old male with liver mass with fibrous septae and NO history of cirrhosis or hepatitis	Fibrolamellar hepatocellular carcinoma
75.	EKG with flattening of T waves and U waves	Hypokalemia
76.	Central pontine myelinolysis	Too-rapid correction of hyponatremia
77.	Polydipsia, polyuria, and constipation	Hypercalcemia

SCORE YOUR ANSWERS: Pre- and Post-Book Self-Assessment of Surgical Knowledge

Pre-test: _____/15

Post-test: _____/15

Cumulative: Pre-test: _____/77

Cumulative: Post-test: _____/77

78. **Factor VIII deficiency**	Hemophilia A
79. **Abdominal pain, fever, hypotension, HYPERkalemia, and HYPOnatremia**	Adrenal insufficiency (addisonian crisis)
80. **Massive urine output and HYPERnatremia**	Diabetes insipidus
81. **Increased urine osmolality, HYPOnatremia, and low serum osmolality**	SIADH
82. **IV antibiotics, fever, diarrhea**	*Clostridium difficile* pseudomembranous colitis
83. **Bleeding gums and wound dehiscence**	Vitamin C deficiency
84. **Fever, central line, and HYPERglycemia**	Central line infection
85. **Appendectomy followed by fever and abdominal pain on postoperative day #7**	Peritoneal abscess
86. **Advancing crepitus, fever, and blood blisters**	Necrotizing fasciitis
87. **High INTRAoperative fever**	Malignant hyperthermia
88. **Confusion, ataxia, and ophthalmoplegia**	Wernicke's encephalopathy
89. **Tracheal deviation, decreased breath sounds, and hyperresonance**	Tension pneumothorax
90. **Hypotension, decreased heart sounds, and JVD**	Pericardial tamponade
91. **Four ribs broken in two places and pulmonary contusion**	Flail chest
92. **Otorrhea (clear) and Battle's sign**	Basilar skull fracture
93. **Ulcer and decreased pain with food**	Duodenal ulcer

SCORE YOUR ANSWERS: Pre- and Post-Book Self-Assessment of Surgical Knowledge

Pre-test: _____/16   Post-test: _____/16

Cumulative: Pre-test: _____/93   Cumulative: Post-test: _____/93

94.	Vomiting, retching, and epigastric pain	Mallory–Weiss tear
95.	Fever on postoperative day #1, with "bronze" weeping, tender wound	Clostridial wound infection
96.	Hematochezia and tenesmus	Rectal cancer
97.	Upper GI bleed, jaundice, and RUQ pain	Hemobilia
98.	Gallstones, epigastric pain radiating to back, and nausea	Gallstone pancreatitis
99.	18-year-old female with bloody nipple discharge	Ductal papilloma
100.	Irritability, diaphoresis, weakness, tremulousness, and palpitations	Insulinoma

SCORE YOUR ANSWERS: Pre- and Post-Book Self-Assessment of Surgical Knowledge

Pre-test: _____/7   Post-test: _____/7

Total number of microvignettes answered correctly:

Pre-test: _____/100   Post-test: _____/100

Chapter 1 | Introduction

OPERATING ROOM FAQs

What if I have to sneeze?	Back up STRAIGHT back; do not turn your head, as the sneeze exits through the sides of your mask!
What if I feel faint?	Do not be a hero—say, "I feel faint. May I sit down?" This is no big deal and is very common (**Note:** It helps to always eat before going to the O.R.)
What should I say when I first enter the O.R.?	Introduce yourself as a student; state that you have been invited to scrub and ask if you need to get out your gloves and/or gown
Should I wear my ID tag into the O.R.?	Yes
Can I wear nail polish?	Check, as some institutions do not allow it
Can I wear my rings and my watch when scrubbed in the O.R.?	No
Can I wear earrings?	No
When scrubbed, is my back sterile?	No
When in the surgical gown, are my underarms sterile?	No; do not put your hands under your arms
How far down my gown is considered part of the sterile field?	Just to your waist
How far up my gown is considered sterile?	Up to the nipples

How do I stand if I am waiting for the case to start?

Hands together in front above your waist

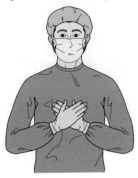

Can I button up a surgical gown (when I am not scrubbed!) with bare hands?

Yes (*Remember:* the back of the gown is NOT sterile)

How many pairs of gloves should I wear when scrubbed?

2 (2 layers)

What is the normal order of sizes of gloves: small pair, then larger pair?

No; usually the order is a larger size followed by a smaller size (e.g., men commonly wear a size #8 covered by a size #7.5; women commonly wear a size #7 covered by a size #6.5)

What items comprise the sterile field in the operating room?

Instrument table, Mayo tray, and anterior drapes on the patient

What is the tray with the instruments called?

Mayo tray

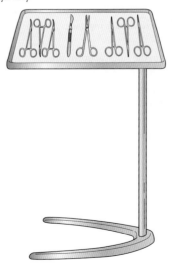

Can I grab things off the Mayo tray?

No; ask the scrub nurse/tech for permission

How do you remove blood with a laparotomy pad ("lap pad")?

Dab; do not wipe, because wiping removes platelet plugs

Can you grab the skin with DeBakey pickups?

NO; pickups for the skin must have teeth (e.g., Adson, rat-tooth) because it is "better to cut the skin than crush it"

How should you cut the sutures after tying a knot?

1. Rest the cutting hand on the noncutting hand
2. Slip the scissors down to the knot and then cant the scissors at a 45° angle so you do not cut the knot itself

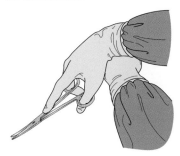

What should you do when you are scrubbed and someone is tying a suture?

Ask the scrub nurse for a pair of suture scissors, so you are ready if you are asked to cut the sutures

SURGERY SIGNS, TRIADS, ETC., YOU SHOULD KNOW

What is the Allen's test?

Test for patency of ulnar artery prior to placing a radial arterial line or performing an ABG: Examiner occludes both ulnar and radial arteries with fingers as patient makes fist; patient opens fist while examiner releases ulnar artery occlusion to assess blood flow to hand (28% of pop. have complete radial artery dominance!)

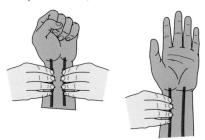

Define the following terms:

Ballance's sign

Constant dullness to percussion in the left flank/LUQ and resonance to percussion in the right flank seen with splenic rupture/hematoma

Battle's sign

Ecchymosis over the mastoid process in patients with basilar skull fractures

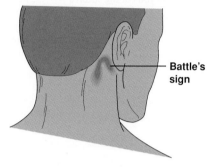

Beck's triad

Seen in patients with cardiac tamponade:
1. JVD
2. Decreased or muffled heart sounds
3. Decreased blood pressure

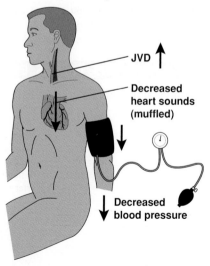

Blumer's shelf

Metastatic disease to the rectouterine (pouch of Douglas) or rectovesical pouch creating a "shelf" that is palpable on rectal examination

Carcinoid triad	Seen with carcinoid syndrome (Think: "**FDR**"): 1. **F**lushing 2. **D**iarrhea 3. **R**ight-sided heart failure
Charcot's triad	Seen with cholangitis: 1. Fever (chills) 2. Jaundice 3. Right upper quadrant pain (Pronounced "char-cohs")
Chvostek's sign	Twitching of facial muscles upon tapping the facial nerve in patients with hypocalcemia (Think: **CH**vostek's = **CH**eek)
Courvoisier's law	Enlarged nontender gallbladder seen with obstruction of the common bile duct, most commonly with pancreatic cancer ***Note:*** Not seen with gallstone obstruction because the gallbladder is scarred secondary to chronic cholelithiasis (Pronounced "koor-vwah-ze-ay")
Cullen's sign	Bluish discoloration of the periumbilical area due to retroperitoneal hemorrhage tracking around to the anterior abdominal wall through fascial planes (e.g., acute hemorrhagic pancreatitis)

Umbilicus

Cushing's triad	Signs of increased intracranial pressure: 1. Hypertension 2. Bradycardia 3. Irregular respirations

Goodsall's rule	Anal fistulae course in a straight path anteriorly and a curved path posteriorly from midline (Think of a dog with a straight anterior nose and a curved posterior tail)

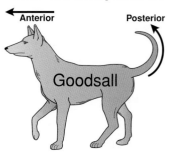

Hamman's sign/crunch	Crunching sound on auscultation of the heart resulting from emphysematous mediastinum; seen with Boerhaave's syndrome, pneumomediastinum, etc.
Howship–Romberg sign	Pain along the inner aspect of the thigh; seen with an obturator hernia as the result of nerve compression
McBurney's point	One third the distance from the anterior iliac spine to the umbilicus on a line connecting the two to find the appendix
Meckel's diverticulum rule of 2s	2% of the population have a Meckel's diverticulum, 2% of those are symptomatic, and they occur within ≈2 feet of the ileocecal valve
Murphy's sign	Cessation of inspiration while palpating under the right costal margin; the patient cannot continue to inspire deeply because it brings an inflamed gallbladder under pressure (seen in acute cholecystitis)
Obturator sign	Pain upon internal rotation of the leg with the hip and knee flexed; seen in patients with appendicitis/pelvic abscess

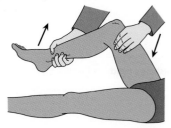

Pheochromocytoma SYMPTOMS triad	Think of the first three letters in the word pheochromocytoma—"**P-H-E**": **P**alpitations **H**eadache **E**pisodic diaphoresis
Psoas sign	Pain elicited by extending the hip with the knee in full extension, seen with appendicitis and psoas inflammation

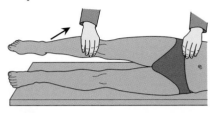

Raccoon eyes	Bilateral black eyes as a result of basilar skull fracture

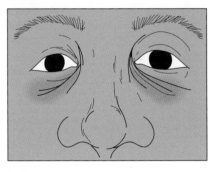

Reynolds' pentad	1. Fever 2. Jaundice 3. Right upper quadrant pain 4. Mental status changes 5. Shock/sepsis Thus, Charcot's triad plus #4 and #5; seen in patients with **suppurative** cholangitis
Rovsing's sign	Palpation of the left lower quadrant resulting in pain in the right lower quadrant; seen in appendicitis
Virchow's node	Metastatic tumor to left supraclavicular node (classically due to gastric cancer)
Morel-Lavallée lesion	Closed "degloving" injury from trauma

Virchow's triad	Risk factors for thrombosis: 1. Stasis 2. Abnormal endothelium 3. Hypercoagulability

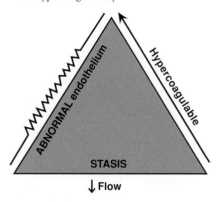

Trousseau's sign	Carpal spasm after occlusion of blood to the forearm with a BP cuff in patients with hypocalcemia
Valentino's sign	Right lower quadrant pain from a perforated peptic ulcer due to succus/pus draining into the RLQ
Whipple's triad	Evidence for insulinoma: 1. Hypoglycemia (<50) 2. CNS and vasomotor symptoms (e.g., syncope, diaphoresis) 3. Relief of symptoms with administration of glucose

Chapter 2 | Surgical Syndromes

What is afferent loop syndrome?	Obstruction of the afferent loop of a Billroth II gastrojejunostomy
What does ARDS stand for?	**A**cute **R**espiratory **D**istress **S**yndrome (poor oxygenation caused by alveolar and capillary inflammation)
What is blind loop syndrome?	Bacterial overgrowth of intestine caused by stasis
What is Boerhaave's syndrome?	Esophageal perforation from emesis heaves
What is Budd–Chiari syndrome?	Thrombosis of hepatic veins

What is carcinoid syndrome?	Syndrome of **"B FDR"**: **B**ronchospasm **F**lushing **D**iarrhea **R**ight-sided heart failure (caused by factors released by carcinoid tumor)
What is compartment syndrome?	Compartmental hypertension caused by edema, resulting in muscle necrosis of the lower extremity, because the fascial compartments do NOT stretch, often seen in the calf; patient may have a distal pulse
What is Cushing's syndrome?	Excessive cortisol production
What is dumping syndrome?	Delivery of a large amount of hyperosmolar chyme into the small bowel, usually after vagotomy and a gastric drainage procedure (pyloroplasty/gastrojejunostomy); results in autonomic instability, abdominal pain, and diarrhea
What is Fitz-Hugh–Curtis syndrome?	Perihepatic gonorrhea infection (perihepatic adhesions)
What is Gardner's syndrome?	GI polyps and associated findings of **S**ebaceous cysts, **O**steomas, and **D**esmoid tumors (**SOD**); polyps have high malignancy potential (Think: A **Gardner** plants **SOD**)
What is HITT syndrome?	**H**eparin-**I**nduced **T**hrombocytopenic **T**hrombosis syndrome: Heparin-induced platelet antibodies cause platelets to thrombosed vessels, often resulting in loss of limb or life
What is Leriche's syndrome?	**C**laudication of buttocks and thighs, **I**mpotence, **A**trophy of legs (seen with iliac occlusive disease) (Think: **CIA**)
What is Mallory–Weiss syndrome?	Postemesis/retching tears in the gastric mucosa (near gastroesophageal junction)
What is Mendelson's syndrome?	Chemical pneumonitis after aspiration of gastric contents
What is Mirizzi's syndrome?	Extrinsic obstruction of the common hepatic bile duct from a gallstone in the gallbladder or cystic duct
What is Munchausen's syndrome?	Self-induced illness; patient desires the attention comfort of the "sick" role
What is Ogilvie's syndrome?	Massive **nonobstructive** colonic dilatation
What is Peutz–Jeghers syndrome?	Benign GI polyps and buccal pigmentation (Think: **P**eutz = **P**igmentation)

What is RED reaction syndrome?	Syndrome of rapid vancomycin infusion, resulting in skin erythema
What is refeeding syndrome?	Hypokalemia, hypomagnesemia, and hypophosphatemia after refeeding a starved patient
What is Rendu–Osler–Weber (ROW) syndrome?	Syndrome of GI tract telangiectasia/A-V malformations
What is short-gut syndrome?	Malnutrition resulting from <200 cm of viable small bowel
What is SIADH?	**S**yndrome of **I**nappropriate **A**nti**D**iuretic **H**ormone (Think: **I**nappropriately **I**ncreased ADH)
What is superior vena cava (SVC) syndrome?	Obstruction of the SVC (e.g., by tumor, thrombosis)
What is thoracic outlet syndrome?	Compression of the structures exiting from the thoracic outlet
What is toxic shock syndrome?	*Staphylococcus aureus* toxin–induced syndrome marked by fever, hypotension, organ failure, and **rash** (desquamation— especially palms and soles)
What is Trousseau's syndrome?	Syndrome of deep venous thrombosis (DVT) associated with carcinoma
What is Zollinger–Ellison syndrome?	Gastrinoma and PUD

Chapter 3 | Surgical Most Commons

What is the most common:

Type of melanoma?	Superficial spreading
Type of breast cancer?	Infiltrating ductal
Site of breast cancer?	Upper outer quadrant
Vessel involved with a bleeding duodenal ulcer?	Gastroduodenal artery
Cause of common bile duct obstruction?	Choledocholithiasis
Cause of small bowel obstruction (SBO) in adults in the United States?	Postoperative peritoneal adhesions
Cause of SBO in children?	Hernias
Cause of emergency abdominal surgery in the United States?	Acute appendicitis

Electrolyte deficiency causing ileus?	Hypokalemia
Cause of blood transfusion resulting in death?	Clerical error (wrong blood types)
Site of distant metastasis of sarcoma?	Lungs (hematogenous spread)
Position of anal fissure?	Posterior
Acute pancreatitis?	Gallstones
Chronic pancreatitis?	Alcohol
Cause of large bowel obstruction?	Colon cancer
Cause of fever <48 postoperative hours?	Atelectasis
Bacterial cause of urinary tract infection (UTI)?	*Escherichia coli*
Abdominal organ injured in blunt abdominal trauma?	Liver (not the spleen, as noted in recent studies!)
Benign tumor of the liver?	Hemangioma
Malignancy of the liver?	Metastasis
Pneumonia in the ICU?	Gram-negative bacteria
Cause of epidural hematoma?	Middle meningeal artery injury
Cause of lower GI bleeding?	Upper GI bleeding
Cancer in females?	Breast cancer
Cancer in males?	Prostate cancer
Type of cancer causing DEATH in males and females?	LUNG cancer
Cause of free peritoneal air?	Perforated peptic ulcer disease
Cause of death ages 1 to 44?	TRAUMA

Chapter 4 | Surgical Percentages

What percentage of people in the United States will develop acute appendicitis?	≈7%
What is the acceptable percentage of normal appendices removed with the preoperative diagnosis of appendicitis?	Up to 20%; it is better to remove some normal appendices than to miss a case of acute appendicitis, which could result in a ruptured appendix

In what percentage of cases does an upper GI bleed stop spontaneously?	≈80%
What percentage of American women develops breast cancer?	12%
What percentage of patients with gallstones will have radiopaque gallstones on abdominal x-ray (AXR)?	≈10%
What percentage of kidney stones is radiopaque on AXR?	≈90%
At 6 weeks, wounds have achieved what percentage of their total tensile strength?	≈90%
What percentage of the population has a Meckel's diverticulum?	2%
One unit of packed RBCs increases the hematocrit by how much?	3%
Additional 1 L/min by nasal cannula increases FIO_2 by how much?	3%

Chapter 5 | Surgical Instruments

How should a pair of scissors/needle driver/clamp be held?	With the thumb and **fourth** finger, using the index finger to steady

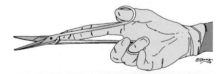

Is it better to hold the skin with a DeBakey or an Adson, or toothed, forceps?	Better to use an Adson, or toothed, pickup because it is better to cut the skin rather than crush it!
What helps steady the scissor or Bovie hand?	Resting it on the opposite hand

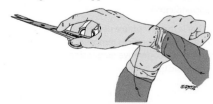

What can be done to guarantee that you do not cut the knot when cutting sutures?

Slide the scissors down to the knot, then turn the scissors at a 45° angle, and cut

How should a pair of forceps be held?

Like a pencil

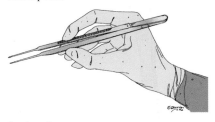

What are forceps also known as?

"Pickups"

Identify the following instruments:

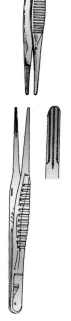

Forceps

DeBakey pickup

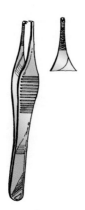

Adson pickup

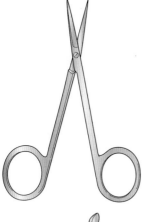

Iris scissors

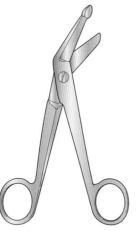

Bandage scissors

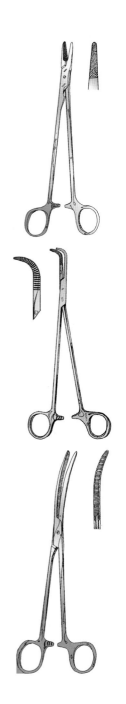

Needle driver

Right-angle clamp

Kelly clamp

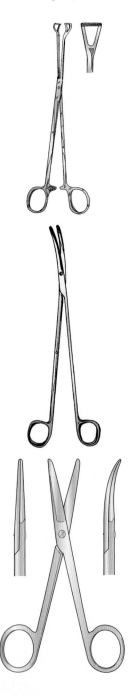

Babcock clamp

Metzenbaum scissors

Mayo scissors (heavy scissors)

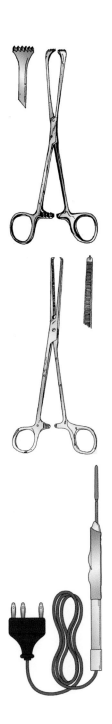

Allis clamp

Kocher clamp, for very thick tissue (e.g., fascia)

Bovie electrocautery

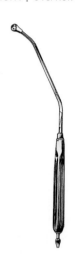

Yankauer suction (sucker)

Define the following scalpel blades:

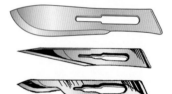

Number 10

Number 11

Number 15

RETRACTORS (YOU WILL GET TO KNOW THEM WELL!)

What does it mean to "toe in" the retractor?

To angle the tip of the retractor in by angling the retractor handle up

Identify the following retractors:

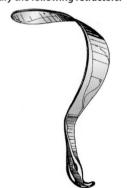

Deaver retractor

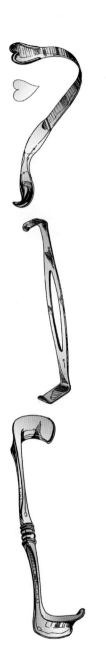

Sweetheart retractor (Harrington)

Army–Navy retractor

Richardson retractor, also known as a "RICH"

What is a "malleable" retractor?

Metal retractor that can be bent to customize to the situation at hand

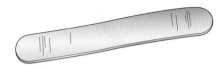

Chapter 6 | Sutures and Stitches

SUTURE MATERIALS

General Information

What is a suture?

Any strand of material used to ligate blood vessels or to approximate tissues

How are sutures sized?

By diameter; stated as a number of 0's: the higher the number of 0's, the smaller the diameter (e.g., 2-0 suture has larger diameter than 5-0 suture)

Which is thicker, 1-0 suture or 3-0 suture?

1-0 suture (pronounced "one oh")

Classification

What are the two most basic suture types?

Absorbable and nonabsorbable

What is an absorbable suture?

Suture that is completely broken down by the body (dissolving suture)

What is a nonabsorbable suture?

Suture is not broken down (permanent suture)

Sutures

Catgut

What are "catgut" sutures made of?

Purified collagen fibers from the intestines of healthy cows or sheep (sorry, no cats)

What are the two types of gut sutures?

Plain and chromic

What is the difference between plain and chromic gut?

Chromic gut is treated with chromium salts (chromium trioxide), which results in more collagen cross-links, making the suture more resistant to breakdown by the body

Vicryl® Suture

What is it?

Absorbable, braided, and multifilamentous copolymer of lactide and glycoside

How long does it retain its strength?

60% at 2 weeks, 8% at 4 weeks

Should you ever use PURPLE-colored Vicryl® for skin closure?

NO—it may cause purple tattooing

PDS®

What is it?

Absorbable, monofilament polymer of polydioxanone (absorbable fishing line)

How long does it maintain its tensile strength?

70% to 74% at 2 weeks, 50% to 58% at 4 weeks, 25% to 41% at 6 weeks

How long does it take to complete absorption?

180 days (6 months)

Other Sutures

What is silk?

Braided protein filaments spun by the silkworm larva; known as a nonabsorbable suture

What is Prolene®?

Nonabsorbable suture (used for vascular anastomoses, hernias, abdominal fascial closure)

What is nylon?

Nonabsorbable "fishing line"

What is monocryl?

Absorbable monofilament

What kind of suture should be used for the biliary tract or the urinary tract?

ABSORBABLE—otherwise the suture will end up as a nidus for stone formation!

WOUND CLOSURE

General Information

What are the three types of wound healing?

1. Primary closure (intention)
2. Secondary intention
3. Tertiary intention (**D**elayed **P**rimary **C**losure: **DPC**)

What is primary intention?

When the edges of a clean wound are closed in some manner immediately (e.g., suture, Steri-Strips®, staples)

What is secondary intention?

When a wound is allowed to remain open and heal by granulation, epithelization, and contraction—used for dirty wounds, otherwise an abscess can form

What is tertiary intention?

When a wound is allowed to remain open for a time and then closed, allowing for débridement and other wound care to reduce bacterial counts prior to closure (i.e., delayed primary closure)

What is another term for tertiary intention?

DPC = **D**elayed **P**rimary **C**losure

Suture Techniques

What is a taper-point needle?

Round body, leaves a round hole in tissue (spreads without cutting tissue)

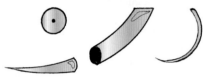

What is it used for?

Suturing of soft tissues other than skin (e.g., GI tract, muscle, nerve, peritoneum, fascia)

What is a conventional cutting needle?

Triangular body with the sharp edge toward the inner circumference; leaves a triangular hole in tissue

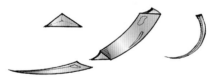

What are its uses?

Suturing of **skin**

What is a simple interrupted stitch?

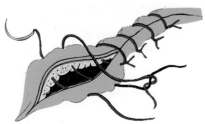

What is a vertical mattress stitch?

Simple stitch is made, the needle is reversed, and a small bite is taken from each wound edge; the knot ends up on one side of the wound

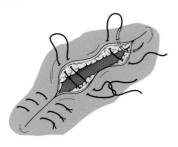

What is the vertical mattress stitch also known as?

Far–far, near–near stitch—oriented perpendicular to wound

What is it used for?

Difficult-to-approximate skin edges; everts tissue well

What is a simple running (continuous) stitch?

Stitches made in succession without knotting each stitch

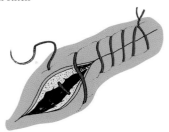

What is a subcuticular stitch?

Stitch (usually running) placed just underneath the epidermis, can be either absorbable or nonabsorbable (pull-out stitch if nonabsorbable)

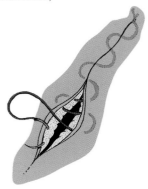

What is a purse-string suture?

Stitch that encircles a tube perforating a hollow viscus (e.g., gastrostomy tube), allowing the hole to be drawn tight and thus preventing leakage

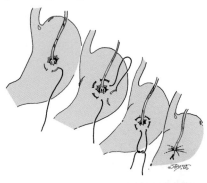

What are metallic skin staples?

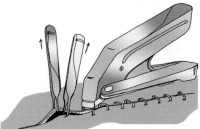

What is a staple removal device?

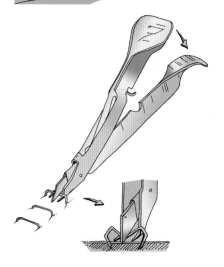

What is a gastrointestinal anastomosis (GIA) device?

Stapling device that lays two rows of small staples in a hemostatic row and **automatically cuts** in between them

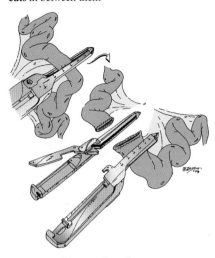

What is a Lembert stitch?

It is a second layer in bowel anastomoses

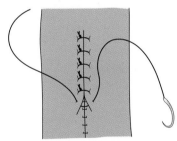

What is a Connell's stitch?

The first mucosa-to-mucosa layer in an anastomosis; basically, a running **U stitch**

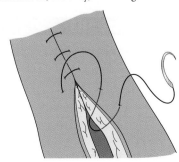

What is a suture ligature (a.k.a. "stick tie")?	Suture is anchored by passing it through the vessel **on a needle** before wrapping it around and occluding the vessel; prevents slippage of knot-use on larger vessels

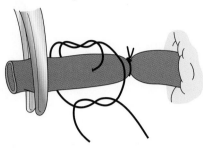

What is a retention suture?	Large suture (#2) that is full thickness through the entire abdominal wall except the peritoneum; used to buttress an abdominal wound at risk for dehiscence and evisceration

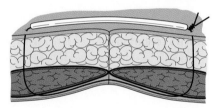

What is a pop-off suture?	Suture that is not permanently swaged to the needle, allowing the surgeon to "pop off" the needle from the suture without cutting the suture

Chapter 7 │ Surgical Knot Tying

KNOTS AND EARS

What is the basic surgical knot?	Square knot

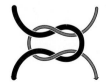

What is the first knot that should be mastered?	Instrument knot

What is a "surgeon's knot"?

Double-wrap throw followed by single-square knot throws

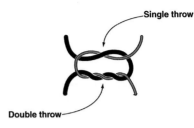

What are the guidelines for the number of minimal throws needed?

Depends on the suture material:
Silk—3
Gut—4
Vicryl®, Dexon®, other braided synthetics—4
Nylon, polyester, polypropylene, PDS, Maxon—6

How long should the ears of the knot be cut?

Some guidelines are:
Silk vessel ties—1 to 2 mm
Abdominal fascia closure—5 mm
Skin sutures, drain sutures—5 to 10 mm (makes them easier to find and remove)

When should skin sutures be removed?

As soon as the wound has healed enough to withstand expected mechanical trauma
Any stitch left in more than ≈10 days will leave a scar
Guidelines are:
Face—3 to 5 days
Extremities—10 days
Joints—10 to 14 days
Back—14 days
Abdomen—7 days

How can strength be added to an incision during and after suture removal?

With Steri-Strips®

In general, in which group of patients should skin sutures be left in longer than normal?

Patients on steroids

How should the sutures be cut?

Use the tips of the scissors to avoid cutting other tissues
Try to remove the cut ends (less foreign material decreases risk of infection)
Rest the scissor-hand on the non–scissor-hand to steady

How is an instrument knot tied?

Always start with a double wrap, known as a "surgeon's knot," and then use a single wrap, pulling the suture in the opposite directions after every "throw"

Does a student need to know a one-hand tie?

No! Master the two-hand tie and the instrument tie

INSTRUMENT TIE

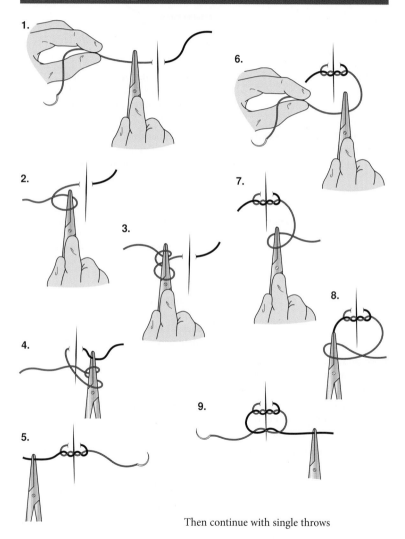

Then continue with single throws

TWO-HAND TIE

What is the basic position for the two-hand tie?

"C" position, formed by the thumb and index finger; the suture will **alternate** over the thumb and then the index finger for each throw

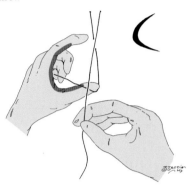

How is a two-hand knot tied?

First, use the index finger to lead

A

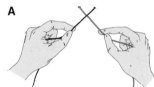

B

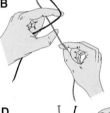

C

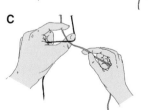

D

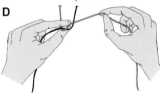

E

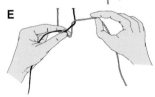

F

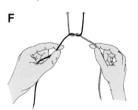

Then use the thumb to lead

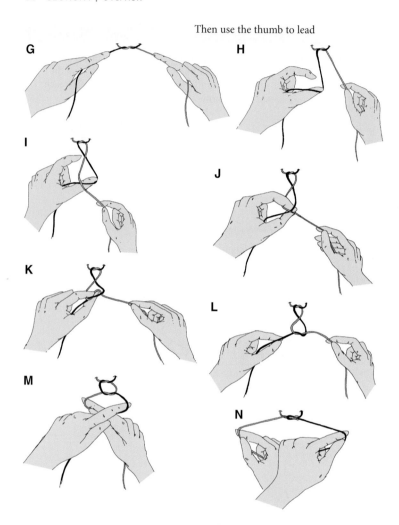

Ask a resident or intern to help you after you have tried for a while.
Open book to this page for guidance.

Chapter 8 | Procedures for the Surgical Ward and Clinic

COMMON PROCEDURES

How do you place a peripheral intravenous (IV) catheter?

1. Place a rubber tourniquet above the site
2. Use alcohol antiseptic
3. Place IV into vein with "flash" of blood
4. Remove inner needle while advancing IV catheter
5. Secure with tape

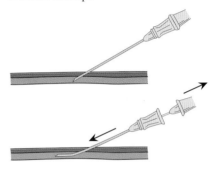

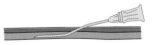

How do you draw blood from the femoral vein?

Remember "**NAVEL**": In the lateral to medial direction—**N**erve, **A**rtery, **V**ein, **E**mpty space, **L**ymphatics—and thus place needle medial to the femoral pulse

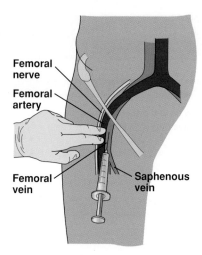

Femoral nerve
Femoral artery
Femoral vein
Saphenous vein

How do you remove staples?

Use a staple remover (see Chapter 6), then place Steri-Strips®

How do you remove stitches?

1. Cut the suture next to the knot
2. Pull end of suture out by holding onto the knot
3. Place Steri-Strips®

How do you place Steri-Strips®?

1. Dry the skin edges of the wound
2. Place adhesive (e.g., benzoin)
3. With the Adson pickup or with your fingers, place strips to gently appose epidermis (**Note:** Avoid any tension or blisters will appear)

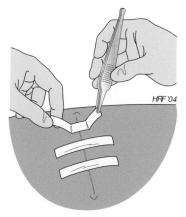

How do you place a Foley catheter?

1. Stay sterile
2. Apply Betadine® to the urethral opening (meatus)
3. Lubricate the catheter
4. Place catheter into urethra
5. As soon as urine returns, inflate balloon with saline (balloon size is given in cc on the catheter)

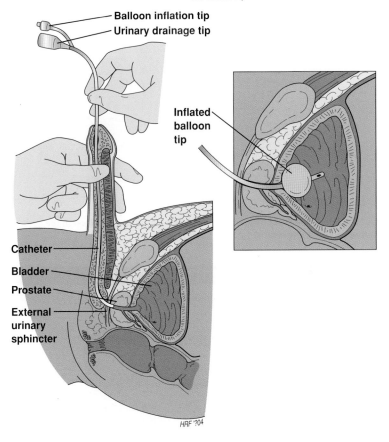

Balloon inflation tip
Urinary drainage tip

Inflated balloon tip

Catheter
Bladder
Prostate
External urinary sphincter

HRF '04

How do you find the urethra in females?

First find the clitoris and clitoral hood: The urethra is just below these structures; wiping a Betadine®-soaked sponge over this area will often result in having the urethra "wink" open

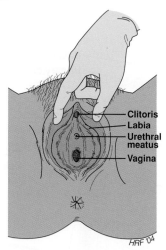

Can you inflate the Foley balloon before you get urine return?

No, you might inflate a balloon in the urethra!

NASOGASTRIC TUBE (NGT) PROCEDURES

How do you determine how much of the NGT should be advanced into the body for the correct position?

Rough guide: from nose, around ear, to 5 cm below the xiphoid

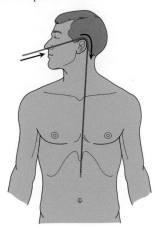

How do you place the NGT in one of the nares (nostrils)?

First place lubrication (e.g., Surgilube®), then place NGT straight back—not up or down!

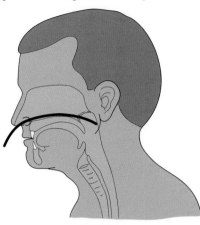

What is the best neck position for advancing the NGT?

Neck FLEXED! Also have the patient drink some water (using a straw)

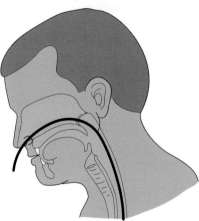

What if there are 3 L/24 hrs drainage from an NGT?

Think DUODENUM—the NGT may be in the duodenum and not in the stomach! Check an x-ray

How can you clinically confirm that an NGT is in the stomach?

Use a Toomey syringe to "inject" air while listening over the stomach with a stethoscope; you will hear the "swish" if the NGT is in place

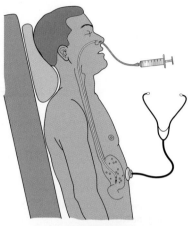

How do you tape an NGT?

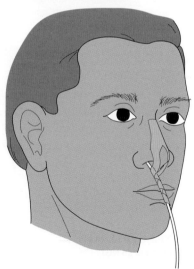

What MUST you obtain and examine before using an NGT for feeding?

LOWER chest/upper abdominal x-ray to absolutely verify placement into the stomach and NOT into the LUNG—patients have died from pulmonary tube feeding!

How do you draw a radial arterial blood gas (ABG)?

Feel for the pulse and advance directly into the artery; ABG syringes do not have to have the plunger withdrawn manually

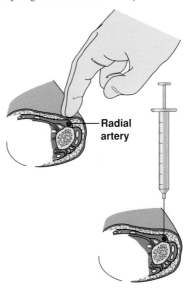

Radial artery

How do you drain an abscess?

By **I**ncision and **D**rainage ("**I & D**"): After using local anesthetic, use a #11 blade to incise and then open the abscess pocket; large abscesses are best drained with removal of a piece of skin; pack the open wound

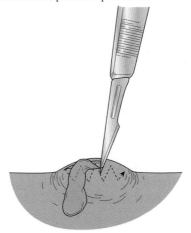

How do you remove an epidermal cyst or sebaceous cyst?

1. Administer local anesthetic
2. Remove the ellipse of skin overlying the cyst, including the pore
3. Remove the cyst with the encompassing sac lining

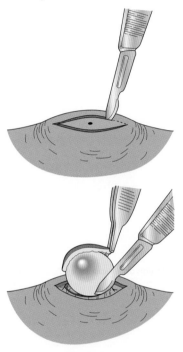

Chapter 9 | Incisions

If a patient has an old incision, is it best to make a subsequent incision next to or through the old incision?

Through the old incision, or excise the old incision, because it has scar tissue that limits the amount of collaterals that would be needed to heal an incision placed next to it

What is used to incise the epidermis?

Scalpel blade

What is used to incise the dermis?

Scalpel or electrocautery

Describe the following incisions:

Kocher   Right subcostal incision for open
                              cholecystectomy:

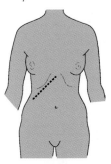

Midline laparotomy   Incision down the middle of abdomen along
                              and through the linea alba:

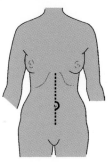

McBurney's   Small, oblique right lower quadrant incision
                              for an appendectomy through McBurney's
                              point (one third from the anterior superior
                              iliac spine to the umbilicus):

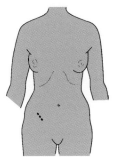

Pfannenstiel ("fan-en-steel")

Low transverse abdominal incision with retraction of the rectus muscles laterally; most often used for gynecologic procedures:

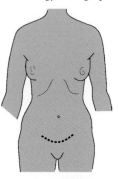

Median sternotomy

Midline sternotomy incision for heart procedures; less painful than a lateral thoracotomy:

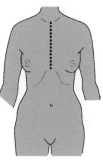

Thoracotomy

Usually through the fourth or fifth intercostal space; may be anterior or posterior lateral incisions

Very painful, but many are performed with muscle sparing (muscle retraction and not muscle transection):

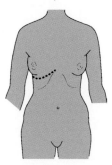

CEA (carotid endarterectomy)

Incision down anterior border of the sternocleidomastoid muscle to expose the carotid:

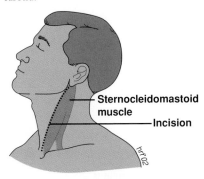

Inguinal hernia repair (open)

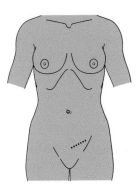

Laparoscopic cholecystectomy

Four trocar incisions:

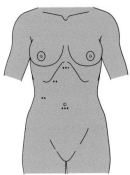

Chapter 10 | Surgical Positions

Define the following positions:

Supine

Patient lying flat, face up

Prone

Patient lying flat, face down

Left lateral decubitus

Patient lying down on his left side (Think: **left** lateral decubitus = **left** side down)

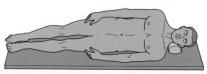

Right lateral decubitus

Patient lying down on his right side (Think: **right** lateral decubitus = **right** side down)

Lithotomy

Patient lying supine with legs spread

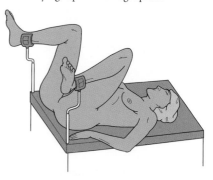

Trendelenburg

Patient supine with head lowered (a.k.a. "headdownenburg"—used during placement of a subclavian vein catheter as the veins distend with blood from gravity flow)

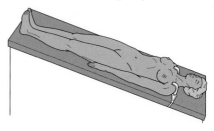

| Reverse Trendelenburg | Patient supine with head elevated (usual position for laparoscopic cholecystectomy to make the intestines fall away from the operative field) |
| **What is the best position for a pregnant patient?** | Left side down to take gravid uterus off the IVC |

Chapter 11 | Surgical Speak

The language of surgery is quite simple if you master a few suffixes.

Define the suffix:

-ectomy	To surgically **remove** part of or an entire structure/organ
-orraphy	Surgical **repair**
-otomy	Surgical **incision into** an organ
-ostomy	Surgically created **opening** between two organs, or organ and skin
-plasty	Surgical "shaping" or formation

Now test your knowledge of surgical speak:

Word for the surgical repair of a hernia	Herniorrhaphy
Word for the surgical removal of the stomach	Gastrectomy
Word for the surgical creation of an opening between the colon and the skin	Colostomy
Word for the surgical formation of a "new" pylorus	Pyloroplasty
Word for the surgical opening of the stomach	Gastrotomy
Surgical creation of an opening (anastomosis) between the common bile duct and jejunum	Choledochojejunostomy
Surgical creation of an opening (anastomosis) between the stomach and jejunum	Gastrojejunostomy

Chapter 12 | Preoperative 101

When can a patient eat prior to major surgery?

Patient should be NPO after midnight, the night before or for at least 8 hours before surgery

What risks should be discussed with all patients and documented on the consent form for a surgical procedure?

Bleeding, infection, anesthesia, scar; other risks are specific to the individual procedure (also MI, CVA, and death if cardiovascular disease is present)

If a patient is on antihypertensive medications, should the patient take them on the day of the procedure?

Yes (remember clonidine "rebound")

If a patient is on an oral hypoglycemic agent (OHA), should the patient take the OHA on the day of surgery?

Not if the patient is to be NPO on the day of surgery

If a patient is taking insulin, should the patient take it on the day of surgery?

No, only half of a long-acting insulin (e.g., Lantus®) and start D5NS IV; check glucose levels often preoperatively, operatively, and postoperatively

Should a patient who smokes cigarettes stop before an operation?

Yes, improvement is seen in just 2 to 4 weeks after smoking cessation

What laboratory test must all women of childbearing age have before entering the O.R.?

β-HCG and CBC because of the possibility of pregnancy and anemia from menses

What is a preoperative colon surgery "bowel prep"?

Bowel prep with colon cathartic (e.g., GoLYTELY®), oral antibiotics (neomycin and erythromycin base), and IV antibiotic before incision (controversial)

Has a preoperative bowel prep been shown conclusively to decrease postoperative infections in colon surgery?

No, there is no data to support its use

What must you always order preoperatively for your patient undergoing a major operation?

1. NPO/IVF
2. Preoperative antibiotics
3. Type and cross blood (PRBCs)

What electrolyte must you check preoperatively if a patient is on hemodialysis?

Potassium

Who gets a preoperative ECG?

Patients age >40 years

Chapter 13 | Surgical Operations You Should Know

Define the following procedures:

Billroth I   Antrectomy with gastroduodenostomy

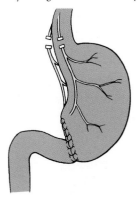

Billroth II   Antrectomy with gastrojejunostomy

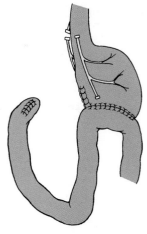

How can the difference between a Billroth I and Billroth II be remembered?   Billroth 1 has one limb; Billroth 2 has two limbs

Describe the following procedures:

Roux-en-Y limb

Jejunojejunostomy forming a Y-shaped figure of small bowel; the free end can then be anastomosed to a second hollow structure (e.g., esophagojejunostomy)

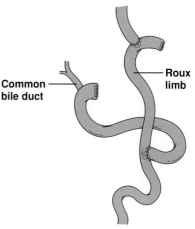

Brooke ileostomy

Standard ileostomy that is **folded on itself** to protrude from the abdomen ≈2 cm to allow easy appliance placement and collection of succus

CEA

Carotid EndArterectomy; removal of atherosclerotic plaque from a carotid artery

APR

AbdominoPerineal Resection; removal of the rectum and sigmoid colon through abdominal and perineal incisions (patient is left with a colostomy); used for low rectal cancers

LAR

Low Anterior Resection; **resection** of **low** rectal tumors through an **anterior** abdominal incision

Hartmann's procedure

1. Proximal colostomy
2. Distal stapled-off colon or rectum that is left in peritoneal cavity

Mucous fistula	Distal end of the colon is brought to the abdominal skin as a stoma (proximal end is brought up to skin as an end colostomy)
Kocher ("koh-ker") maneuver	Dissection of the duodenum from the right-sided peritoneal attachment to allow mobilization and visualization of the back of the duodenum/pancreas

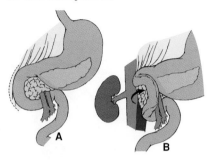

Cattel maneuver	Mobilization of the ascending colon to the midline. If combined with a Kocher maneuver, exposes the vena cava (Think: **C**attel = **K**ocher = right sided)
Seldinger technique	Placement of a central line by first placing a wire in the vein, followed by placing the catheter over the wire
Cricothyroidotomy	Emergent surgical airway through the cricoid membrane
Hepaticojejunostomy	Anastomosis between a jejunal Roux limb and the hepatic bile ducts

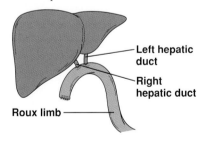

Puestow procedure

Side-to-side anastomosis of the pancreas and jejunum (pancreatic duct is filleted open)

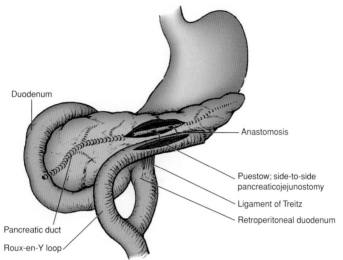

Duodenum

Anastomosis

Puestow; side-to-side pancreaticojejunostomy

Ligament of Treitz

Retroperitoneal duodenum

Pancreatic duct

Roux-en-Y loop

Enterolysis	Lysis of peritoneal adhesions
LOA	**L**ysis **Of A**dhesions (enterolysis)
Appendectomy	Removal of the appendix
Lap appy	Laparoscopic removal of the appendix
Cholecystectomy	Removal of the gallbladder
Lap chole	Laparoscopic removal of the gallbladder
Nissen	Nissen fundoplication; 360° wrap of the stomach by the fundus of the stomach around the distal esophagus to prevent reflux

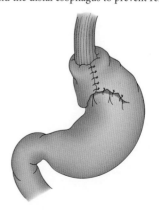

Lap Nissen	Nissen fundoplication with laparoscopy
Simple mastectomy	Removal of breast and nipple without removal of nodes
Choledochojejunostomy	Anastomosis of the common bile duct to the jejunum (end to side)

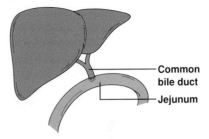

Graham patch	Placement of omentum with stitches over a gastric or duodenal perforation (i.e., omentum is used to plug the hole)
Heineke-Mikulicz pyloroplasty	Longitudinal incision through all layers of the pylorus, sewing closed in a transverse direction to make the pylorus nonfunctional (used after truncal vagotomy)

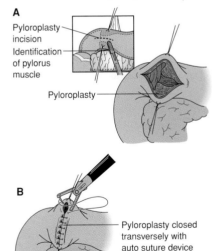

Pringle maneuver

Temporary occlusion of the porta hepatis (for temporary control of liver blood flow when liver parenchyma is actively bleeding)

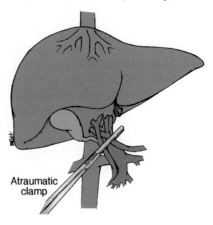

Atraumatic clamp

Modified radical mastectomy

Removal of the breast, nipple, **and axillary lymph nodes** (no muscle is removed)

Lumpectomy and radiation

Removal of breast mass and axillary lymph nodes; normal surrounding breast tissue is spared; patient then undergoes postoperative radiation treatments

I & D

Incision and Drainage of pus; the wound is then packed and left open

Exploratory laparotomy

Laparotomy to explore the peritoneal cavity looking for the cause of pain, peritoneal signs, obstruction, hemorrhage, etc.

TURP

TransUrethral Resection of the Prostate; removal of obstructing prostatic tissue via scope in the urethral lumen

Fem-pop bypass

FEMoral artery to POPliteal artery bypass using synthetic graft or saphenous vein; used to bypass blockage in the femoral artery

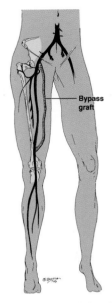

Ax-Fem

Long prosthetic graft tunneled under the skin placed from the **AX**illary artery to the **FEM**oral artery (Extra-anatomic bypass)

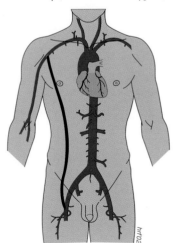

Triple A repair

Repair of an **AAA** (**A**bdominal **A**ortic **A**neurysm): Open aneurysm and place prosthetic graft; then close old aneurysm sac around graft

CABG

Coronary Artery Bypass Grafting; via saphenous vein graft or internal mammary artery bypass grafts to coronary arteries from aorta (cardiac revascularization)

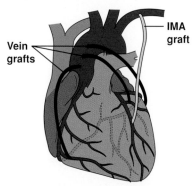

Hartmann's pouch

Oversewing of a rectal stump (or distal colonic stump) after resection of a colonic segment; patient is left with a proximal colostomy

PEG

Percutaneous Endoscopic Gastrostomy: Endoscope is placed in the stomach, which is then inflated with air; a needle is passed into the stomach percutaneously, wire is passed through the needle traversing the abdominal wall, and the gastrostomy is then placed by using the Seldinger technique over the wire

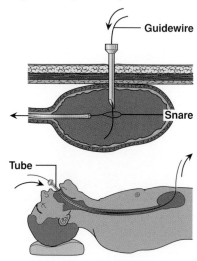

Hemicolectomy	Removal of a colonic segment (i.e., partial colectomy)
Truncal vagotomy	Transection of the vagus nerve trunks; must provide drainage procedure to stomach (e.g., gastrojejunostomy or pyloroplasty) because after truncal vagotomy, the **pylorus does not relax**

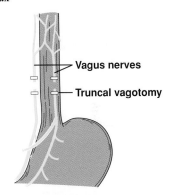

Vagus nerves

Truncal vagotomy

Antrectomy	Removal of stomach antrum
Whipple procedure	Pancreaticoduodenectomy:

    Cholecystectomy

    Truncal vagotomy

    Pancreaticoduodenectomy—removal of the head of the pancreas and duodenum

    Choledochojejunostomy

    Pancreaticojejunostomy (anastomosis of distal pancreas remnant to the jejunum)

    Gastrojejunostomy (anastomosis of stomach to jejunum)

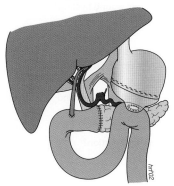

Excisional biopsy	Biopsy with complete excision of all suspect tissue (mass)
Incisional biopsy	Biopsy with incomplete removal of suspect tissue (incises tissue from mass)
Tracheostomy	Placement of airway tube into trachea surgically or percutaneously

Chapter 14 | Wounds

Define the following terms:

Primary wound closure	Suture wound closed immediately (a.k.a. "first intention")
Secondary wound closure	Wound is left open and heals over time **without sutures** (a.k.a. "secondary intention"); it heals by granulation, contraction, and epithelialization over weeks (leaves a larger scar)
Delayed primary closure (DPC)	Suture wound closed 3 to 5 days AFTER incision (classically 5 days)
How long before a sutured wound epithelializes?	24 to 48 hours
After a primary closure, when should the dressing be removed?	POD #2
When can a patient take a shower after a primary closure?	Anytime after POD #2 (after wound epithelializes)
What is a wet-to-dry dressing?	Damp (not wet) gauze dressing placed over a granulating wound and then allowed to dry to the wound; removal allows for "microdébridement" of the wound
What inhibits wound healing?	Infection, ischemia, diabetes mellitus, malnutrition, anemia, steroids, cancer, radiation, and smoking
What reverses the deleterious effects of steroids on wound healing?	Vitamin A
What is an abdominal wound dehiscence?	Opening of the fascial closure (not skin); treat by returning to the O.R. for immediate fascial reclosure
What is Dakin solution?	Dilute sodium hypochlorite (**bleach**) used on contaminated wounds

What is negative-pressure wound therapy (a.k.a. "wound vac")?

Occlusive dressing with sponge and negative pressure system used to accelerate wound healing in acute and chronic wounds

What are the components of a negative pressure wound therapy (NPWT) system?

1. Negative pressure unit
2. Occlusive dressing
3. Foam sponge

What are the potential advantages of negative-pressure wound therapy?

Draws wound edges together, removes exudates and infectious materials, reduces edema, promotes perfusion, and facilitates formation of granulation tissue

Chapter 15 | Drains and Tubes

What is the purpose of drains?

1. Withdrawal of fluids
2. Apposition of tissues to remove a potential space by suction
3. Monitor fluid output

What is a Jackson–Pratt (JP) drain?

Closed drainage system attached to a suction bulb ("grenade")

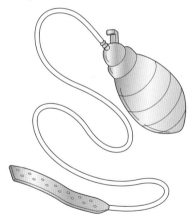

What are the "three S's" of Jackson–Pratt drain removal?

1. Stitch removal
2. Suction discontinuation
3. Slow, steady pull (cover with 4 × 4 to reduce splashing)

What is a Penrose drain?

Open drainage system composed of a thin rubber hose; associated with increased infection rate in clean wounds

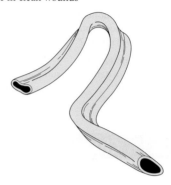

Define the following terms:

G-tube

Gastrostomy tube; used for drainage or feeding

J-tube

Jejunostomy tube; used for feeding; may be a small-needle catheter (remember to flush after use or it will clog) or a large, red rubber catheter

Cholecystostomy tube

Tube placed surgically or percutaneously with ultrasound guidance to drain the gallbladder

T-tube

Tube placed in the common bile duct with an ascending and descending limb that forms a "T"

Drains percutaneously; placed after common bile duct exploration

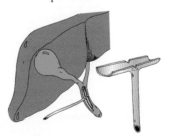

CHEST TUBES

What is a thoracostomy tube?

Chest tube

What is the purpose of a chest tube?

To appose the parietal and visceral pleura by draining blood, pus, fluid, chyle, or air

How is a chest tube inserted?

1. Administer local anesthetic
2. Incise skin in the fourth or fifth intercostal space between the mid- and anterior-axillary lines
3. Perform blunt Kelly-clamp dissection **over** the rib into the pleural space
4. Perform finger exploration to confirm intrapleural placement
5. Place tube posteriorly and superiorly

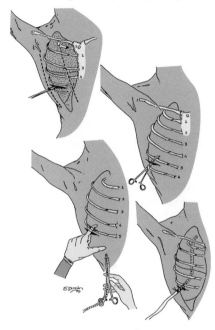

Is the chest tube placed under or over the rib?

Over to avoid the vessels and nerves

What are the goals of chest tube insertion?

Drain the pleural cavity
Appose parietal and visceral pleura to seal any visceral pleural holes

In most cases, where should the chest tube be positioned?

Posteriorly into the apex

How can you tell on CXR if the last hole on the chest tube is in the pleural cavity?

Last hole is cut through the radiopaque line in the chest tube and is seen on CXR as a break in the line, which should be within the pleural cavity

What are the centimeter measurements on a chest tube?

Centimeters from the last hole on the chest tube

What is the chest tube connected to?

Suction, water seal, collection system (three-chambered box, e.g., Pleur-evac®)

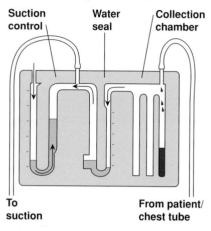

Suction control | **Water seal** | **Collection chamber**

To suction | **From patient/ chest tube**

What are the three chambers of the Pleur-evac®?

1. Collection chamber
2. Water seal
3. Suction control

Describe how each chamber of the Pleur-evac® box works as the old three-bottle system:

   Collection chamber

Collects fluid, pus, blood, or chyle and measures the amount; connects to the water seal bottle and to the chest tube

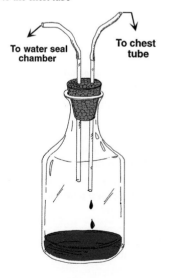

To water seal chamber | **To chest tube**

Water seal chamber

One-way valve—allows air to be removed from the pleural space; does not allow air to enter pleural cavity; connects to the suction control bottle and to the collection chamber

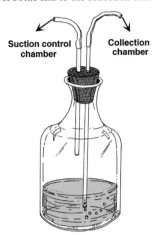

Suction control | **Collection**
chamber | **chamber**

Suction control chamber

Controls the amount of suction by the height of the water column; sucking in room air releases excessive suction; connects to wall suction and to the water seal bottle

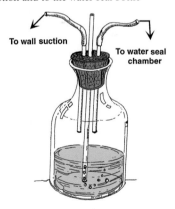

To wall suction

To water seal chamber

Give a good example of a water seal:

Place a straw in a cup of water—you can blow air out but if you suck in, the straw fills with water and thus forms a one-way valve for air just like the chest tube water seal

How is a chest tube placed on water seal?

By removing the suction; a tension pneumothorax (PTX) cannot form because the one-way valve (water seal) allows release of air buildup

Should a chest tube ever be clamped off?

No, except to "run the system" **momentarily**

What does it mean to "run the system" of a chest tube?

To see if the air leak is from a leak in the pleural cavity (e.g., hole in lung) or from a leak in the tubing

Momentarily occlude the chest tube and if the air leak is still present, it is from the tubing or tubing connection, not from the chest

How can you tell if the chest tube is "tidaling"?

Take off suction and look at the water seal chamber: Fluid should move with respiration/ventilation (called "tidaling"); this decreases and ceases if the pleura seals off the chest tube

How can you check for an air leak?

Look at the water seal chamber on suction:
If bubbles pass through the water seal fluid, a large air leak (i.e., air leaking into chest tube) is present; if no air leak is evident on suction, remove suction and ask the patient to cough
If air bubbles through the water seal, a small air leak is present

What is the usual course for removing a chest tube placed for a PTX?

1. Suction until the PTX resolves and the air leak is gone
2. Water seal for 24 hours
3. Remove the chest tube if no PTX or air leak is present after 24 hours of water seal

How fast is a small, stable PTX absorbed?

≈1% daily; therefore, a 10% PTX by volume will absorb in ≈10 days

How should a chest tube be removed?

1. Cut the stitch
2. Ask the patient to exhale or inhale maximally
3. Rapidly remove the tube (split second) and at same time, place petroleum jelly gauze covered by 4 × 4's and then tape
4. Obtain a CXR

What is a Heimlich valve?

One-way flutter valve for a chest tube

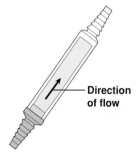

Direction of flow

NASOGASTRIC TUBES (NGT)

How should an NGT be placed?

1. Use lubrication and have suction up on the bed
2. Use anesthetic to numb nose
3. Place head in flexion
4. Ask patient to drink a small amount of water when the tube is in the back of the throat and to swallow the tube; if the patient can talk without difficulty and succus returns, the tube should be in the stomach (Get an x-ray if there is any question about position)

How should an NGT be removed?

Give patient a tissue, discontinue suction, untape nose, remove quickly, and tell patient to blow nose

What test should be performed before feeding via any tube?

High abdominal x-ray to confirm placement into the GI tract and NOT the lung!

How does an NGT work?

Sump pump, dual lumen tube—the large clear tube is hooked to suction, and the small blue tube allows for air sump (i.e., circuit sump pump with air in the blue tube and air and succus sucked out through the large clear lumen)

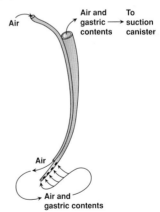

How can you check to see if the NGT is working?

Blue port will make a sucking noise; always keep the blue port opening above the stomach

Should an NGT be placed on continuous or intermittent suction?

Continuous low suction—side holes disengage if they are against mucosa because of the sump mechanism and multiple holes

What happens if the NGT is clogged/not functional?	Tube will not decompress the stomach and will keep the low esophageal sphincter (LES) open (i.e., a setup for aspiration)
How should an NGT be unclogged?	Saline-flush the clear port, reconnect to suction, and flush air down the blue sump port
What is the common cause of excessive NGT drainage?	Tip of the NGT is inadvertently placed in the duodenum and drains the pancreatic fluid and bile; an x-ray should be taken and the tube repositioned into the stomach
What is the difference between a feeding tube (Dobbhoff tube) and an NGT?	A feeding tube is a thin tube weighted at the end that is not a sump pump but a simple catheter; usually placed past the pylorus, which is facilitated by the weighted end and peristalsis

FOLEY CATHETER

What is a Foley catheter?	Catheter into the bladder, allowing accurate urine output determination
What is a coudé catheter?	Foley catheter with a small, curved tip to help maneuver around a large prostate

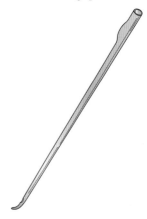

If a Foley catheter cannot be inserted, what are the next steps?	1. Anesthetize the urethra with a sterile local anesthetic (e.g., lidocaine jelly) 2. Try a **larger** Foley catheter 3. Try coudé catheter 4. Consult Urology

What if a patient has a urethral injury and a Foley cannot be placed?

Suprapubic catheter will need to be placed

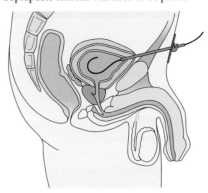

CENTRAL LINES

What are they?

Catheters placed into the major veins (central veins) via subclavian, internal jugular, or femoral vein approaches

What major complications result from placement?

PTX (always obtain postplacement CXR), bleeding, malposition (e.g., into the neck from subclavian approach), dysrhythmias

In long-term central lines, what does the "cuff" do?

Allows ingrowth of fibrous tissue, which:
1. Holds the line in place
2. Forms a barrier to the advance of bacteria

What is a Hickman® or Hickman-type catheter?

External central line tunneled under the skin with a "cuff"

What is a Port-A-Cath®?

Central line that has a port buried under the skin, which must be accessed through the skin (percutaneously)

What is a "cordis"?

Large central line catheter; used for massive fluid resuscitation or for placing a Swan–Ganz catheter

If you try to place a subclavian central line unsuccessfully, what must you do before trying the other side?

Get a CXR—a bilateral pneumothorax can be fatal!

How can diameter in mm be determined from a French measurement?

Divide the French size by π, or 3.14 (e.g., a 15 French tube has a diameter of 5 mm)

Chapter 16 | Surgical Anatomy Pearls

What is the drainage of the left testicular vein?

Left renal vein

What is the drainage of the right testicular vein?

IVC

Which artery bleeds in bleeding duodenal ulcers?

Gastroduodenal artery

What is Morison's pouch?

Hepatorenal recess; the most posterior cavity within the peritoneal cavity

Where are the blood vessels on a rib?

Vein, Artery, and Nerve (**VAN**) are underneath the rib (thus, place chest tubes and thoracentesis needles above the rib!)

What is the order of the femoral vessels?

Femoral vein is medial to the femoral artery (Think: **"NAVEL"** for the order of the right femoral vessels—**N**erve, **A**rtery, **V**ein, **E**mpty space, **L**ymphatics)

What is Hesselbach's triangle?

The area bordered by:
1. Inguinal ligament
2. Epigastric vessels
3. Lateral border of the rectus sheath

What nerve is located on top of the spermatic cord?

Ilioinguinal nerve

What is Calot's triangle?

The area bordered by:
1. Cystic duct
2. Common hepatic duct
3. Cystic artery
(Pronounced "kal-ohs")

What is Calot's node?

Lymph node found in Calot's triangle

What separates the right and left lobes of the liver?

Cantle's line—a line drawn from the IVC to just left of the gallbladder fossa

What is the gastrinoma triangle?

Triangle where >90% of gastrinomas are located, bordered by:
1. Junction of the second and third portions of the duodenum
2. Cystic duct
3. Pancreatic neck

Which artery is responsible for anterior spinal syndrome?

Artery of Adamkiewicz (pronounced "ah-dahm'kē-ā'vich")

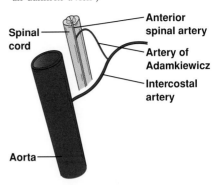

Where is McBurney's point?

One third the distance from the anterior superior iliac spine to the umbilicus (estimate of the position of the appendix)

How can you find the appendix after you find the cecum?

Trace the taeniae back as they converge on the origin of the appendix

What are the white lines of Toldt?

Lateral peritoneal reflections of the ascending and descending colon

What is the strongest layer of the small bowel?

Submucosa (NOT the serosa, think: **SU**bmucosa = **SU**perior)

Which parts of the GI tract do not have a serosa?

Esophagus
Middle and distal rectum

What are the plicae circulares?

Plicae = folds, circulares = circular; thus, the circular folds of mucosa of the small bowel

What are the major structural differences between the jejunum and ileum?

Jejunum—long vasa rectae; large plicae circulares; thicker wall
Ileum—shorter vasa rectae; smaller plicae circulares; thinner wall (Think: **I**leum = **I**nferior vasa rectae, **I**nferior plicae circulares, and **I**nferior wall)

What are the major anatomic differences between the colon and the small bowel?

Colon has taeniae coli, haustra, and appendices epiploicae (fat appendages), whereas the small intestine is smooth

How far up does the diaphragm extend?

To the nipples in men (fourth intercostal space; thus, the abdomen extends to the level of the nipples)

Which dermatome is at the umbilicus?

T10

What are the major layers of an artery?

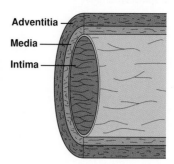

Adventitia

Media

Intima

Chapter 17 | Fluids and Electrolytes

What are the two major body fluid compartments?
1. Intracellular
2. Extracellular

What are the two subcompartments of extracellular fluid?
1. Interstitial fluid (in between cells)
2. Intravascular fluid (plasma)

What percentage of body weight is in fluid?
60%

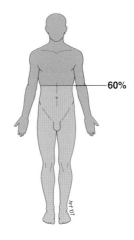

—60%

What percentage of body fluid is intracellular?
66%

What percentage of body fluid is extracellular?
33%

What is the composition of body fluid?
Fluids = 60% total body weight:
    Intracellular = 40% total body weight
    Extracellular = 20% total body weight
(Think: 60, 40, 20)

On average, what percentage of ideal body weight does blood account for in adults?
≈7%

How many liters of blood are in a 70-kg man?
$0.07 \times 70 = 5$ L

What is the physiologic response to hypovolemia?

Sodium/H_2O retention via renin → aldosterone, water retention via ADH, vasoconstriction via angiotensin II and sympathetic nervous system, low urine output and tachycardia (early), hypotension (late)

THIRD SPACING

What is it?

Fluid accumulation in the interstitium of tissues, as in edema (think of the intravascular and intracellular spaces as the first two spaces)

When does "third spacing" occur postoperatively?

Third-spaced fluid tends to mobilize back into the intravascular space around POD #3

What are the classic signs of third spacing?

Tachycardia
Decreased urine output

What is the treatment?

IV hydration with isotonic fluids

What are the surgical causes of the following conditions:

  Metabolic acidosis

Loss of bicarbonate: diarrhea, ileus, fistula, high-output ileostomy, carbonic anhydrase inhibitors
Increase in acids: lactic acidosis (ischemia), ketoacidosis, renal failure, necrotic tissue

  Hypochloremic alkalosis

NGT suction, loss of gastric HCl through vomiting/NGT

  Metabolic alkalosis

Vomiting, NG suction, diuretics, alkali ingestion, mineralocorticoid excess

  Respiratory acidosis

Hypoventilation (e.g., CNS depression), drugs (e.g., morphine), PTX, pleural effusion, parenchymal lung disease, acute airway obstruction

  Respiratory alkalosis

Hyperventilation (e.g., anxiety, pain, fever, wrong ventilator settings)

What is the "classic" acid–base finding with significant vomiting or NGT suctioning?

Hypokalemic and hypochloremic metabolic alkalosis

Why hypokalemia with NGT suctioning?

Loss in gastric fluid—loss of HCl causes alkalosis, driving K^+ into cells

What is the treatment for hypokalemic and hypochloremic metabolic alkalosis?

IVF, Cl^-/K^+ replacement (e.g., NS with KCl)

What is paradoxic alkalotic aciduria?	Seen in severe hypokalemic, hypovolemic, and hypochloremic metabolic alkalosis with paradoxic metabolic alkalosis of serum and acidic urine
How does paradoxic alkalotic aciduria occur?	H^+ is lost in the urine in exchange for Na^+ in an attempt to restore volume
With paradoxic alkalotic aciduria, why is H^+ preferentially lost?	H^+ is exchanged preferentially into the urine instead of K^+ because of the low concentration of K^+
What can be followed to assess fluid status?	Urine output, base deficit, lactic acid, vital signs, weight changes, skin turgor, jugular venous distention (JVD), mucosal membranes, rales (crackles), central venous pressure, PCWP, chest x-ray findings
With hypovolemia, what changes occur in vital signs?	Tachycardia, tachypnea, initial rise in diastolic blood pressure because of clamping down (peripheral vasoconstriction) with subsequent decrease in both systolic and diastolic blood pressures, pulse pressure variability during inspiration on positive pressure ventilation
How can the estimated levels of daily secretions from bile, gastric, and small bowel sources be remembered?	Alphabetically and numerically: **BGS** and **123** or **B1, G2, S3,** because **B**ile, **G**astric, and **S**mall bowel produce roughly **1** L, **2** L, and **3** L, respectively!

COMMON IV REPLACEMENT FLUIDS (ALL VALUES ARE PER LITER)

What comprises normal saline (NS)?	154 mEq of Cl^- 154 mEq of Na^+
What comprises 1/2 NS?	77 mEq of Cl^- 77 mEq of Na^+
What comprises 1/4 NS?	39 mEq of Cl^- 39 mEq of Na^+
What comprises Lactated Ringer's (LR)?	130 mEq Na^+ 109 mEq Cl^- 28 mEq lactate 4 mEq K^+ 3 mEq Ca^+
What comprises D5W?	5% dextrose (50 g) in H_2O
What accounts for tonicity?	Mainly electrolytes; thus, NS and LR are both isotonic, whereas 1/2 NS is hypotonic to serum

What happens to the lactate in LR in the body?	Converted into bicarbonate; thus, LR cannot be used as a maintenance fluid because patients would become alkalotic
IVF replacement by anatomic site:	
Gastric (NGT)	D5 1/2 NS + 20 KCl
Biliary	LR ± sodium bicarbonate
Pancreatic	LR ± sodium bicarbonate
Small bowel (ileostomy)	LR
Colonic (diarrhea)	LR ± sodium bicarbonate

CALCULATION OF MAINTENANCE FLUIDS

What is the 4/2/1 rule?	Maintenance IV fluids for hourly rate: **4** mL/kg for the first 10 kg **2** mL/kg for the next 10 kg **1** mL/kg for every kg over 20
What is the maintenance rate for a 70-kg man?	Using 4/2/1: $4 \times 10 \text{ kg} = 40$ $2 \times 10 \text{ kg} = 20$ $1 \times 50 \text{ kg} = 50$ Total = 110 mL/hr maintenance rate
What is the common adult maintenance fluid?	D5 1/2 NS with 20 mEq KCl/L
What is the common pediatric maintenance fluid?	D5 1/4 NS with 20 mEq KCl/L (use 1/4 NS because of the decreased ability of children to concentrate urine)
Why should sugar (dextrose) be added to maintenance fluid?	To inhibit muscle breakdown
What is the best way to assess fluid status?	Urine output (unless the patient has cardiac or renal dysfunction, in which case central venous pressure or wedge pressure is often used)
What is the minimal urine output for an adult on maintenance IV?	30 mL/hr (0.5 cc/kg/hr)
What are the common isotonic fluids?	NS, LR
What is a bolus?	Volume of fluid given IV rapidly (e.g., 1 L over 1 hour); used for increasing intravascular volume, and isotonic fluids should be used (i.e., NS or LR)
After a laparotomy, when should a patient's fluid be "mobilized"?	Classically, POD #3; the patient begins to "mobilize" the third-space fluid back into the intravascular space

ELECTROLYTE IMBALANCES

Hyperkalemia

What is the normal range for potassium level?

3.5 to 5.0 mEq/L

What are the surgical causes of hyperkalemia?

Iatrogenic overdose, blood transfusion, renal failure, diuretics, acidosis, tissue destruction (injury/hemolysis)

What are the ECG findings?

Peaked T waves, depressed ST segment, prolonged PR, wide QRS, bradycardia, ventricular fibrillation

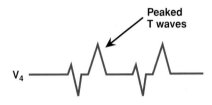

What are the critical values?

$K^+ >6.5$

What is the nonacute treatment?

Furosemide (Lasix®), sodium polystyrene sulfonate (Kayexalate®)

What is the acronym for the treatment of acute symptomatic hyperkalemia?

"CB DIAL K":
    Calcium
    Bicarbonate

    Dialysis
    Insulin/dextrose
    Albuterol
    Lasix

    Kayexalate

What is "pseudohyperkalemia"?

Spurious hyperkalemia as a result of falsely elevated K^+ in sample from sample hemolysis

What acid–base change lowers the serum potassium?

Alkalosis (thus, give bicarbonate for hyperkalemia)

What nebulizer treatment can help lower K^+ level?

Albuterol

Hypokalemia

What are the surgical causes?

Diuretics, certain antibiotics, steroids, alkalosis, diarrhea, intestinal fistulae, NG aspiration, vomiting, insulin, insufficient supplementation, amphotericin

What are the signs/symptoms?	Weakness, tetany, nausea, vomiting, **ileus**, paresthesia
What are the ECG findings?	**Flattening of T waves, U waves,** ST segment depression, PAC, PVC, atrial fibrillation
What is a U wave?	

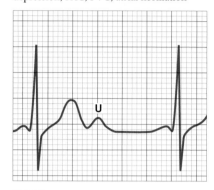

What is the rapid treatment?	KCl IV
What is the most common electrolyte-mediated ileus in the surgical patient?	Hypokalemia
What electrolyte deficiency can actually cause hypokalemia?	Low magnesium
What electrolyte must you replace first before replacing K⁺?	Magnesium
Why does hypomagnesemia make replacement of K⁺ with hypokalemia nearly impossible?	Hypomagnesemia inhibits K^+ reabsorption from the renal tubules

Hypernatremia

What is the normal range for sodium level?	135 to 145 mEq/L
What are the surgical causes?	Inadequate hydration, diabetes insipidus, diuresis, vomiting, diarrhea, diaphoresis, tachypnea, iatrogenic (e.g., TPN and 3% hypertonic saline)
What are the signs/symptoms?	Seizures, confusion, stupor, pulmonary or peripheral edema, tremors, respiratory paralysis
What is the usual treatment supplementation slowly over days?	D5W, 1/4 NS, or 1/2 NS

How fast should you lower the sodium level in hypernatremia?	Guideline is <12 mEq/L per day
What is the major complication of lowering the sodium level too fast?	Seizures due to cerebral edema (NOT central pontine myelinolysis)

Hyponatremia

What are the surgical causes of the following types:	
Hypovolemic	Diuretic excess, hypoaldosteronism, vomiting, NG suction, burns, pancreatitis, diaphoresis
Euvolemic	SIADH, CNS abnormalities, drugs
Hypervolemic	Renal failure, CHF, liver failure (cirrhosis), iatrogenic fluid overload (dilutional)
What are the signs/symptoms?	Seizures, coma, nausea, vomiting, ileus, lethargy, confusion, weakness
What are the treatments of the following types:	
Hypovolemic	NS IV, correct underlying cause
Euvolemic	SIADH: furosemide and NS acutely, fluid restriction
Hypervolemic	Dilutional: fluid restriction and diuretics
How fast should you increase the sodium level in hyponatremia?	Guideline is <12 mEq/L per day
What may occur if you correct hyponatremia too quickly?	Central pontine myelinolysis!
What are the signs of central pontine myelinolysis?	1. Confusion 2. Spastic quadriplegia 3. Horizontal gaze paralysis
What is the most common cause of mild postoperative hyponatremia?	Fluid overload
How can the sodium level in SIADH be remembered?	**SIADH** (**S**odium **I**s **A**lways **D**own **H**ere) = Hyponatremia

How can you remember the complications of correcting sodium abnormality too quickly?

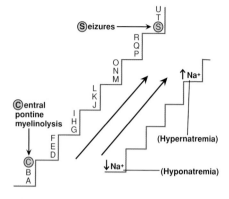

"Pseudohyponatremia"

What is it?

Spurious lab value of hyponatremia as a result of hyperglycemia, hyperlipidemia, or hyperproteinemia

Hypercalcemia

What are the causes?

"CHIMPANZEES":
1. **C**alcium supplementation IV
2. **H**yperparathyroidism (1°/3°) hyperthyroidism
3. **I**mmobility/**I**atrogenic (thiazide diuretics)
4. **M**ets/**M**ilk-alkali syndrome
5. **P**aget's disease (bone)
6. **A**ddison's disease/**A**cromegaly
7. **N**eoplasm (colon, lung, breast, prostate, multiple myeloma)
8. **Z**ollinger–Ellison syndrome (as part of MEN I)
9. **E**xcessive vitamin D
10. **E**xcessive vitamin A
11. **S**arcoid

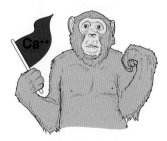

What are the signs/symptoms?	Hypercalcemia—"Stones, bones, abdominal groans, and psychiatric overtones"; polydipsia; polyuria; constipation
What are the ECG findings?	Short QT interval, prolonged PR interval
What is the acute treatment of hypercalcemic crisis?	Volume expansion with NS, diuresis with furosemide (not thiazides)
What are other options for lowering Ca$^+$ level?	Steroids, calcitonin, bisphosphonates (pamidronate, etc.), mithramycin, dialysis (last resort)

Hypocalcemia

How can the calcium level be determined with hypoalbuminemia?	(4—measured albumin level) × 0.8, then add this value to the measured calcium level
What are the surgical causes?	Short bowel syndrome, intestinal bypass, vitamin D deficiency, sepsis, acute pancreatitis, osteoblastic metastasis, aminoglycosides, diuretics, renal failure, hypomagnesemia, rhabdomyolysis
What is Chvostek's sign?	Facial muscle spasm with tapping of facial nerve (Think: **CH**vostek = **CH**eek)
What is Trousseau's sign?	Carpal spasm after occluding blood flow in forearm with blood pressure cuff
What are the signs/symptoms?	Chvostek's and Trousseau's signs, perioral paresthesia (early), increased deep tendon reflexes (late), confusion, abdominal cramps, laryngospasm, stridor, seizures, tetany, psychiatric abnormalities (e.g., paranoia, depression, hallucinations)
What are the ECG findings?	Prolonged QT and ST intervals (peaked T waves are also possible, as in hyperkalemia)
What is the acute treatment?	Calcium gluconate IV
What is the chronic treatment?	Calcium PO, vitamin D
What is the possible complication of infused calcium if the IV infiltrates?	**Tissue necrosis**; never administer peripherally unless absolutely necessary (calcium gluconate is less toxic than calcium chloride during an infiltration)
What is the best way to check the calcium level in the ICU?	Check ionized calcium

Hypermagnesemia

What is the normal range for magnesium level?	1.5 to 2.5 mEq/L
What is the surgical cause?	TPN, renal failure, IV over supplementation
What are the signs/symptoms?	Respiratory failure, CNS depression, decreased deep tendon reflexes
What is the treatment?	Calcium gluconate IV, insulin plus glucose, dialysis (similar to treatment of hyperkalemia), furosemide (Lasix®)

Hypomagnesemia

What are the surgical causes?	TPN, hypocalcemia, gastric suctioning, aminoglycosides, renal failure, diarrhea, vomiting
What are the signs/symptoms?	Increased deep tendon reflexes, tetany, asterixis, tremor, Chvostek's sign, ventricular ectopy, vertigo, tachycardia, dysrhythmias
What is the acute treatment?	$MgSO_4$ IV
What is the chronic treatment?	Magnesium oxide PO (side effect: diarrhea)
What is the other electrolyte abnormality that hypomagnesemia may make it impossible to correct?	Hypokalemia (always fix hypomagnesemia with hypokalemia)

Hyperglycemia

What are the surgical causes?	Diabetes (poor control), infection, stress, TPN, drugs, lab error, drawing over IV site, somatostatinoma, glucagonoma
What are the signs/symptoms?	Polyuria, hypovolemia, confusion/coma, polydipsia, ileus, DKA (Kussmaul breathing), abdominal pain, hyporeflexia
What is the treatment?	Insulin
What is the Weiss protocol?	Sliding scale insulin
What is the goal glucose level in the ICU?	140 to 180 mg/dL (it was lower but is now higher due to episodes of hypoglycemia)

Hypoglycemia

What are the surgical causes?	Excess insulin, decreased caloric intake, insulinoma, drugs, liver failure, adrenal insufficiency, gastrojejunostomy

What are the signs/symptoms?	Sympathetic response (diaphoresis, tachycardia, palpitations), confusion, coma, headache, diplopia, neurologic deficits, seizures
What is the treatment?	Glucose (IV or PO)

Hypophosphatemia

What are the signs/symptoms?	Weakness, cardiomyopathy, neurologic dysfunction (e.g., ataxia), rhabdomyolysis, hemolysis, poor pressor response
What is the complication of severe hypophosphatemia?	Respiratory failure
What are the causes?	GI losses, inadequate supplementation, medications, sepsis, alcohol abuse, renal loss
What is the critical value?	<1.0 mg/dL
What is the treatment?	Supplement with sodium phosphate or potassium phosphate IV (depending on potassium level)

Hyperphosphatemia

What are the signs/symptoms?	Calcification (ectopic), heart block
What are the causes?	Renal failure, sepsis, chemotherapy, hyperthyroidism
What is the treatment?	Aluminum hydroxide (binds phosphate)

Miscellaneous

This ECG pattern is consistent with which electrolyte abnormality?	Hyperkalemia: peaked T waves

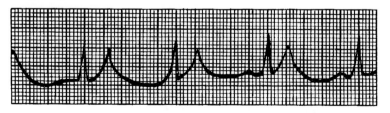

If hyperkalemia is left untreated, what can occur?

Ventricular tachycardia/fibrillation → death

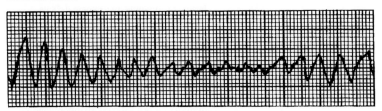

Which electrolyte is an inotrope?

Calcium

What are the major cardiac electrolytes?

Potassium (dysrhythmias), magnesium (dysrhythmias), calcium (dysrhythmias/inotrope)

What is the most common cause of electrolyte-mediated ileus?

Hypokalemia

What is a colloid fluid?

Protein-containing fluid (albumin)

An elderly patient goes into CHF (congestive heart failure) on POD #3 after a laparotomy. What is going on?

Mobilization of the "third-space" fluid into the intravascular space, resulting in fluid overload and resultant CHF (but also must rule out MI)

What fluid is used to replace NGT (gastric) aspirate?

D5 1/2 NS with 20 KCl

What electrolyte is associated with succinylcholine?

Hyperkalemia

RAPID-FIRE REVIEW

Name the most likely diagnosis:

28-year-old female s/p total abdominal colectomy and ileostomy now with increased ileostomy output and U waves on EKG

Hypokalemia

51-year-old male with alcoholic cirrhosis has a sodium level of 127. The intern corrects the sodium to 140 in 1 hour with hypertonic saline and reveals neurologic signs and symptoms

Central pontine myelinolysis

70-year-old male s/p (status post) fall with a subdural develops hypernatremia with copious amounts of urine	Diabetes insipidus
80-year-old female s/p fall with a subdural hematoma develops hyponatremia and increase in urine osmolality with normal urine output	SIADH

Chapter 18 | Blood and Blood Products

Define the following terms:

PT	**P**rothrombin **T**ime: Tests extrinsic coagulation pathway
PTT	**P**artial **T**hromboplastin **T**ime: Tests intrinsic coagulation pathway
INR	**I**nternational **N**ormalized **R**atio (reports PT results)
Packed red blood cells (PRBCs)	One unit equals ≈300 mL (±50 mL); no platelets or clotting factors; can be mixed with NS to infuse faster
Platelets	Replace platelets with units of platelets (6 to 10 units from single donor or random donors)
Fresh frozen plasma (FFP)	Replaces **clotting factors;** (no RBCs/WBCs/platelets)
Cryoprecipitate (cryo)	Replaces fibrinogen, von Willebrand factor (vWF), and some clotting factors
Which electrolyte is most likely to fall with the infusion of stored blood? Why?	Ionized calcium; the citrate preservative used for the storage of blood binds serum calcium
What changes occur in the storage of PRBCs?	$\downarrow$Ca$^+$, $\uparrow$K$^+$, $\downarrow$2,3-DPG, $\uparrow$H$^+$ ($\downarrow$pH), $\downarrow$PMNs
What is the rough formula for converting Hgb to Hct?	Hgb × 3 = Hct
One unit of PRBC increases Hct by how much?	≈3% to 4%

Which blood type is the "universal" donor for PRBCs?	O negative
What is Kcentra® (prothrombin complex concentrate)?	Factors 2, 7, 9, and 10—reverses warfarin (Coumadin®) in life-threatening bleeding
Which blood type is the "universal" donor for FFP?	AB
What is a type and screen?	Patient's blood type is determined and the blood is screened for antibodies; a type and cross from that sample can then be ordered if needed later
What is a type and cross?	Patient's BLOOD is sent to the blood bank and cross-matched for **specific donor units for possible blood transfusion**
What is thrombocytopenia?	Low platelet count (<100,000)
What can be given to help correct platelet dysfunction from uremia, aspirin, or bypass?	DDAVP (desmopressin)
What common medication causes platelets to irreversibly malfunction?	Aspirin (inhibits cyclooxygenase)
What is Plavix®?	Clopidogrel—irreversibly inhibits platelet $P2Y_{12}$ ADP receptor (blocks fibrin crosslinking of platelets)
What platelet count is associated with spontaneous bleeding?	<20,000
What should the platelet count be before surgery?	>50,000
When should "prophylactic" platelet transfusions be given?	With platelets <10,000 (old recommendation was 20,000)
How to reverse the effect of clopidogrel (Plavix®)?	No reversal known. Many treat with platelet transfusion
What is microcytic anemia "until proven otherwise" in a man or postmenopausal woman?	Colon cancer
For how long can packed RBCs be stored?	≈6 weeks (42 days)
What is the most common cause of transfusion hemolysis?	ABO incompatibility as a result of **clerical error**
What is the risk of receiving a unit of blood infected with HIV?	≈1 in 1,000,000
What are the symptoms of a transfusion reaction?	**Fever,** chills, nausea, hypotension, lumbar pain, chest pain, abnormal bleeding

What is the treatment for transfusion hemolysis?	**Stop** transfusion; provide fluids; perform diuresis (Lasix) to protect kidneys; alkalinize urine (bicarbonate); give pressors as needed
What component of the blood transfusion can cause a fever?	WBCs
What is the transfusion "trigger" Hgb?	<7.0
What is the widely considered "optimal" Hgb in a patient with a history of heart disease or stroke?	FOCUS trial = Liberal (<10 Hgb) versus restrictive (<8 Hgb) Trigger = No difference in mortality or morbidity
When should aspirin administration be discontinued preoperatively?	At 1 week because platelets live 7 to 10 days (must use judgment if patient is at risk for stroke or MI; it may be better to continue and use excellent surgical hemostasis in these patients)
What can move the oxyhemoglobin dissociation curve to the right?	Acidosis; 2,3-DPG; fever; elevated PCO_2 (to the right means greater ability to release the O_2 to the tissues)
What is the normal life of RBCs?	120 days
What is the normal life of platelets?	7 to 10 days
How can the clotting factor for hemophilia A be remembered?	Think: "**Eight**" sounds like "**A**"
How do you remember which factors are deficient with hemophilia A and hemophilia B?	Think alphabetically and chronologically: **A** before **B**—**8** before **9** Hemophilia **A** = factor **VIII** Hemophilia **B** = factor **IX**

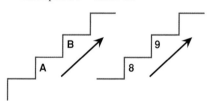

What is von Willebrand's disease?	Deficiency of vWF and factor VIII:C
What is used to correct von Willebrand's disease?	DDAVP or cryoprecipitate
What coagulation is abnormal with the following disorders:	
Hemophilia A	PTT (elevated)
Hemophilia B	PTT (elevated)
von Willebrand's disease	Bleeding time

What is the usual "therapeutic" PT?	With Coumadin®, usually shoot for an INR of 2.0 to 3.0
What is the acronym basis for the word WARFARIN?	**W**isconsin **A**lumni **R**esearch **F**oundation-**ARIN**
What is the most common inherited hypercoagulable state?	Factor V Leiden (Think: **LE**iden = **LE**ader)

RAPID-FIRE REVIEW

List the blood product or medication(s) that you would give for each of the following patients:

18-year-old female in high-speed motorcycle collision with subdural hematoma and flail chest; platelets = 189,000; fibrinogen = 400; ionized calcium = 2.8; PT 23 (INR = 3.4); PTT = 35	FFP (fresh frozen plasma)
44-year-old male involved in a fall from scaffolding going to the operating room for exploratory laparotomy for significant free air on CT scan; platelets = 25,000; PT = 13.1; PTT = 38; fibrinogen = 200	Platelets
Patient s/p prostate resection develops diffuse oozing; platelets = 200,000; PT = 13; PTT = 39	Amicar® (epsilon-aminocaproic acid) (an antifibrinolytic)
56-year-old female 1 hour s/p CABG × 4 on bypass with continued mediastinal bleeding; surgeons confirm excellent surgical hemostasis; the patient is warm, platelets 178,000; PT = 12.9; PTT = 78	Protamine
67-year-old patient with liver failure and s/p fall in the operating room for an exploratory laparotomy; the patient develops progressive oozing; the PT and PTT are normalized; platelets = 300,000; fibrinogen = 49.7	Cryoprecipitate—provides fibrinogen

Patient with liver failure and poor nutrition with elevated PT that is refractory to multiple transfusions of FFP	Vitamin K, prothrombin complex concentrate (PCC)
8-year-old male with hemophilia A with spontaneous bruising and nosebleed	Factor VIII
7-year-old male with hemophilia B with large right knee hemarthrosis	Factor IX
23-year-old female with von Willebrand's disease who develops bleeding complications	First try DDAVP; then cryoprecipitate

Chapter 19 | Surgical Hemostasis

What motto is associated with surgical hemostasis?	"All bleeding stops"
What is the most immediate method to obtain hemostasis?	Pressure (finger)
What is a "Bovie"?	Electrocautery (designed by Bovie with Cushing for neurosurgery in the 1920s)
Where should a Bovie be applied to a clamp or pickup to coagulate a vessel?	**Anywhere** on the clamp/pickup

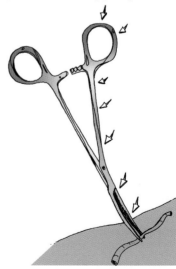

Should you ever "blindly" place a clamp in a wound to stop bleeding?

No, you may injure surrounding tissues such as nerves

What is a figure-of-eight suture?

Suture ligature placed twice in the tissue prior to being tied

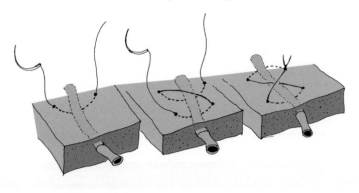

Chapter 20 | Common Surgical Medications

ANTIBIOTICS

What is an "antibiogram?"

List of bacteria and the antibiotic sensitivities at a specific hospital

Which antibiotics are commonly used for anaerobic infections?

Metronidazole, clindamycin, cefoxitin, cefotetan, imipenem, ticarcillin-clavulanic acid, Augmentin® (amoxicillin-clavulanic acid), Zosyn® (piperacillin-tazobactam)

Which antibiotics are commonly used for gram-negative infections?

Gentamicin and other aminoglycosides, ciprofloxacin, aztreonam, third-generation cephalosporins, sulfamethoxazole-trimethoprim

Which antibiotic, if taken with alcohol, will produce a disulfiram-like reaction?

Metronidazole (Flagyl®) (disulfiram is Antabuse®)

What is the drug of choice for treating amoebic infections?

Metronidazole (Flagyl®)

Which antibiotic is associated with cholestasis?

Ceftriaxone (Rocephin®)

Which antibiotic cannot be given to children or pregnant women?

Ciprofloxacin (interferes with the growth plate)

Is rash (only) in response to penicillins a contraindication to cephalosporins?	No, but breathing problems, urticaria, and edema in response to penicillins are contraindications to the cephalosporins

Describe the following medications:

Augmentin®	Amoxicillin and clavulanic acid
Unasyn®	Ampicillin and sulbactam
Zosyn®	Piperacillin and tazobactam: extended spectrum penicillin with β-lactamase inhibitor
Cefazolin (Ancef®)	First-generation cephalosporin; surgical prophylaxis for **skin flora**
Ceftazidime (Ceftaz®)	Third-generation cephalosporin; strong activity against *Pseudomonas*
Clindamycin	Strong activity against gram-negative **anaerobes** such as *Bacteroides fragilis*; adequate gram-positive activity
Gentamicin	Aminoglycoside used to treat aerobic **gram-negative** bacteria; nephrotoxic, ototoxic; blood peak/trough levels should be monitored
Metronidazole (Flagyl®)	Used for serious **anaerobic** infections (e.g., diverticulitis); also used to treat amebiasis; patient must abstain from alcohol use during therapy
Vancomycin	Used to treat methicillin-resistant *Staphylococcus aureus* (MRSA), nephrotoxicity, and red-man syndrome; used orally to treat *Clostridium difficile* pseudomembranous colitis (poorly absorbed from the gut); with IV administration, peak levels should be maintained >15
Ciprofloxacin (Cipro®)	Quinolone antibiotic with activity against gram-negative bacteria, including *Pseudomonas*
Aztreonam (Azactam®)	Monobactam with gram-negative spectrum
Amphotericin	IV antifungal antibiotic associated with renal toxicity, hypokalemia
Fluconazole (Diflucan®)	Antifungal agent (IV or PO) NOT associated with renal toxicity
Nystatin	PO and topical antifungal

STEROIDS

Can steroids be stopped abruptly?	No, steroids should never be stopped abruptly; always taper
Which patients need stress-dose steroids before surgery?	Those who are on steroids, were on steroids in the past year, have suspected hypoadrenalism, or are about to undergo adrenalectomy
What is the "stress dose" for steroids?	**100** mg of hydrocortisone IV every 8 hours and then taper (adults)
Which vitamin helps counteract the deleterious effects of steroids on wound healing?	Vitamin A

HEPARIN

What is its action?	Heparin binds with and activates antithrombin III
What are its uses?	Prophylaxis/treatment—DVT, pulmonary embolism, stroke, atrial fibrillation, acute arterial occlusion, cardiopulmonary bypass
What are the side effects?	Bleeding complications; can cause thrombocytopenia
What reverses the effects?	**Protamine IV (1:100, 1** mg of protamine to every **100** units of heparin)
What laboratory test should be used to follow effect?	aPTT—activated partial thromboplastin time
What is the standard lab target for therapeutic heparinization?	1.5 to 2.5 times control or measured antifactor Xa level
Who is at risk for a protamine anaphylactic reaction?	Patients with type 1 diabetes mellitus, s/p prostate surgery
What is the half-life of heparin?	≈90 minutes (1 to 2 hours)
How long before surgery should it be discontinued?	From 4 to 6 hours preoperatively
Does heparin dissolve clots?	No; it stops the progression of clot formation and allows the body's own fibrinolytic systems to dissolve the clot
What is LMWH?	Low-Molecular-Weight Heparin

WARFARIN (COUMADIN®)

ACRONYM basis for name?	**W**isconsin **A**lumni **R**esearch **F**oundation
Describe its action:	**Inhibits vitamin K–dependent clotting factors II, VII, IX, and X** (i.e., 2, 7, 9, and 10 [Think: **2 + 7 = 9** and **10**]), produced in the liver
What are its uses?	Long-term anticoagulation (PO)
What are its associated risks?	Bleeding complications, teratogenic in pregnancy, skin necrosis, dermatitis
What laboratory test should be used to follow its effect?	PT (prothrombin time) as reported as INR
What is INR?	**I**nternational **N**ormalized **R**atio
What is the classic therapeutic INR?	INR of 2 to 3
What is the half-life of effect?	40 hours; thus, it takes ≈2 days to observe a change in the PT
What is PCC?	**P**rothrombin **C**omplex **C**oncentrate (a.k.a. "Kcentra®"; has factors 2, 7, 9, 10)
What reverses the action?	**PCC cessation,** vitamin K, fresh frozen plasma
How long before surgery should it be discontinued?	From 3 to 5 days preoperatively and IV heparin should be started; heparin should be discontinued from 4 to 6 hours preoperatively and can be restarted postoperatively; Coumadin® can be restarted in a few days
How can warfarin cause skin necrosis when first started?	Initially depressed protein C and S result in a HYPERcoagulable state; avoid by using heparin concomitantly when starting

MISCELLANEOUS AGENTS

What is an antibiotic option for colon/appendectomy coverage if the patient is allergic to penicillin?	1. IV ciprofloxacin (Cipro®) AND 2. IV clindamycin or IV Flagyl®
If the patient does not respond to a dose of furosemide, should the dose be repeated, increased, or decreased?	Dose should be doubled if there is no response to the initial dose
What medication is used to treat promethazine-induced dystonia?	Diphenhydramine hydrochloride IV (Benadryl®)

What type of antihypertensive medication is contraindicated in patients with renal artery stenosis?	ACE inhibitors
What medications are used to stop seizures?	Benzodiazepines (e.g., lorazepam [Ativan®]); phenytoin [Dilantin®])

NARCOTICS

What medication reverses the effects of narcotic overdose?	Naloxone (Narcan®), 0.4 mg IV
What is the half-life of naloxone?	0.5 to 1.5 hours. May need to redose when narcotic half-life is longer

MISCELLANEOUS

What reverses the effects of benzodiazepines?	Flumazenil (Romazicon®), 0.2 mg IV
What is Toradol®?	Ketorolac = IV NSAID
What are the risks of Toradol®?	GI bleed, renal injury, platelet dysfunction
Why give patients IV Cipro® if they are eating a regular diet?	No reason—500 mg of Cipro® PO gives the same serum level as 400 mg Cipro® IV! And PO is much cheaper!
What is clonidine "rebound"?	Abruptly stopping clonidine can cause the patient to have severe "rebound" hypertension (also seen with β-blockers)

RAPID-FIRE REVIEW

Give the medical treatment for each surgical disease process:

Pheochromocytoma	α-Blocker
Zollinger–Ellison syndrome	Omeprazole
Carcinoid	Cyproheptadine
Desmoid tumors	Tamoxifen
Bleeding esophageal varices	Somatostatin
Diabetes insipidus	DDAVP
Malignant hyperthermia	Dantrolene
Necrotizing migratory erythema	Octreotide
Pancreatic fistula	Somatostatin

β-Blocker overdose	Glucagon
Benzodiazepine overdose	Flumazenil
Narcotic overdose	Narcan
Melanoma metastasis	Interferon
Heparin overdose	Protamine

Name the most likely diagnosis:

| 56-year-old male on IV heparin with atrial fibrillation develops thrombocytopenia | HIT (heparin-induced thrombocytopenia) |

Chapter 21 | Complications

ATELECTASIS

What is it?	Collapse of the alveoli
What are the signs?	Fever, decreased breath sounds with rales, tachypnea, tachycardia, and increased density on CXR
What is its claim to fame?	Most common cause of fever during PODs #1 to #2
What prophylactic measures can be taken?	Preoperative smoking cessation, incentive spirometry, good pain control
What is the treatment?	Postoperative **incentive spirometry,** deep breathing, coughing, early ambulation, NT suctioning, and chest PT

POSTOPERATIVE RESPIRATORY FAILURE

What is it?	Respiratory impairment with increased respiratory rate, shortness of breath, dyspnea
What is the treatment?	Supplemental O_2, chest PT; suctioning, intubation, and ventilation, if necessary
What is the initial workup?	ABG, CXR, EKG, pulse oximetry, and auscultation
What are the indications for intubation and ventilation?	Cannot protect airway (unconscious), excessive work of breathing, progressive **hypoxemia** (PaO_2 <55 despite supplemental O_2), progressive **acidosis** (pH <7.3 and PCO_2 >50), RR >35

What is the treatment of postoperative wheezing?	Albuterol nebulizer
Why may it be dangerous to give a patient with chronic COPD supplemental oxygen?	This patient uses relative hypoxia for respiratory drive, and supplemental O_2 may remove this drive!

PULMONARY EMBOLISM

What is a pulmonary embolism (PE)?	DVT that embolize to the pulmonary arterial system
What is DVT?	**D**eep **V**enous **T**hrombosis—a clot forming in the pelvic or lower extremity veins
What are the signs/symptoms of DVT?	Lower extremity pain, swelling, tenderness, Homans' sign, PE Up to 50% can be asymptomatic!
What is Homans' sign?	Calf pain with dorsiflexion of the foot classically seen with DVT, but actually found in fewer than 1/3 of patients with DVT
What test is used to evaluate for DVT?	Duplex ultrasonography
What is Virchow's triad?	1. Stasis 2. Endothelial injury 3. Hypercoagulable state (risk factors for thrombosis)
What are the signs/symptoms of PE?	Shortness of breath, tachypnea, hypotension, CP, occasional fever, loud pulmonic component of S2, hemoptysis with pulmonary infarction
What are the associated lab findings?	ABG—decreased PO_2 and PCO_2 (from hyperventilation)
What diagnostic test is indicated?	CT angiogram
What are the associated CXR findings?	1. Westermark's sign (wedge-shaped area of decreased pulmonary vasculature resulting in hyperlucency) 2. Opacity with base at pleural edge from pulmonary infarction
What are the associated EKG findings?	>50% are abnormal; classic finding is cor pulmonale (S1Q3T3, RBBB, and right-axis deviation); EKG most commonly shows flipped T waves or ST depression

What is a "saddle" embolus?

PE that "straddles" the pulmonary artery and is in the lumen of both the right and left pulmonary arteries

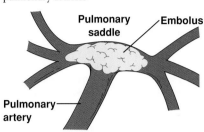

What is the treatment if the patient is stable?

Anticoagulation (heparin/Lovenox®) followed by long-term (3–6 months) Coumadin® or a DOAC

What is a DOAC?

Direct **O**ral **A**nti**C**oagulants—they DIRECTLY inhibit a single clotting factor

Name two DOACs?

Apixaban (Eliquis®), rivaroxaban (Xarelto®)

What is an IVC filter?

Metallic filter placed into IVC via jugular vein to catch emboli prior to lodging in the pulmonary artery

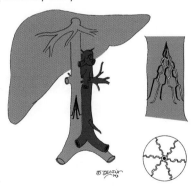

Where did Dr. Greenfield get the idea for the IVC filter?

Oil pipeline filters!

When is an IVC filter indicated?

If anticoagulation is contraindicated or patient has further PE on adequate anticoagulation or is high risk (e.g., pelvic and femur fractures)

What is the treatment if the patient's condition is unstable?

Consider thrombolytic therapy; consult thoracic surgeon for possible Trendelenburg operation; consider catheter suction embolectomy

What is the Trendelenburg operation?	Pulmonary artery embolectomy
What is a "retrievable" IVC filter?	IVC filter that can be removed ("retrieved")
What prophylactic measures can be taken for DVT/PE?	LMWH (Lovenox®) 40 mg SQ QD; **or** 30 mg SQ b.i.d.; subQ heparin (5,000 units subQ every 8 hours); and SCD boots

ASPIRATION PNEUMONIA

What is it?	Pneumonia following aspiration of vomitus
What are the signs/symptoms?	Respiratory failure, CP, increased sputum production, fever, cough, mental status changes, tachycardia, cyanosis, infiltrate on CXR
What is the treatment?	Bronchoscopy, antibiotics if pneumonia develops, intubation if respiratory failure occurs, ventilation with PEEP if ARDS develops
What is Mendelson's syndrome?	Chemical pneumonitis secondary to aspiration of stomach contents (i.e., gastric acid)
Are prophylactic antibiotics indicated for aspiration pneumonitis?	NO

GASTROINTESTINAL COMPLICATIONS

Gastric Dilatation

What are the risk factors?	Abdominal surgery, gastric outlet obstruction, splenectomy, narcotics
What are the signs/symptoms?	Abdominal distension, hiccups, electrolyte abnormalities, nausea
What is the treatment?	NGT decompression
What do you do if you have a patient with high NGT output?	Check high abdominal x-ray and, if the NGT is in duodenum, pull back the NGT into the stomach

Postoperative Pancreatitis

What is it?	Pancreatitis resulting from manipulation of the pancreas during surgery or low blood flow during the procedure (i.e., cardiopulmonary bypass), gallstones, hypercalcemia, medications, idiopathic

What lab tests are performed?	Amylase and lipase
What is the initial treatment?	Same as that for the other causes of pancreatitis (e.g., NPO, aggressive fluid resuscitation, ± NGT PRN)

Constipation

What are the postoperative causes?	Narcotics, immobility
What is the treatment?	OBR
What is OBR?	**O**rtho **B**owel **R**outine: docusate sodium (daily), dicacodyl suppository if no bowel movement occurs, Fleet® enema if suppository is ineffective

Short Bowel Syndrome

What is it?	Malabsorption and diarrhea resulting from extensive bowel resection (<200 cm of small bowel remaining)
What is the initial treatment?	TPN early, followed by many small meals chronically

Blind Loop Syndrome

What is it?	Bacterial overgrowth in the small intestine
What are the causes?	Anything that disrupts the normal flow of intestinal contents (i.e., causes stasis)
What are the surgical causes of B12 deficiency?	Blind loop syndrome, gastrectomy (decreased secretion of intrinsic factor), and excision of the terminal ileum (site of B12 absorption)

Postvagotomy Diarrhea

What is it?	Diarrhea after a truncal vagotomy
What is the cause?	It is thought that after truncal vagotomy, a rapid transport of bile salts to the colon results in osmotic inhibition of water absorption in the colon, leading to diarrhea

Dumping Syndrome

What is it?	Delivery of **hyperosmotic** chyme to the small intestine causing massive fluid shifts into the bowel (normally the stomach will decrease the osmolality of the chyme prior to its emptying)

With what conditions is it associated?	Any procedure that bypasses the pylorus or compromises its function (i.e., gastroenterostomies or pyloroplasty); thus, "dumping" of chyme into small intestine
What are the signs/symptoms?	Postprandial diaphoresis, tachycardia, abdominal pain/distention, emesis, increased flatus, dizziness, weakness
What is the medical treatment?	Small, multiple, low-fat/carbohydrate meals that are high in protein content
What is the surgical treatment?	Conversion to Roux-en-Y (± reversed jejunal interposition loop)

ENDOCRINE COMPLICATIONS

Diabetic Ketoacidosis (DKA)

What is it?	Deficiency of body insulin, resulting in hyperglycemia, formation of ketoacids, osmotic diuresis, and metabolic acidosis
What are the signs of DKA?	Polyuria, tachypnea, dehydration, confusion, abdominal pain, "ketone breath"
What is the treatment?	Insulin drip, IVF rehydration, K^+ supplementation, ± bicarbonate IV
What electrolyte must be monitored closely in DKA?	Potassium and HYPOkalemia (Remember correction of acidosis and GLC/insulin drive K^+ into cells and are treatment for HYPERkalemia!)
What must you rule out in a diabetic with DKA?	Infection (perirectal abscess is classically missed!)

Addisonian Crisis

What is it?	Acute adrenal insufficiency in the face of a stressor (i.e., surgery, trauma, infection)
How can you remember what it is?	Think: **ADD**isonian = **Ad**renal **D**own
What is the cause?	Postoperatively, inadequate cortisol release usually results from steroid administration in the past year
What are the signs/symptoms?	Tachycardia, nausea, vomiting, diarrhea, **abdominal pain,** ± fever, progressive lethargy, **hypotension, eventual hypovolemic shock**
What is its clinical claim to infamy?	Tachycardia and hypotension refractory to IVF and pressors!

Which lab values are classic?

Decreased Na⁺, increased K⁺ (secondary to decreased aldosterone)

How can the electrolytes with ADDisonian = ADrenal Down be remembered?

Think: **DOWN** the alphabetical electrolyte stairs

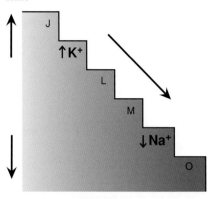

What is the treatment?

IVFs (D5NS), hydrocortisone IV, fludrocortisone PO

What is fludrocortisone?

Mineralocorticoid replacement (aldosterone)

SIADH

What is it?

Syndrome of Inappropriate AntiDiuretic Hormone (ADH) secretion (think of **inappropriate increase** in ADH secretion)

What does ADH do?

ADH increases NaCl and H_2O resorption in the kidney, increasing intravascular volume (released from posterior pituitary)

What are the causes?

Mainly lung/CNS: CNS trauma, oat-cell lung cancer, small-cell lung carcinoma, pancreatic cancer, duodenal cancer, pneumonia/lung abscess, increased PEEP, stroke, general anesthesia, idiopathic, postoperative, morphine

What are the associated lab findings?

Low sodium, low chloride, low serum osmolality; increased urine osmolality

How can the serum sodium level in SIADH be remembered?

Remember, **SIADH = S**odium **I**s **A**lways **D**own **H**ere = hyponatremia

What is the treatment?

Treat the primary cause and restrict fluid intake

Diabetes Insipidus (DI)

What is it?	Failure of ADH renal fluid conservation resulting in dilute urine in large amounts (Think: **DI** = **D**ecreased ADH)
What is the source of ADH?	POSTERIOR pituitary
What are the two major types?	1. Central (neurogenic) DI 2. Nephrogenic DI
What is the mechanism of the two types?	1. Central DI = decreased production of ADH 2. Nephrogenic DI = decreased ADH effect on kidney
What are the classic causes of central DI?	**BRAIN** injury, tumor, surgery, and infection
What are the classic causes of nephrogenic DI?	Amphotericin B, hypercalcemia, and chronic kidney infection
What lab values are associated with DI?	HYPERnatremia, decreased urine sodium, decreased urine osmolality, and increased serum osmolality
What is the treatment?	Fluid replacement; follow NA^+ levels and urine output; central DI warrants vasopressin; nephrogenic DI may respond to thiazide diuretics

CARDIOVASCULAR COMPLICATIONS

Myocardial Infarction (MI)

What is the most dangerous period for a postoperative MI following a previous MI?	6 months after an MI
What are the risk factors for postoperative MI?	History of MI, angina, QS on EKG, S3, JVD, CHF, aortic stenosis, advanced age, extensive surgical procedure, MI within 6 months, EKG changes
How do postoperative MIs present?	Often without chest pain New-onset **CHF,** new-onset **cardiac dysrhythmia,** hypotension, chest pain, tachypnea, tachycardia, nausea/vomiting, bradycardia, neck pain, arm pain
What EKG findings are associated with cardiac ischemia/MI?	Flipped T waves, ST elevation, ST depression, dysrhythmias (e.g., new-onset AFib, PVC, V-tach)
Which lab tests are indicated?	Troponin I, cardiac isoenzymes (elevated CK-MB fraction)

How can the treatment of postoperative MI be remembered?	"BEMOAN": **BE**ta-blocker (as tolerated) **M**orphine **O**xygen **A**spirin **N**itrates
When do postoperative MIs occur?	Two thirds occur on PODs #2 to #5 (often silent and present with **dyspnea** or **dysrhythmia**)

Postoperative CVA

What is a CVA?	CerebroVascular Accident (stroke)
What are the signs/symptoms?	Aphasia, motor/sensory deficits usually lateralizing
What is the workup?	Head CT scan; must rule out hemorrhage if anticoagulation is going to be used; carotid Doppler ultrasound study to evaluate for carotid occlusive disease
What is the treatment?	ASA, ± heparin if feasible postoperatively; thrombolytic therapy is not usually postoperative option
What is the perioperative prevention?	Avoid hypotension; continue aspirin therapy preoperatively in high-risk patients, if feasible; preoperative carotid Doppler study in high-risk patients

MISCELLANEOUS

Postoperative Renal Failure

What is it?	Increase in serum creatinine and decrease in creatinine clearance; usually associated with decreased urine output
Define the following terms:	
Anuria	<50 cc urine output in 24 hours
Oliguria	50 to 400 cc of urine output in 24 hours
What is the differential diagnosis?	
Prerenal	**Inadequate blood perfusing the kidney:** inadequate fluids, hypotension, cardiac pump failure (CHF)
Renal	**Kidney parenchymal dysfunction:** acute tubular necrosis, nephrotoxic contrast or drugs

Postrenal	**Obstruction to outflow of urine from kidney:** Foley catheter obstruction/stone, ureteral/urethral injury, BPH, bladder dysfunction (e.g., medications, spinal anesthesia)
What is the workup?	Lab tests: electrolytes, BUN, Cr, urine lytes, FENa, urinalysis, renal ultrasound
What is FENa?	**F**ractional **E**xcretion of **Na**$^+$ (sodium)
What is the formula for FENa?	"YOU NEED PEE" = **UNP** $(\mathbf{U}_{Na^+} \times \mathbf{P}_{Cr}/\mathbf{P}_{Na^+} \times \mathbf{U}_{Cr}) \times 100$ (**U** = urine, Cr = creatinine, **Na**$^+$ = sodium, **P** = plasma)
Define the lab results with prerenal versus renal failure:	
BUN/Cr ratio	Prerenal: >20:1 Renal: <20:1
Specific gravity	Prerenal: >1.020 (as the body tries to retain fluid) Renal: <1.020 (kidney has decreased ability to concentrate urine)
FENa	Prerenal: <1% Renal: >2%
Urine Na$^+$ (sodium)	Prerenal: <20 Renal: >40
Urine osmolality	Prerenal: >450 mOsm/kg Renal: <300 mOsm/kg
What are the indications for dialysis?	Fluid overload, refractory hyperkalemia, BUN >130, acidosis, uremic complication (encephalopathy, pericardial effusion)
What acronym helps you remember the indications for dialysis?	"AEIOU": **A**cidosis **E**lectrolytes **I**ntoxication Volume **O**verload **U**remic complication

DIC

What is it?	Activation of the coagulation cascade leading to **thrombosis** and **consumption** of clotting factors and platelets and activation of fibrinolytic system (fibrinolysis), resulting in **bleeding**

What is the treatment?	**Removal of the cause;** otherwise supportive: IVFs, O_2, platelets, FFP, cryoprecipitate (fibrin), epsilon-aminocaproic acid, as needed in predominantly thrombotic cases
	Use of heparin is indicated in cases that are predominantly thrombotic with antithrombin III supplementation as needed

Abdominal Compartment Syndrome

What is it?	Increased intra-abdominal pressure usually seen after laparotomy or after massive IVF resuscitation (e.g., burn patients)
What are the signs/symptoms?	Tight distended abdomen, decreased urine output, increased airway pressure, **increased intra-abdominal pressure**
How to measure intra-abdominal pressure?	Read intrabladder pressure (Foley catheter hooked up to manometry after instillation of 50 to 100 cc of water)
What is normal intra-abdominal pressure?	<15 mm Hg
What intra-abdominal pressure indicates need for treatment?	≥25 mm Hg, especially if there are signs of compromise
What is the treatment?	Release the pressure by decompressive laparotomy (leaving fascia open)

Urinary Retention

What is it?	Enlarged urinary bladder resulting from medications or spinal anesthesia
How is it diagnosed?	Physical exam (palpable bladder), bladder residual volume upon placement of a Foley catheter
What is the treatment?	Foley catheter
With massive bladder distention, how much urine can be drained immediately?	Most would clamp after 1 L and then drain the rest over time to avoid a vasovagal reaction
What is the classic sign of urinary retention in an elderly patient?	Confusion

Pseudomembranous Colitis

What are the signs/symptoms?	**Diarrhea,** fever, hypotension/tachycardia
How is it diagnosed?	*Clostridium difficile* toxin in stool, fecal WBC, flex sig (mucous pseudomembrane visible in the lumen of the colon = hence the name)
What is the treatment?	1. Flagyl® (PO or IV) 2. PO vancomycin if refractory to Flagyl®
What is the indication for emergent colectomy?	Toxic megacolon

RAPID-FIRE REVIEW

What is the correct diagnosis?

During placement of a central line, a 42-year-old female with breast cancer becomes acutely short of breath; her breath sounds are decreased on the ipsilateral side of the line placement	Pneumothorax
56-year-old female s/p gastrojejunostomy for duodenal trauma (pyloric exclusion) now presents 1 year post op with tachycardia, dizziness, and abdominal pain after eating	Dumping syndrome
28-year-old female s/p spinal anesthesia for a tubal ligation develops back pain, fever, and increased WBCs on POD #3	Epidural abscess
65-year-old smoker with severe COPD treated intermittently with antibiotics, prednisone, and albuterol undergoes a colectomy; post op, the patient develops hypotension, dizziness, and fever with normal hematocrit and abdominal exam	Adrenal crisis—adrenal insufficiency

59-year-old female smoker POD #4 from AAA repair develops hypotension and tachycardia with multiple PVCs	Myocardial infarction
56-year-old alcoholic female receives D5 1/2 NS IV bolus in the ER; she develops confusion, ataxia, and inability of gaze laterally	Wernicke's encephalopathy
39-year-old female 3 years s/p Billroth II for perforated gastric ulcer presents with intermittent upper abdominal pain relieved by a large amount of bilious vomiting	Afferent limb syndrome

Chapter 22 | Common Causes of Ward Emergencies

What can cause hypotension?	Hypovolemia (iatrogenic, hemorrhage), sepsis, MI, cardiac dysrhythmia, hypoxia, false reading (e.g., wrong cuff/arterial line twist or clot), pneumothorax, PE, cardiac tamponade, medications (e.g., morphine)
How do you act?	ABCs, examine, recheck BP, IV access, IV bolus, labs (e.g., HCT), EKG, pulse ox/vital signs monitoring, CXR, supplemental oxygen, check medications/history, give IV antibiotics "stat" if sepsis likely, compress all bleeding sites
What are the common causes of postoperative hypertension?	**Pain** (from catecholamine release), anxiety, hypercapnia, hypoxia (which may also cause hypotension), pre-existing condition, bladder distention
What can cause hypoxia/ shortness of breath?	Atelectasis, pneumonia, mucous plug, pneumothorax, **PE,** MI/dysrhythmia, venous blood in ABG syringe, sat% machine malfunction/probe malposition, iatrogenic (wrong ventilator settings), severe anemia/hypovolemia, low cardiac output, CHF, ARDS, fluid overload

How do you act?	ABCs, physical exam, vital signs/pulse oximetry monitoring, supplemental oxygen, IV access, ABG, EKG, CXR
What can cause mental status change?	**Hypoxia** until ruled out, hypotension (e.g., cardiogenic shock), hypovolemia, iatrogenic (narcotics/benzodiazepines), drug reaction, alcohol withdrawal, drug withdrawal, seizure, ICU psychosis, CVA, sepsis, metabolic derangements, intracranial bleeding, **urinary retention in the elderly**
What are the signs of alcohol withdrawal?	**Confusion,** tachycardia/autonomic instability, seizure, hallucinations
What are the causes of tachycardia?	Hypovolemia/third spacing, pain, alcohol withdrawal, anxiety/agitation, urinary retention, cardiac dysrhythmia (e.g., sinoventricular tachycardia, atrial fibrillation with rapid rate), MI, PE, β-blocker withdrawal, anastomotic leak
What are the causes of decreased urine output?	Hypovolemia, urinary retention, Foley catheter malfunction, cardiac failure, MI, acute tubular necrosis (ATN), ureteral/urethral injury, abdominal compartment syndrome, sepsis
How do you act initially in a case of decreased urine output?	Examine vital signs, check or place Foley catheter, irrigate Foley catheter, IV fluid bolus

RAPID-FIRE REVIEW

What is the correct diagnosis?

57-year-old male develops confusion and wide swings in heart rate and systolic blood pressure POD #2 after an appendectomy for a perforated appendix; sats = 99%, HCT stable, electrolytes normal, chest x-ray normal	Alcohol withdrawal
34-year-old in the ICU s/p laparotomy with fascia closed, decreased urine output, increased peak airway pressure, decreased CVP, normal chest x-ray, normal EKG	Abdominal compartment syndrome

A 77-year-old male s/p laparoscopic cholecystectomy returns to the clinic with a palpable lower abdominal mass, confusion, and weak urine stream

Urinary retention

Name the diagnostic modality:

74-year-old female s/p ex lap now POD #4 with acute onset of shortness of breath; ABG reveals hypoxia and hypocapnia

Chest CTA to rule out pulmonary embolism

Chapter 23 | Surgical Respiratory Care

What is the most common cause of fever in the first 48 hours postoperatively?

Atelectasis

What is absorption atelectasis?

Elevated inhaled oxygen replaces the nitrogen in the alveoli resulting in collapse of the air sac (atelectasis); nitrogen keeps alveoli open by "stenting" them

What is incentive spirometry?

Patient can document tidal volume and will have an "incentive" to increase it

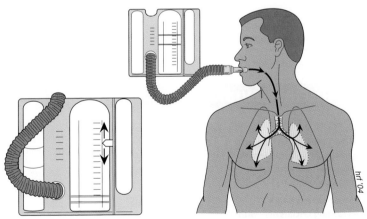

What is oxygen-induced hypoventilation?

Some patients with COPD have low oxygen as the main stimulus for the respiratory drive; if given supplemental oxygen, they will have a decreased respiratory drive and hypoventilation

Why give supplemental oxygen to a patient with a pneumothorax?

Pneumothorax is almost completely nitrogen—thus increasing the oxygen in the alveoli increases the nitrogen gradient and results in faster absorption of the pneumothorax!

What is a nonrebreather mask?

100% oxygen with a reservoir bag

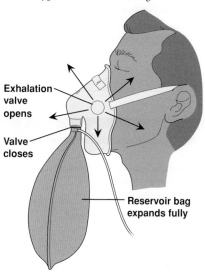

Exhalation valve opens

Valve closes

Reservoir bag expands fully

How do you figure out the PaO$_2$ from an O$_2$ sat?

PaO$_2$ of 40, 50, 60 roughly equals 70, 80, 90 in sats

How much do you increase the FiO$_2$ by each liter added to the nasal cannula?

$\approx$3%

RAPID-FIRE REVIEW

Name the most likely diagnosis:

POD #1 after bariatric gastric bypass a 34-year-old female develops fever and crackles on chest auscultation

Atelectasis

18-year-old male with necrotizing fasciitis now with acute onset of respiratory failure, PaO$_2$ to FiO$_2$ ratio of 145, normal heart echo, bilateral pulmonary edema on CXR

Moderate ARDS

Chapter 24 | Surgical Nutrition

What is the motto of surgical nutrition?	"If the gut works, use it"
What are the normal daily dietary requirements for adults of the following:	
Protein	1 g/kg/day
Calories	30 kcal/kg/day
What is the calorie content of the following substances:	
Fat	9 kcal/g
Protein	4 kcal/g
Carbohydrate	4 kcal/g
What is the formula for converting nitrogen requirement/loss to protein requirement/loss?	Nitrogen $\times$ 6.25 = protein
What is RQ?	**R**espiratory **Q**uotient; ratio of CO_2 produced to O_2 consumed
What is the normal RQ?	0.8
What can be done to decrease the RQ?	More fat, less carbohydrates
What dietary change can be made to decrease CO_2 production in a patient in whom CO_2 retention is a concern?	Decrease carbohydrate calories and increase calories from **fat**
What lab tests are used to monitor nutritional status?	Blood levels of: **Prealbumin** ($t_{1/2} \approx$ 2–3 days)—acute change determination Transferrin ($t_{1/2} \approx$ 8–9 days) Albumin ($t_{1/2} \approx$ 14–20 days)—more chronic determination Total lymphocyte count Anergy Retinol-binding protein ($t_{1/2} \approx$ 12 hours)
Where is iron absorbed?	Duodenum (some in proximal jejunum)
Where is vitamin B12 absorbed?	Terminal ileum
What are the surgical causes of vitamin B12 deficiency?	Gastrectomy, excision of terminal ileum, blind loop syndrome
Where are bile salts absorbed?	Terminal ileum

Where are fat-soluble vitamins absorbed?	Terminal ileum
Which vitamins are fat soluble?	**K, A, D, E ("KADE")**
What are the signs of the following disorders:	
Vitamin A deficiency	Poor wound healing
Vitamin B12/folate deficiency	Megaloblastic anemia
Vitamin C deficiency	Poor wound healing, bleeding gums
Vitamin K deficiency	Decrease in vitamin K–dependent clotting factors (II, VII, IX, and X); bleeding; elevated PT
Chromium deficiency	Diabetic state
Zinc deficiency	Poor wound healing, alopecia, dermatitis, taste disorder
Fatty acid deficiency	Dry, flaky skin; alopecia
What vitamin increases the PO absorption of iron?	PO vitamin C (ascorbic acid)
What vitamin lessens the deleterious effects of steroids on wound healing?	Vitamin A
What are the common indications for total parenteral nutrition (TPN)?	NPO >7 days Enterocutaneous fistulas Short bowel syndrome Prolonged ileus
What is TPN?	**T**otal **P**arenteral **N**utrition = IV nutrition
What is the major nutrient of the gut (small bowel)?	Glutamine
What is "refeeding syndrome"?	Decreased serum **potassium, magnesium,** and **phosphate** after refeeding (via TPN or enterally) a starving patient
What are the vitamin K–dependent clotting factors?	2, 7, 9, 10 (Think: 2 + 7 = 9, and then 10)
What is an elemental tube feed?	Very low residue tube feed in which almost all the tube feed is absorbed
Where is calcium absorbed?	Duodenum (actively) Jejunum (passively)
What is the major nutrient of the colon?	**Butyrate** (and other short-chain fatty acids)
What must bind B12 for absorption?	Intrinsic factor from the gastric parietal cells

What sedative medication has caloric value?	Propofol delivers 1 kcal/cc in the form of lipid!
Why may all the insulin placed in a TPN bag not get to the patient?	Insulin will bind to the IV tubing
How can serum bicarbonate be increased in patients on TPN?	Increase acetate (which is metabolized into bicarbonate)
What are "trophic" tube feeds?	Very low rate of tube feeds (usually 10–25 cc/hr), which are thought to keep mucosa alive and healthy
What is the best lab to check adequacy of nutritional status?	Prealbumin

RAPID-FIRE REVIEW

56-year-old male alcoholic with new-onset NGT feeds develops hypokalemia, hypophosphatemia, and hypomagnesemia	Refeeding syndrome

Chapter 25 | Shock

What is the definition of shock?	Inadequate tissue perfusion
What are the different types (5)?	1. Hypovolemic 2. Septic 3. Cardiogenic 4. Neurogenic 5. Anaphylactic
What are the signs of shock?	Pale, diaphoretic, cool skin Hypotension, tachycardia, tachypnea Decreased mental status and pulse pressure Poor capillary refill Poor urine output
What are the best indicators of tissue perfusion?	Urine output, mental status
What lab tests help assess tissue perfusion?	Lactic acid (elevated with inadequate tissue perfusion), base deficit, pH from ABG (acidosis associated with inadequate tissue perfusion)

HYPOVOLEMIC SHOCK

What is the definition?

Decreased intravascular volume

What are the common causes?

Hemorrhage
Burns
Bowel obstruction
Crush injury
Pancreatitis

What are the signs?

Early—Orthostatic hypotension, mild
tachycardia, anxiety, diaphoresis,
vasoconstriction (decreased pulse
pressure with increased diastolic
pressure)

Late—Changed mental status, decreased BP,
marked tachycardia

What are the signs/symptoms with:

Class I hemorrhage (<15% or 750 cc blood loss)

Mild anxiety, normal vital signs

Class II hemorrhage (15%–30% or 750–1,500 cc blood loss)

Normal systolic BP with decreased pulse
pressure, tachycardia, tachypnea, anxiety

Class III hemorrhage (30%–40% or 1,500–2,000 cc blood loss)

Tachycardia (heart rate >120), tachypnea
(respiratory rate >30), **decreased systolic BP,**
decreased pulse pressure, confusion

Class IV hemorrhage (>40% or >2,000 cc blood loss)

Decreased systolic BP, tachycardia (heart
rate >140), tachypnea (respiratory rate >35),
decreased pulse pressure, confused and
lethargic, no urine output

What is the treatment?

1. Stop the bleeding
2. Volume: blood products as needed

How is the effectiveness of treatment evaluated:

Bedside indicator

Urine output, BP, heart rate, mental status,
extremity warmth, capillary refill, body
temperature

Labs

pH, base deficit, and lactate level

Why does decreased pulse pressure occur with early hypovolemic shock?

Pulse pressure (systolic–diastolic BP)
decreases because of vasoconstriction,
resulting in an elevated diastolic BP

What is the most common vital sign change associated with early hypovolemic shock?

Tachycardia

What type of patient does not mount a normal tachycardic response to hypovolemic shock?	Patients on β-blockers, spinal shock (loss of sympathetic tone), endurance athletes
Should vasopressors be used to treat hypovolemic shock?	No

SEPTIC SHOCK

What is the definition?	Documented infection and hypotension
What are the signs/symptoms?	Initial—vasodilation, resulting in warm skin and full pulses; normal urine output Delayed—vasoconstriction and poor urine output; mental status changes; hypotension
What percentage of blood cultures is positive in patients with bacterial septic shock?	Only ≈50%!
What are the associated findings?	Fever, hyperventilation, tachycardia
What is the treatment?	1. Volume (IVF) 2. Antibiotics (empiric, then by cultures) 3. Drainage of infection 4. Pressors PRN

CARDIOGENIC SHOCK

What is the definition?	Cardiac insufficiency; left ventricular failure (usually), resulting in inadequate tissue perfusion
What are the causes?	MI, papillary muscle dysfunction, massive cardiac contusion, cardiac tamponade, tension pneumothorax, cardiac valve failure

NEUROGENIC SHOCK

What is the definition?	Inadequate tissue perfusion from loss of sympathetic vasoconstrictive tone

What are the common causes?	Spinal cord injury:
	  Complete transection of spinal cord
	  Partial cord injury with spinal shock
	  Spinal anesthesia

What are the signs/symptoms?	**Hypotension** and **bradycardia,** neurologic deficit

Why are heart rate and BP decreased?	Loss of sympathetic tone (but hypovolemia [e.g., hemoperitoneum] must be ruled out)
What are the associated findings?	Neurologic deficits suggesting cord injury
What MUST be ruled out in any patient where neurogenic shock is suspected?	Hemorrhagic shock!
What is the treatment?	**IV fluids** (vasopressors reserved for hypotension refractory to fluid resuscitation)
What is spinal shock?	Complete flaccid paralysis immediately following spinal cord injury; may or may not be associated with circulatory shock
What is the lowest reflex available to the examiner?	Bulbocavernosus reflex: checking for contraction of the anal sphincter upon compression of the glans penis or clitoris
What is the lowest level voluntary muscle?	External anal sphincter
What are the classic findings associated with neurogenic shock?	Hypotension Bradycardia or lack of compensatory tachycardia

MISCELLANEOUS

What is the acronym for treatment options for anaphylactic shock?	"**BASE**": **B**enadryl **A**minophylline **S**teroids **E**pinephrine

RAPID-FIRE REVIEW

What is the treatment?

15-year-old s/p trampoline injury with tetraplegia (a.k.a. "quadriplegia") with hypotension; no other injuries on CT scans	Neurogenic shock; treat with IV fluids and then vasopressors as needed

Chapter 26 | Surgical Infection

Define:

Bacteremia	Bacteria in the blood
SIRS	**S**ystemic **I**nflammatory **R**esponse **S**yndrome (fever, tachycardia, tachypnea, leukocytosis)
Define SIRS criteria	2 or more of the following: Temperature <36°C or >38°C Tachypnea >20 bpm Heart rate >90 bpm Leukocytes <4k or >12k
Sepsis	Documented infection and SIRS
Septic shock	Sepsis and hypotension
Cellulitis	**Blanching erythema** from superficial dermal/epidermal infection (usually strep > staph)
Abscess	Collection of pus within a cavity
Superinfection	New infection arising while a patient is receiving antibiotics for the original infection at a different site (e.g., *Clostridium difficile* colitis)
Nosocomial infection	Infection originating in the hospital
Empiric	Use of antibiotic based on previous sensitivity information or previous experience awaiting culture results in an established infection
Prophylactic	Antibiotics used to prevent an infection
What is the most common nosocomial infection?	Urinary tract infection (UTI)
What is the most common nosocomial infection causing death?	Respiratory tract infection (pneumonia)

URINARY TRACT INFECTION (UTI)

What diagnostic tests are used?	Urinalysis, culture, urine microscopy for WBC
What constitutes a POSITIVE urine analysis?	Positive nitrite (from bacteria) Positive leukocyte esterase (from WBC) >10 WBC/HPF Presence of bacteria (supportive)
What number of colony-forming units (CFU) confirms the diagnosis of UTI?	On urine culture, classically 100,000 or 10^5 CFU

What are the common organisms?	*Escherichia coli, Klebsiella, Proteus (Enterococcus, Staphylococcus aureus)*
What is the treatment?	Antibiotics with gram-negative spectrum (e.g., sulfamethoxazole/trimethoprim [Bactrim™], gentamicin, ciprofloxacin, aztreonam); use antibiogram, then check culture and sensitivity
What is the treatment of bladder candidiasis?	1. Remove or change Foley catheter 2. Administer systemic fluconazole or amphotericin bladder washings

CENTRAL LINE INFECTIONS

What are the signs of a central line infection?	**Unexplained hyperglycemia,** fever, mental status change, hypotension, tachycardia → **shock,** pus, and erythema at central line site
What is a central line–associated bloodstream infection (CLABSI)?	1. Central line in place >2 days 2. +Blood culture 3. No other source of infection
What is the most common cause of "catheter-related bloodstream infections"?	Coagulase-negative *staphylococci* (33%), followed by enterococci, *S. aureus,* gram-negative rods
When should central lines be changed?	When they are infected; there is NO advantage to changing them every 7 days in nonburn patients
What central line infusion increases the risk of infection?	Hyperal (TPN)
What is the treatment for central line infection?	1. Remove central line (send for culture) ± IV antibiotics 2. Place NEW central line in a different site
When should peripheral IV short angiocatheters be changed?	Every 72 to 96 hours

WOUND INFECTION (SURGICAL SITE INFECTION)

What is it?	Infection in an operative wound
When do these infections arise?	Classically, PODs #5 to #7
What are the signs/symptoms?	**Pain** at incision site, erythema, drainage, induration, warm skin, fever
What is the treatment?	Remove skin sutures/staples, rule out fascial dehiscence, pack wound open, send wound culture, administer antibiotics

What are the most common bacteria found in postoperative wound infections?	*S. aureus* (20%) *E. coli* (10%) *Enterococcus* (10%) Other causes: *Staphylococcus epidermidis, Pseudomonas,* anaerobes, other gram-negative organisms, *Streptococcus*
Which bacteria causes fever and wound infection in the first 24 hours after surgery?	1. *Streptococcus* 2. *Clostridium* (bronze-brown weeping tender wound)

CLASSIFICATION OF OPERATIVE WOUNDS

What is a "clean" wound?	Elective, nontraumatic wound without acute inflammation; usually closed primarily without the use of drains
What is the infection rate of a clean wound?	<1.5%
What is a clean-contaminated wound?	Operation on the GI or respiratory tract without unusual contamination or entry into the biliary or urinary tract
Without infection present, what is the infection rate of a clean-contaminated wound?	<3%
What is a contaminated wound?	Acute inflammation, traumatic wound, GI tract spillage, or a major break in sterile technique
What is the infection rate of a contaminated wound?	≈5%
What is a dirty wound?	Pus present, perforated viscus, or dirty traumatic wound
What is the infection rate of a dirty wound?	≈33%
What factors influence the development of infections?	Foreign body (e.g., suture, drains, grafts) Decreased blood flow (poor delivery of PMNs and antibiotics) Strangulation of tissues with excessively tight sutures Necrotic tissue or excessive local tissue destruction (e.g., too much Bovie) Long operations (>2 hours) Hypothermia in O.R. Hematomas or seromas Dead space that prevents the delivery of phagocytic cells to bacterial foci Poor approximation of tissues

What is the treatment?	Incision and drainage—an abscess must be drained (**Note:** fluctuation is a sign of a *subcutaneous* abscess; most abdominal abscesses are drained percutaneously) Antibiotics for deep abscesses
What are the indications for antibiotics after drainage of a subcutaneous abscess?	Diabetes mellitus, surrounding cellulitis, prosthetic heart valve, or an immunocompromised state

Peritoneal Abscess

What is a peritoneal abscess?	Abscess within the peritoneal cavity
What are the causes?	Postoperative status after a laparotomy, ruptured appendix, peritonitis, any inflammatory intraperitoneal process, anastomotic leak
What are the signs/symptoms?	Fever (classically spiking), abdominal pain, mass
How is the diagnosis made?	Abdominal CT scan (or ultrasound)
When should an abdominal CT scan be obtained looking for a postoperative abscess?	After POD #7 (otherwise, abscess will not be "organized" and will look like a normal postoperative fluid collection)
What CT scan findings are associated with abscess?	Fluid collection with fibrous rind, **gas** in fluid collection
What is the treatment?	Percutaneous CT–guided drainage
What is an option for drainage of pelvic abscess?	Transrectal drainage (or transvaginal)
All abscesses must be drained except which type?	Amebiasis!

NECROTIZING FASCIITIS

What is it?	Bacterial infection of underlying fascia (spreads rapidly along fascial planes)
What are the causative agents?	Classically, group A *Streptococcus pyogenes,* but most often polymicrobial with anaerobes/gram-negative organisms
What are the signs/symptoms?	Fever, pain, crepitus, cellulitis, skin discoloration, blood blisters (hemorrhagic bullae), weeping skin, increased WBCs, subcutaneous air on x-ray, septic shock

What is the LRINEC score for necrotizing fasciitis?	Laboratory **R**isk **I**ndicator for **NEC**rotizing fasciitis
What are the values for the LRINEC associated with necrotizing fasciitis?	C-reactive protein >150, WBC >15, HGB <13.5, sodium <135, creatinine >1.6, glucose >180
How is the diagnosis made?	In the O.R. with surgical incisions (fat/muscle peels away easily from the fascia)
What is the treatment?	IVF, IV antibiotics, and aggressive early extensive surgical débridement, cultures, tetanus prophylaxis
What antibiotics?	Triple therapy: for example, Zosyn®, vancomycin, clindamycin
Why clindamycin?	Binds staph/strep exotoxin
Is necrotizing fasciitis an emergency?	YES, patients must be taken to the O.R. immediately!

CLOSTRIDIAL MYOSITIS

What is it?	Clostridial muscle infection
What is another name for this condition?	Gas gangrene
What is the most common causative organism?	*Clostridium perfringens*
What are the signs/symptoms?	Pain, fever, shock, crepitus, foul-smelling brown fluid, subcutaneous air on x-ray
What is the treatment?	IV antibiotics, aggressive surgical débridement of involved muscle, tetanus prophylaxis

HIDRADENITIS SUPPURATIVA

What is it?	Infection/abscess formation in **apocrine** sweat glands
In what three locations does it occur?	Perineum/buttocks, inguinal area, axillae (site of apocrine glands)
What is the most common causative organism?	*S. aureus*
What is the treatment?	Antibiotics Incision and drainage (excision of skin with glands for chronic infections)

PSEUDOMEMBRANOUS COLITIS

What is it?	Antibiotic-induced colonic overgrowth of *C. difficile*
What are the signs/symptoms?	**Diarrhea** (bloody in 10% of patients), ± fever, ± increased WBCs, ± abdominal cramps, ± abdominal distention
What causes the diarrhea?	Exotoxin released by *C. difficile*
How is the diagnosis made?	Assay stool for **exotoxin titer**
What is the treatment?	PO metronidazole (Flagyl®; DNA PCR test 93% sensitive) or PO vancomycin (97% sensitive); discontinuation of causative agent **Never** give antiperistaltics

PROPHYLACTIC ANTIBIOTICS

What must a prophylactic antibiotic cover for procedures on the large bowel/abdominal trauma/appendicitis?	Anaerobes (and gram negatives)
When is the appropriate time to administer prophylactic antibiotics?	Must be in adequate levels in the blood stream **prior to surgical incision!**

PAROTITIS

What is it?	Infection of the parotid gland
What is the most common causative organism?	*Staphylococcus*
What are the signs?	Hot, red, tender parotid gland and increased WBCs
What is the treatment?	Antibiotics, operative drainage as necessary

MISCELLANEOUS

What is a "stitch" abscess?	Subcutaneous abscess centered around a subcutaneous stitch, which is a "foreign body"; treat with drainage and stitch removal
Which bacteria can be found in the stool (colon)?	Anaerobic—*Bacteroides fragilis* Aerobic—*E. coli*
Which bacteria are found in infections from human bites?	*Streptococcus viridans*, *S. aureus*, *Peptococcus*, **Eikenella** (treat with Augmentin®)

What are the most common ICU pneumonia bacteria?	Gram-negative organisms
What is Fournier's gangrene?	Perineal infection starting classically in the scrotum in patients with diabetes; treat with triple antibiotics and wide debridement—a surgical emergency!
Does adding antibiotics to peritoneal lavage solution lower the risk of abscess formation?	No ("Dilution is the solution to pollution")
Which antibiotic is used to treat amoeba infection?	Metronidazole (Flagyl®)
Which bacteria commonly infect prosthetic material and central lines?	*S. epidermis*
What is the antibiotic of choice for *Actinomyces*?	Penicillin G (exquisitely sensitive)
What is a furuncle?	Staphylococcal abscess that forms in a hair follicle (Think: **F**ollicle = **F**uruncle)
What is a carbuncle?	Subcutaneous staphylococcal abscess (usually an extension of a furuncle), most commonly seen in patients with diabetes (i.e., rule out diabetes)
What is a felon?	Infection of the finger pad (Think: **F**elon = **F**inger printing)
What microscopic finding is associated with *Actinomyces*?	Sulfur granules
What organism causes tetanus?	*Clostridium tetani*
What are the signs of tetanus?	Lockjaw, muscle spasm, laryngospasm, convulsions, respiratory failure
What are the appropriate prophylactic steps in tetanus-prone (dirty) injury in the following patients:	
Three previous immunizations	None (tetanus toxoid only if >5 years since last toxoid)
Two previous immunizations	Tetanus toxoid
One previous immunization	Tetanus immunoglobulin IM and tetanus toxoid IM (at different sites!)
No previous immunizations	Tetanus immunoglobulin IM and tetanus toxoid IM (at different sites!)
What is Fitz-Hugh–Curtis syndrome?	RUQ pain from gonococcal perihepatitis in women

RAPID-FIRE REVIEW

Name the most likely diagnosis:

Midline laparotomy wound that drains continuous straw-colored fluid	Fascial dehiscence
POD #1 with bright red wound infection	Streptococcus infection
POD #1 with painful wound and weeping bronze-colored fluid	Clostridial wound infection
67-year-old male POD #5 s/p AAA repair with bloody diarrhea	Ischemic colitis
80-year-old male s/p appendectomy with fever, right-sided face pain, and elevated WBCs	Parotitis

Chapter 27 | Fever

What is postoperative fever?	Temperature >38.5°C or 101.5°F
What are the five classic W's of postoperative fever?	1. Wind—atelectasis 2. Water—urinary tract infection (UTI) 3. Wound—wound infection 4. Walking—DVT/thrombophlebitis 5. Wonder drugs—drug fever
Give the classic postoperative timing for the following causes of postoperative fever:	
Atelectasis (Wind)	First 24 to 48 hours
UTI (Water)	Anytime after POD #3
Wound infection (Wound)	Usually after POD #5 (but it can be anytime!)
DVT/PE/thrombophlebitis (Walking)	PODs #7 to #10
Drug fever (Wonder drugs)	Anytime
What is the most common cause of fever on PODs #1 to #2?	Atelectasis (most likely cytokine release from tissue damage!)
What is a "fever" workup?	Physical exam (look at wound), CXR, urinalysis, blood cultures, CBC

What causes fever before 24 postoperative hours?	Atelectasis, cytokine release, β-hemolytic streptococcal or clostridial wound infections, anastomotic leak
What causes fever from PODs #3 to #5?	UTI, pneumonia, IV site infection, wound infection
What is an anesthetic cause of fever INTRAoperatively?	Malignant hyperthermia—treat with **dantrolene**
What causes fever from PODs #5 to #10?	Wound infection, pneumonia, abscess, infected hematoma, *Clostridium difficile* colitis, anastomotic leak **DVT, peritoneal abscess, drug fever** PE, abscess, parotitis
What causes wound infection on PODs #1 to #2?	*Streptococcus* Clostridia (painful bronze-brown weeping wound)
What can cause fever at any time?	1. IV site infection 2. Central line infection 3. Medications

RAPID-FIRE REVIEW

What is the correct diagnosis?

38-year-old female diabetic with cellulitis on broad-spectrum antibiotics for 2 weeks develops fever, massive diarrhea, and abdominal pain	*C. difficile* colitis
27-year-old female who following menses develops rash, hypotension, and fever	Toxic shock syndrome

Chapter 28 | Surgical Prophylaxis

What medications provide protection from postoperative GI bleeding?	H_2 blockers, PPI (proton-pump inhibitor)
What measures provide protection from postoperative atelectasis/pneumonia?	Incentive spirometry, coughing, **smoking cessation**, ambulation
What treatments provide protection from postoperative DVT?	Low-molecular-weight heparin (LMWH), subcutaneous low-dose unfractionated heparin, sequential compression device (SCD) for lower extremities, early ambulation

What measures provide protection from wound infection?	Shower the night before surgery with chlorhexidine scrub **Never use a razor** for hair removal (electric shavers only) Ensure adequate skin prep in O.R. Do not close the skin in a contaminated case Ensure preoperative antibiotics in the bloodstream **before incision**
Why not use a razor to remove hair?	Micro cuts are a nidus for bacteria and subsequent wound infection
How long should "prophylactic antibiotics" be given?	<24 hours
What measures prevent ventilator-associated pneumonia (VAP)?	Head of bed >30°, handwashing, patient oral hygiene, avoidance of gastric overdistention
What treatment provides protection from Wernicke's encephalopathy?	**Rally pack** (a.k.a. "banana bag" because the fluid is yellow with the vitamins in it); pack includes thiamine, folate, and magnesium
To avoid Wernicke's encephalopathy in alcoholics, when do you give the glucose?	AFTER thiamine administration!
What is Wernicke's encephalopathy?	Condition resulting from thiamine deficiency in patients with alcoholism, causing a **triad** of symptoms; think **"COA"**: 1. **C**onfusion 2. **O**phthalmoplegia 3. **A**taxia
What treatment decreases the risk of perioperative adrenal crisis in a patient on chronic steroids?	"Stress-dose" steroids: 100 mg hydrocortisone administered preoperatively, continued postoperatively q8 hours, and then tapered off

Chapter 29 | Surgical Radiology

CHEST

Which CXR is better: P-A or A-P?	P-A, less magnification of the heart (heart is closer to the x-ray plate)
Classically, how much pleural fluid can the diaphragm hide on upright CXR?	It is said that the diaphragm can overshadow up to 500 cc

How can CXR confirm that the last hole on a chest tube is in the pleural cavity?

Last hole is through the radiopaque line on the chest tube; thus, look for the break in the radiopaque line to be within the rib cage/pleura

How can a loculated pleural effusion be distinguished from a free-flowing pleural effusion?

Ipsilateral decubitus CXR; if fluid is not loculated (or contained), it will layer out

How do you recognize a pneumothorax on CXR?

Air without lung markings is seen outside the white pleural line—best seen in the apices on an upright CXR

What x-ray should be obtained before feeding via a nasogastric or nasoduodenal tube?

Low CXR to ensure the tube is in the GI tract and not in the lung

What C-spine views are used to rule out bony injury?

CT scan

What is used to look for ligamentous C-spine injury?

Lateral flex and extension C-spine films, MRI

How should a CT scan be read?

Cross section with the patient in supine position looking up from the feet

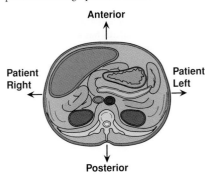

ABDOMEN

How can you tell the difference between a small bowel obstruction (SBO) and an ileus?

In SBO, there is a transition point (cut-off sign) between the distended proximal bowel and the distal bowel of normal caliber (may be gasless), whereas the bowel in ileus is *diffusely* distended

What is the significance of an air–fluid level?

Seen in obstruction or ileus on an upright x-ray; intraluminal bowel diameter increases, allowing for separation of fluid and gas

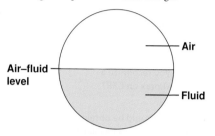

What are the normal calibers of the small bowel, transverse colon, and cecum?

Use the "**3, 6, 9 rule**":
 Small bowel <3 cm
 Transverse colon <6 cm
 Cecum <9 cm

What percentage of kidney stones is radiopaque?

≈90%

What percentage of gallstones is radiopaque?

≈10%

What percentage of patients with acute appendicitis has a radiopaque fecalith?

≈5%

What is the "parrot's beak" or "bird's beak" sign?

Evidence of sigmoid volvulus on barium enema; evidence of achalasia on barium swallow

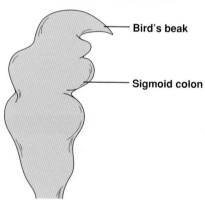

What is a "cut-off sign"?

Seen in obstruction, bowel distention, and distended bowel that is "cut off" from normal bowel

What are "sentinel loops"?

Distention or air–fluid levels (or both) near a site of abdominal inflammation (e.g., seen in RLQ with appendicitis)

What is loss of the psoas shadow?	Loss of the clearly defined borders of the psoas muscle on AXR; loss signifies inflammation or ascites
What is loss of the peritoneal fat stripe (a.k.a. "preperitoneal fat stripe")?	Loss of the lateral peritoneal/preperitoneal fat interface; implies inflammation
What is "thumbprinting"?	Nonspecific colonic mucosal edema resembling thumb indentations on AXR
What is pneumatosis intestinalis?	Gas within the intestinal wall (usually means **dead gut**) that can be seen in patients with congenital variant or chronic steroids
What is free air?	Air free within the peritoneal cavity (air or gas should be seen only within the bowel or stomach); results from bowel or stomach perforation

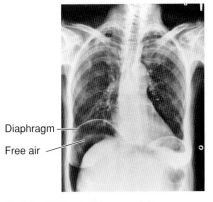

Diaphragm —

Free air —

What is the best position for the detection of FREE AIR (free intraperitoneal air)?	**Upright CXR**—air below the right diaphragm
If you cannot get an upright CXR, what is the second-best plain x-ray for free air?	Left lateral decubitus, because it prevents confusion with gastric air bubble; with free air **both** sides of the bowel wall can be seen; can detect as little as 1 cc of air
How long after a laparotomy can there be free air on AXR?	Usually ≤7 days
What is Chilaiditi's sign?	Transverse colon over the liver simulating free air on x-ray
When should a postoperative abdominal/pelvic CT scan for a peritoneal abscess be performed?	POD #7 or later, to give time for the abscess to form

What is the best test to evaluate the biliary system and gallbladder?	Ultrasound (U/S)
What is the normal diameter of the common bile duct with gallbladder present?	<4 mm until age 40, then add 1 mm per decade (e.g., 7 mm at age 70)
What is the normal common bile duct diameter after removal of the gallbladder?	8 to 10 mm
What U/S findings are associated with acute cholecystitis?	Gallstones, thickened gallbladder wall (>3 mm), distended gallbladder (>4 cm A-P), impacted stone in gallbladder neck, pericholecystic fluid
What type of kidney stone is not seen on AXR?	Uric acid (Think: Uric acid = **U**nseen)
What is a C-C mammogram?	**C**ranio-**C**audal mammogram, in which the breast is compressed top to bottom
What is an MLO mammogram?	**M**edio**L**ateral **O**blique mammogram, in which the breast is compressed in a 45° angle from the axilla to the lower sternum

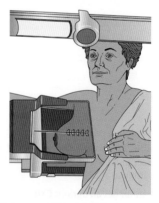

What are the best studies to evaluate for a pulmonary embolus?	Spiral thoracic CT scan, V/Q scan, pulmonary angiogram (gold standard)

RAPID-FIRE REVIEW

Name the diagnostic modality:

40-year-old female s/p MVC with pelvic fracture develops right lower extremity swelling	Extremity duplex scan (duplex is ultrasound and Doppler ultrasound) to look for DVT

Chapter 30 | Anesthesia

Define the following terms:

Local anesthesia

Anesthesia of a small confined area of the body (e.g., lidocaine for an elbow laceration)

Epidural anesthesia

Anesthetic agents injected into the epidural space

Spinal anesthesia

Anesthetic agents injected into the thecal sac

Regional anesthesia

Anesthetic agents injected around from a **region** of the body (e.g., radial nerve block)

General anesthesia

Triad:
1. Unconsciousness/amnesia
2. Analgesia
3. Muscle relaxation

GET or GETA

General EndoTracheal Anesthesia

Give examples of the following terms:

Local anesthetic

Lidocaine, bupivacaine (Marcaine®)

Regional anesthetic

Lidocaine, bupivacaine (Marcaine®)

General anesthesia

Isoflurane, sevoflurane, desflurane

Dissociative agent

Ketamine

What is cricoid pressure?

Manual pressure on cricoid cartilage occluding the esophagus and thus decreasing the chance of aspiration of gastric contents during intubation (a.k.a. "Sellick's maneuver")

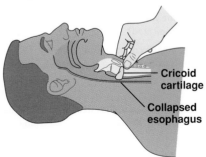

What is "rapid-sequence" anesthesia induction?	1. Oxygenation and short-acting induction agent 2. Paralytic 3. Cricoid pressure 4. Intubation 5. Inhalation anesthetic (rapid: boom, boom, boom → to lower the risk of aspiration during intubation)
Give examples of induction agents	Propofol, etomidate, ketamine
What are contraindications of the depolarizing agent succinylcholine?	Patients with burns, neuromuscular diseases/paraplegia, eye trauma, or increased ICP
Why is succinylcholine contraindicated in these patients?	Depolarization can result in life-threatening **hyperkalemia**
Why doesn't lidocaine work in an abscess?	Lidocaine does not work in an **acidic** environment
What will reverse rocuronium?	Sugammadex—a "selective relaxant binding agent"
Why does lidocaine burn on injection and what can be done to decrease the burning sensation?	Lidocaine is acidic, which causes the burning; add sodium bicarbonate to decrease the burning sensation
Why does some lidocaine come with epinephrine?	Epinephrine vasoconstricts the small vessels, resulting in a decrease in bleeding and blood flow in the area; this prolongs retention of lidocaine and its effects
In what locations is lidocaine with epinephrine contraindicated?	Fingers, toes, penis, etc., because of the possibility of ischemic injury/necrosis resulting from vasoconstriction
What are the contraindications to nitrous oxide?	Nitrous oxide is poorly soluble in serum and thus expands into any air-filled body pockets; avoid in patients with middle ear occlusions, **pneumothorax, small bowel obstruction,** etc.
What is the feared side effect of bupivacaine (Marcaine®)?	Cardiac dysrhythmia after intravascular injection leading to fatal refractory dysrhythmia
What is the treatment of life-threatening respiratory depression with narcotics?	**IV Narcan®** (naloxone)
What are the side effects of epidural analgesia?	**Orthostatic hypotension,** decreased motor function, urinary retention (lumbar epidurals)

MALIGNANT HYPERTHERMIA (MH)

What is it?	Inherited predisposition to an anesthetic reaction, causing uncoupling of the excitation–contraction system in skeletal muscle, which in turn causes **malignant hyperthermia**; hypermetabolism is fatal if untreated
What is the incidence?	Very rare
What are the causative agents?	Volatile anesthetics, succinylcholine
What are the signs/symptoms?	**Increased body temperature;** hypoxia; acidosis; tachycardia, ↑ PCO_2 (↑ end tidal CO_2)
What is the earliest sign of MH?	Rising end tidal CO_2
What is the treatment?	**IV dantrolene,** body cooling, discontinuation of volatile anesthetics

MISCELLANEOUS

What are the antidotes to the nondepolarizing neuromuscular blocking agents?	Neostigmine
What is the antidote to reverse succinylcholine?	Time; endogenous blood pseudocholinesterase (patients deficient in this enzyme may be paralyzed for hours!)
What are the early signs of local anesthetic toxicity?	Tinnitus, perioral/tongue numbness, metallic taste, blurred vision, muscle twitches, drowsiness
What are the signs of local anesthetic toxicity with large overdose?	Seizures, coma, respiratory arrest Loss of consciousness Apnea
What is used to reverse narcotics?	Naloxone (Narcan®)
What is used to reverse benzodiazepines?	Flumazenil

RAPID-FIRE REVIEW

What is the correct diagnosis?

48-year-old female undergoes a hysterectomy and develops an acute increase in end tidal CO_2 in the middle of the operation and then develops a very high fever, cardiac arrhythmia, acidosis, and hyperkalemia

Malignant hyperthermia

Chapter 31 | Surgical Ulcers

Define the following terms:

Peptic ulcer
General term for gastric/duodenal ulcer disease

Gastric ulcer
Ulcer in the stomach

Curling's ulcer
Gastric ulcer after burn injury (Think: Curling's—curling iron burn—burn)

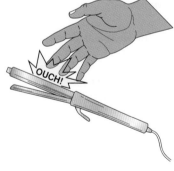

OUCH!

Cushing's ulcer
Peptic ulcer after neurologic insult (Think: Cushing—famous neurosurgeon)

Dieulafoy's ulcer
Pinpoint gastric mucosal defect bleeding from underlying arterial vessel malformation

Marjolin's ulcer
Squamous cell carcinoma ulceration overlying chronic osteomyelitis or burn scar

Aphthous ulcer
GI tract ulcer seen in Crohn's disease

Marginal ulcer	Mucosal ulcer seen at a site of GI tract anastomosis
Decubitus ulcer	Skin/subcutaneous ulceration from pressure necrosis, classically on the buttocks/sacrum
Venous stasis ulcer	Skin ulceration on **medial malleolus** caused by venous stasis of a lower extremity
LE arterial insufficiency ulcer	Skin ulcers usually located on the toes/feet

RAPID-FIRE REVIEW

Name the most likely diagnosis:

22-year-old female s/p TBI with massive upper GI bleed	Cushing's ulcer
40-year-old female with a 60% TBSA burn develops massive upper GI bleed	Curling's ulcer
45-year-old male with long-term left lower leg swelling develops a nonhealing sore over the left medial malleolus	Venous stasis ulcer

Chapter 32 | Surgical Oncology

Define:

Surgical oncology	Surgical treatment of tumors
XRT	Radiation therapy
In situ	Not invading basement membrane
Benign	Nonmalignant tumor—does not invade or metastasize
Malignant	Tumors with anaplasia that invade and metastasize
Adjuvant RX	Treatment that aids or assists surgical treatment = chemo or XRT
Neoadjuvant RX	Chemo, XRT, or both BEFORE surgical resection
Brachytherapy	XRT applied directly or very close to the target tissue (e.g., implantable radioactive seeds)

Metachronous tumors	Tumors occurring at different times
Synchronous tumors	Tumors occurring at the same time
What do the T, M, and N stand for in TMN staging?	**T**—Tumor size **M**—Mets (distant) **N**—Nodes
What tumor marker is associated with colon cancer?	CEA
What tumor marker is associated with hepatoma?	α-Fetoprotein
What tumor marker is associated with pancreatic carcinoma?	CA 19-9
What is paraneoplastic syndrome?	Syndrome of dysfunction not directly associated with tumor mass or metastasis (autoimmune or released substance)
What are the most common cancers in women?	1. Breast 2. Lung 3. Colorectal
What are the most common cancers in men?	1. Skin cancer 2. Prostrate 3. Lung 4. Colorectal
What is the most common cancer causing death in both men and women?	Lung!

Chapter 33 | GI Hormones and Physiology

CHOLECYSTOKININ (CCK)

What is its source?	Duodenal mucosal cells
What stimulates its release?	Fat, protein, amino acids, HCl
What inhibits its release?	Trypsin and chymotrypsin
What are its actions?	Empties gallbladder
	Opens ampulla of Vater
	Slows gastric emptying
	Stimulates pancreatic acinar cell growth and release of exocrine products

SECRETIN

What is its source?	Duodenal cells (specifically the argyrophilic S cells)
What stimulates its release?	pH <4.5 (acid), fat in the duodenum
What inhibits its release?	High pH in the duodenum
What are its actions?	Releases pancreatic bicarbonate/enzymes/ H_2O
	Releases bile/bicarbonate
	Decreases lower esophageal sphincter (LES) tone
	Decreases release of gastric acid

GASTRIN

What is its source?	Gastric antrum G cells
What stimulates its release?	Stomach peptides/amino acids
	Vagal input
	Calcium
What inhibits its release?	pH <3.0
	Somatostatin

What are its actions?	Release of HCl from parietal cells Trophic effect on mucosa of the stomach and small intestine

SOMATOSTATIN

What is its source?	Pancreatic D cells
What stimulates its release?	Food
What are its actions?	Globally inhibits GI function

MISCELLANEOUS

What is the purpose of the colon?	Reabsorption of H_2O and storage of stool
What is the main small bowel nutritional source?	Glutamine
What is the main nutritional source of the colon?	Butyrate (short-chain fatty acid)
Where is calcium absorbed?	Duodenum actively, jejunum passively
Where is iron absorbed?	Duodenum
Where is vitamin B12 absorbed?	Terminal ileum
Which hormone primarily controls gallbladder contraction?	CCK
What supplement does a patient need after removal of the terminal ileum or stomach?	Vitamin B12
What is the blood supply to the liver?	75% from the portal vein, rich in products of digestion 25% from the hepatic artery, rich in O_2 (but each provide for 50% of oxygen)

RAPID-FIRE REVIEW

What is the correct diagnosis?	
Necrotizing migratory erythema	Glucagonoma
Name the diagnostic modality:	
30-year-old female with history of duodenal ulcers and jejunal ulcers refractory to PPI, watery diarrhea	Gastric level and secretin stimulation test for gastrin, CT scan for work up for gastrinoma (Zollinger–Ellison syndrome)

Chapter 34 | Acute Abdomen and Referred Pain

What is an "acute abdomen"?

Acute abdominal pain so severe that the patient seeks medical attention (**Note:** Not the same as a "surgical abdomen," because most cases of acute abdominal pain do not require surgical treatment)

What are peritoneal signs?

Signs of peritoneal irritation: extreme tenderness, percussion tenderness, rebound tenderness, voluntary guarding, motion pain, **involuntary** guarding/rigidity (late)

Define the following terms:

Rebound tenderness

Pain upon releasing the palpating hand pushing on the abdomen

Motion pain

Abdominal pain upon moving, pelvic rocking, moving of stretcher, or heel strike

Voluntary guarding

Abdominal muscle contraction with palpation of the abdomen

Involuntary guarding

Rigid abdomen as the muscles "guard" involuntarily

Colic

Intermittent severe pain (usually because of intermittent contraction of a hollow viscus against an obstruction)

What conditions can mask abdominal pain?

Steroids, diabetes, paraplegia

What is the most common cause of acute abdominal surgery in the United States?

Acute appendicitis (7% of the population will develop it sometime during their lives)

What should the acute abdomen physical exam include?

Inspection (e.g., surgical scars, distention)
Auscultation (e.g., bowel sounds, bruits)
Palpation (e.g., tenderness, R/O hernia, CVAT, rectal, pelvic exam, rebound, voluntary guard, motion tenderness)
Percussion (e.g., liver size, spleen size)

What should go first, auscultation or palpation?

Auscultation

What is the best way to have a patient localize abdominal pain?

"Point with **one** finger to where the pain is worse"

What is the classic position of a patient with peritonitis?

Motionless (often with knees flexed)

What is the classic position of a patient with a kidney stone?

Cannot stay still, restless, writhing in pain

What is the best way to examine a scared child or histrionic adult's abdomen?	Use stethoscope to palpate abdomen
What lab tests are used to evaluate the patient with an acute abdomen?	CBC with **differential**, chem-10, lipase, type and screen, urinalysis, LFTs
What is a "left shift" on CBC differential?	Sign of inflammatory response: Immature neutrophils (bands) *Note:* Many call >80% of WBCs as neutrophils a "left shift"
What lab test should every woman of childbearing age with an acute abdomen receive?	Human chorionic gonadotropin (β-hCG) to rule out pregnancy/ectopic pregnancy
Which x-rays are used to evaluate the patient with an acute abdomen?	Upright chest x-ray, upright abdominal film, supine abdominal x-ray (if patient cannot stand, left lateral decubitus abdominal film)
How is free air ruled out if the patient cannot stand?	Left lateral decubitus—free air collects over the liver and does not get confused with the gastric bubble
What diagnosis must be considered in every patient with an acute abdomen?	**Appendicitis!**

What are the differential diagnoses by quadrant?

RUQ	Cholecystitis, hepatitis, PUD, perforated ulcer, pancreatitis, liver tumors, gastritis, hepatic abscess, choledocholithiasis, cholangitis, pyelonephritis, nephrolithiasis, appendicitis (**especially during pregnancy**); thoracic causes (e.g., pleurisy/pneumonia), PE, pericarditis, MI (especially inferior MI)
LUQ	PUD, perforated ulcer, gastritis, splenic injury, abscess, reflux, dissecting aortic aneurysm, thoracic causes, pyelonephritis, nephrolithiasis, hiatal hernia (strangulated paraesophageal hernia), Boerhaave's syndrome, Mallory–Weiss tear, splenic artery aneurysm, colon disease
LLQ	**Diverticulitis,** sigmoid volvulus, perforated colon, colon cancer, urinary tract infection, small bowel obstruction, inflammatory bowel disease, nephrolithiasis, pyelonephritis, fluid accumulation from aneurysm or perforation, referred hip pain, gynecologic causes, appendicitis (rare)

RLQ	**Appendicitis!** And same as LLQ; also mesenteric lymphadenitis, cecal diverticulitis, Meckel's diverticulum, intussusception
What is the differential diagnosis of epigastric pain?	PUD, gastritis, MI, pancreatitis, biliary colic, gastric volvulus, Mallory–Weiss tear
What are nonsurgical causes of abdominal pain?	Gastroenteritis, DKA, sickle cell crisis, rectus sheath hematoma, acute porphyria, PID, kidney stone, pyelonephritis, hepatitis, pancreatitis, pneumonia, MI, *Clostridium difficile* colitis, IBD
What is the unique differential diagnosis for the patient with AIDS and abdominal pain?	In addition to all common abdominal conditions:

In addition to all common abdominal conditions:
- **C**MV (most **C**ommon)
- Kaposi's sarcoma
- Lymphoma
- TB
- *Mycobacterium Avium* Intracellulare (**MAI**)

What causes pain limited to specific dermatomes?	Early zoster before vesicles erupt
What is referred pain?	Pain felt at a site distant from a disease process

Name the classic locations of referred pain:

Cholecystitis	Right subscapular pain (also epigastric)
Appendicitis	Early: periumbilical Rarely: testicular pain
Diaphragmatic irritation (from spleen, perforated ulcer, or abscess)	Shoulder pain (+ Kehr's sign on the left)
Pancreatitis/cancer	Back pain
Rectal disease	Pain in the small of the back
Nephrolithiasis	Testicular pain/flank pain
Rectal pain	Midline small of back pain
Small bowel	Periumbilical pain
Uterine pain	Midline small of back pain

Give the classic diagnosis for the following cases:

"Abdominal pain out of proportion to exam"	Rule out mesenteric ischemia

Hypotension and pulsatile abdominal mass	Ruptured AAA; go to the O.R.
Fever, LLQ pain, and change in bowel habits	Diverticulitis
Classically, what two endocrine problems can cause abdominal pain?	1. Addisonian crisis 2. **D**iabetic **K**eto**A**cidosis (**DKA**)

RAPID-FIRE REVIEW

Name the most likely diagnosis:

22-year-old female with acute onset of lower abdominal pain, hypotension, tachycardia, adnexal mass, and free fluid on vaginal ultrasound	Ectopic pregnancy rupture
21-year-old female with fever, leukocytosis, lower abdominal pain, + chandelier sign	**P**elvic **I**nflammatory **D**isease (**PID**)
54-year-old male smoker with c/o right-sided abdominal pain, hematuria, and a mass in the right side of his abdomen	Renal cell carcinoma
Abdominal pain "out of proportion to exam"	Mesenteric ischemia
67-year-old male with hypotension, abdominal pain, and an abdominal mass that pulsates	Ruptured abdominal aortic aneurysm
67-year-old female smoker with a history of 25-lb weight loss over 3 months due to abdominal pain after eating; nontender abdomen on exam	Chronic mesenteric ischemia

Chapter 35 | Hernias

What is hernia?	(**L. *rupture***) Protrusion of a peritoneal sac through a musculoaponeurotic barrier (e.g., abdominal wall); a fascial defect
What is the incidence?	5% to 10% lifetime; 50% are indirect inguinal, 25% are direct inguinal, and ≈5% are femoral
What are the precipitating factors?	Increased intra-abdominal pressure: straining at defecation or urination (rectal cancer, colon cancer, prostatic enlargement, constipation), obesity, pregnancy, ascites, valsavagenic (coughing) COPD; an abnormal congenital anatomic route (i.e., patent processus vaginalis)
Why should hernias be repaired?	To avoid complications of incarceration/strangulation, bowel necrosis, SBO, pain
What is more dangerous: a small or large hernia defect?	Small defect is more dangerous because a tight defect is more likely to strangulate if incarcerated
Define the following descriptive terms:	
Reducible	Ability to return the displaced organ or tissue/hernia contents to their usual anatomic site
Incarcerated	Swollen or fixed within the hernia sac (incarcerated = imprisoned); may cause intestinal obstruction (i.e., an irreducible hernia)
Strangulated	Incarcerated hernia with resulting ischemia; will result in signs and symptoms of ischemia and intestinal obstruction or bowel necrosis (Think: strangulated = choked)

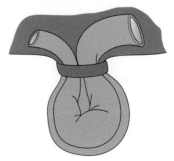

Complete	Hernia sac and its contents protrude all the way through the defect
Incomplete	Defect present without sac or contents protruding completely through it
What is reducing a hernia "en masse"?	Reducing the hernia contents and hernia sac

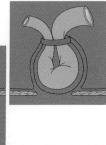
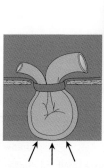

Define the following types of hernias:

Sliding hernia	Hernia sac partially formed by the wall of a viscus (i.e., bladder/cecum)

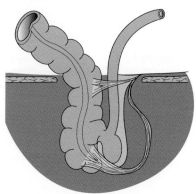

Littre's hernia	Hernia involving a Meckel's diverticulum (Think alphabetically: Littre's Meckel's = LM)
Spigelian hernia	Hernia through the linea semilunaris (or spigelian fascia); also known as spontaneous lateral ventral hernia (Think: Spigelian = Semilunaris)
Internal hernia	Hernia in or involving intra-abdominal structure

Petersen's hernia

Seen after bariatric gastric bypass—internal herniation of small bowel through the mesenteric defect from the Roux limb

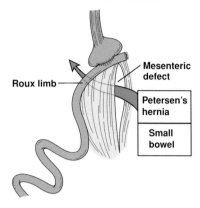

Obturator hernia

Hernia through obturator canal (females > males)

Pantaloon hernia

Hernia sac exists as **both a direct and indirect** hernia straddling the inferior epigastric vessels and protruding through the floor of the canal as well as the internal ring (two sacs separated by the inferior epigastric vessels [the pant crotch] like a pair of pantaloon pants)

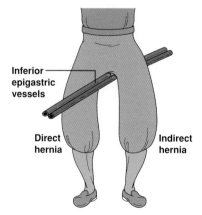

Incisional hernia

Hernia through an incisional site; most common cause is a wound infection

Ventral hernia

Incisional hernia in the ventral abdominal wall

Parastomal hernia

Hernia adjacent to an ostomy (e.g., colostomy)

Richter's hernia	Incarcerated or strangulated hernia involving only **one sidewall of the bowel,** which can spontaneously reduce, resulting in gangrenous bowel and perforation within the abdomen without signs of obstruction

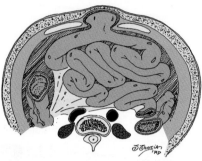

Epigastric hernia	Hernia through the linea alba above the umbilicus
Umbilical hernia	Hernia through the umbilical ring, in adults associated with ascites, pregnancy, and obesity
Femoral hernia	Hernia medial to femoral vessels (under inguinal ligament)
Indirect inguinal	Inguinal hernia lateral to Hesselbach's triangle
Direct inguinal	Inguinal hernia within Hesselbach's triangle
Hiatal hernia	Hernia through esophageal hiatus
What are the boundaries of Hesselbach's triangle?	1. Inferior epigastric vessels 2. Inguinal ligament (Poupart's) 3. Lateral border of the rectus sheath Floor consists of internal oblique and the transversus abdominis muscle
What are the layers of the abdominal wall?	Skin Subcutaneous fat Scarpa's fascia External oblique Internal oblique Transversus abdominis Transversalis fascia Preperitoneal fat Peritoneum ***Note:*** All three muscle layer aponeuroses form the anterior rectus sheath, with the posterior rectus sheath being deficient below the arcuate line

What is the differential diagnosis for a mass in a healed C-section incision?	Hernia, ENDOMETRIOMA

GROIN HERNIAS

What is the differential diagnosis of a groin mass?	Lymphadenopathy, hematoma, seroma, abscess, hydrocele, femoral artery aneurysm, EIC, undescended testicle, sarcoma, hernias, testicle torsion

Direct Inguinal Hernia

What is it?	Hernia within the floor of Hesselbach's triangle, that is, the hernia sac does not traverse the internal ring (Think: **directly** through the abdominal wall)
What is the cause?	Acquired defect from mechanical breakdown over the years
What is the incidence?	≈1% of all men; frequency increases with advanced age
What nerve runs with the spermatic cord in the inguinal canal?	Ilioinguinal nerve

Indirect Inguinal Hernia

What is it?	Hernia through the internal ring of the inguinal canal, traveling down toward the external ring; it may enter the scrotum upon exiting the external ring (i.e., if complete); think of the hernia sac traveling indirectly through the abdominal wall from the internal ring to the external ring

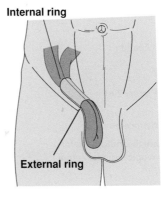

Internal ring

External ring

What is the cause?	Patent processus vaginalis (i.e., congenital)
What is the incidence?	≈5% of all men; most common hernia in both men **and** women
How is an inguinal hernia diagnosed?	Relies mainly on history and physical exam with index finger invaginated into the external ring and palpation of hernia; examine the patient standing up if diagnosis is not obvious (*Note:* if swelling occurs below the inguinal ligament, it is possibly a femoral hernia)
What is the differential diagnosis of an inguinal hernia?	Lymphadenopathy, psoas abscess, ectopic testis, hydrocele of the cord, saphenous varix, lipoma, varicocele, testicular torsion, femoral artery aneurysm, abscess
What is the risk of strangulation?	Higher with indirect than direct inguinal hernia, but highest in femoral hernias
What is the treatment?	Emergent herniorrhaphy is indicated if strangulation is suspected or acute incarceration is present; otherwise, elective herniorrhaphy is indicated to prevent the chance of incarceration/strangulation

Inguinal Hernia Repairs

Define the following procedures:

Bassini	**Sutures** approximate reflection of inguinal ligament (Poupart's) to the transversus abdominis aponeurosis/conjoint tendon
McVay	**Cooper's** ligament sutured to transversus abdominis aponeurosis/conjoint tendon
Lichtenstein	"Tension-free repair" using mesh
Plug and patch	Placing a plug of mesh in hernia defect and then overlaying a patch of mesh over inguinal floor (requires few if any sutures in mesh!)
High ligation	Ligation and transection of indirect hernia sac without repair of inguinal floor (used only in **children**)
TAPP procedure	**T**rans**A**bdominal **P**re**P**eritoneal inguinal hernia repair
TEPA procedure	**T**otally **E**xtra**P**eritoneal **A**pproach
What are the indications for laparoscopic inguinal hernia repair?	1. Bilateral inguinal hernias 2. Recurring hernia 3. Need to resume full activity as soon as possible

Classic Intraoperative Inguinal Hernia Questions

What is the first identifiable subcutaneous named layer?	Scarpa's fascia (thin in adults)
What is the name of the subcutaneous vein that is ligated?	Superficial epigastric vein
What happens if you cut the ilioinguinal nerve?	Numbness of inner thigh or lateral scrotum; usually goes away in 6 months
From what abdominal muscle layer is the cremaster muscle derived?	Internal oblique muscle
From what abdominal muscle layer is the inguinal ligament (a.k.a. "Poupart's ligament") derived?	External oblique muscle aponeurosis
To what does the inguinal (Poupart's) ligament attach?	Anterior-superior iliac spine to the pubic tubercle
Which nerve travels on the spermatic cord?	Ilioinguinal nerve
Why do some surgeons deliberately cut the ilioinguinal nerve?	First they obtain preoperative consent and cut so as to remove the risk of entrapment and postoperative pain
What is in the spermatic cord (6)?	1. Cremasteric muscle fibers 2. Vas deferens 3. Testicular artery 4. Testicular pampiniform venous plexus 5. ± Hernia sac 6. Genital branch of the genitofemoral nerve
What is the hernia sac made of?	Peritoneum (direct) or a patent processus vaginalis (indirect)
What attaches the testicle to the scrotum?	Gubernaculum
What is the most common organ in an inguinal hernia sac in men?	Small intestine
What is the most common organ in an inguinal hernia sac in women?	Ovary/fallopian tube
What lies in the inguinal canal in females instead of the VAS?	Round ligament

Where in the inguinal canal does the hernia sac lie in relation to the other structures?

Anteromedially

What is a "cord lipoma"?

Preperitoneal fat on the cord structures (pushed in by the hernia sac); not a real lipoma; remove surgically, if feasible

What is a small outpouching of testicular tissue off the testicle?

Testicular appendage (a.k.a. "the appendix testes"); remove with electrocautery

What action should be taken if a suture is placed through the femoral artery or vein during an inguinal herniorrhaphy?

Remove the suture as soon as possible and apply pressure (i.e., do not tie the suture down!)

What nerve is found on top of the spermatic cord?

Ilioinguinal nerve

What nerve travels within the spermatic cord?

Genital branch of the genitofemoral nerve

What are the borders of Hesselbach's triangle?

1. Epigastric vessels
2. Inguinal ligament
3. Lateral border of the rectus

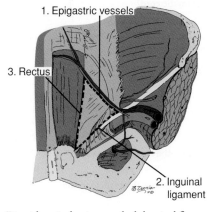

What type of hernia goes through Hesselbach's triangle?

Direct hernia due to a weak abdominal floor

What is a "relaxing incision"?

Incision(s) in the rectus sheath to relax the conjoint tendon so that it can be approximated to the reflection of the inguinal ligament without tension

What is a conjoint tendon?

Aponeurotic attachments of the "conjoining" of the internal oblique and transversus abdominis to the pubic tubercle

Define inguinal anatomy:

1. Inguinal ligament (Poupart's ligament)
2. Transversus aponeurosis
3. Conjoint tendon

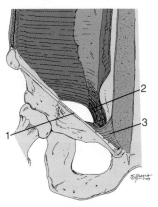

How tight should the new internal inguinal ring be?

Should allow entrance of the tip of a Kelly clamp but not a finger (the new external inguinal ring should not be tight and should allow entrance of a finger)

What percentage of the strength of an inguinal floor repair does an external oblique aponeurosis represent?

ZERO

Femoral Hernia

What is it?

Hernia traveling beneath the inguinal ligament down the femoral canal medial to the femoral vessels (Think: **FM** radio, or **F**emoral hernia = **M**edial)

What are the boundaries of the femoral canal?

1. Cooper's ligament posteriorly
2. Inguinal ligament anteriorly
3. Femoral vein laterally
4. Lacunar ligament medially

What factors are associated with femoral hernias?

Women, pregnancy, and exertion

What percentage of all hernias is femoral?

5%

What percentage of patients with a femoral hernia is female?

85%!

What are the complications?

Approximately 1/3 incarcerate (due to narrow, unforgiving neck)

What is the most common hernia in women?	Indirect inguinal hernia
What is the repair of a femoral hernia?	McVay (Cooper's ligament repair), mesh plug repair

ESOPHAGEAL HIATAL HERNIAS

Define type I and type II hiatal hernias:	Type I = sliding Type II = paraesophageal

Sliding Esophageal Hiatal Hernia

What is it?

Both the stomach and GE junction herniate into the thorax via the esophageal hiatus; also known as type I hiatal hernia

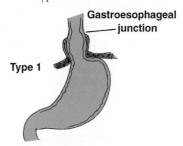

What is the incidence?

>90% of all hiatal hernias

What are the symptoms?

Most patients are asymptomatic, but the condition can cause reflux, dysphagia (from inflammatory edema), esophagitis, and pulmonary problems secondary to aspiration

How is it diagnosed?

UGI series, manometry, esophagogastroduodenoscopy (EGD) with biopsy for esophagitis

What is the treatment?

85% of cases treated medically with antacids, H_2 blockers/PPIs, head elevation after meals, small meals, and no food prior to sleeping; 15% of cases require surgery for persistent symptoms despite adequate medical treatment

What is the surgical treatment?

Laparoscopic Nissen fundoplication (LAP NISSEN) involves wrapping the fundus around the LES and suturing it in place

Paraesophageal Hiatal Hernia

What is it?

Herniation of all or part of the stomach through the esophageal hiatus into the thorax without displacement of the gastroesophageal junction; also known as type II hiatal hernia

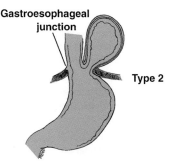

Gastroesophageal junction

Type 2

What are the complications?

Hemorrhage, incarceration, obstruction, and strangulation

What is the treatment?

Surgical, because of frequency and severity of potential complications

RAPID-FIRE REVIEW

Name the most likely diagnosis:

28-year-old male with groin mass, vomiting, air–fluid levels on abdominal x-ray

Incarcerated inguinal hernia

29-year-old female with a mass below inguinal ligament

Femoral hernia

Chapter 36 | Laparoscopy

What is laparoscopy?

Minimally invasive surgical technique using gas to insufflate the peritoneum and instruments manipulated through ports introduced through small incisions with video camera guidance

What gas is used and why?	CO_2 because of better solubility in blood and, thus, less risk of gas embolism; noncombustible
What are the classic findings with a CO_2 gas embolus?	Triad: 1. Hypotension 2. Decreased end tidal CO_2 (low flow to lung) 3. Mill-wheel murmur
What prophylactic measure should every patient get when having a laparoscopic procedure?	**SCD** boots—**S**equential **C**ompression **D**evice (and most add an OGT to decompress the stomach; Foley catheter is usually used for pelvic procedures)
What are the cardiovascular effects of a pneumoperitoneum?	**Increased afterload** and **decreased preload** (but the CVP and PCWP are deceivingly elevated!)
What is the effect of CO_2 insufflation on end tidal CO_2 levels?	Increased as a result of absorption of CO_2 into the bloodstream; the body compensates with increased ventilation and blows the extra CO_2 off and thus there is no acidosis
What are the advantages over laparotomy?	Shorter hospitalization, less pain and scarring, lower cost, decreased ileus
What is the Veress needle?	Needle with spring-loaded, retractable, blunt inner-protective tube that protrudes from the needle end when it enters peritoneal cavity; used for blind entrance and then insufflation of CO_2 through the Veress needle
How can it be verified that the Veress needle is in the peritoneum?	Syringe of saline; saline should flow freely without pressure through the needle "drop test"
What is the Hasson technique?	No Veress needle—cut down and place trocar under **direct visualization**
What is the cause of postlaparoscopic shoulder pain?	Referred pain from CO_2 on diaphragm and diaphragm stretch
What is FRED®?	**F**og **R**eduction **E**limination **D**evice: sponge with antifog solution used to coat the camera lens
How do you get the spleen out through a trocar site after a laparoscopic splenectomy?	Morcellation in a bag, then remove piecemeal

Chapter 37 | Trauma

What widely accepted protocol does trauma care in the United States follow?	Advanced Trauma Life Support (ATLS) precepts of the American College of Surgeons
What are the three main elements of the ATLS protocol?	1. Primary survey/resuscitation 2. Secondary survey 3. Definitive care
How and when should the patient history be obtained?	It should be obtained while completing the primary survey; often the rescue squad, witnesses, and family members must be relied upon

PRIMARY SURVEY

What are the five steps of the primary survey?	Think: **"ABCDEs":**
	    Airway (and C spine stabilization)
	    Breathing
	    Circulation
	    Disability
	    Exposure and **E**nvironment

What principles are followed in completing the primary survey?	Life-threatening problems discovered during the primary survey are **always** addressed **before** proceeding to the next step

Airway

What are the goals during assessment of the airway?	Securing the airway and protecting the spinal cord
In addition to the airway, what MUST be considered during the airway step?	Spinal immobilization
What comprises spinal immobilization?	Use of a full backboard and rigid cervical collar
In an alert patient, what is the quickest test for an adequate airway?	Ask a question: If the patient can speak, the airway is intact
What is the first maneuver used to establish an airway?	Chin lift, jaw thrust, or both; if successful, often an oral or nasal airway can be used to temporarily maintain the airway
If these methods are unsuccessful, what is the next maneuver used to establish an airway?	Endotracheal intubation

If all other methods are unsuccessful, what is the definitive airway?

Cricothyroidotomy, a.k.a. "surgical airway": Incise the cricothyroid membrane between the cricoid cartilage inferiorly and the thyroid cartilage superiorly and place an endotracheal or tracheostomy tube into the trachea

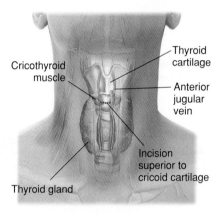

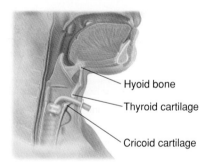

What must always be kept in mind during difficult attempts to establish an airway?

Spinal immobilization and adequate oxygenation; if at all possible, patients must be adequately ventilated with 100% oxygen using a bag and mask before any attempt to establish an airway

Breathing

What are the goals in assessing breathing?

Securing oxygenation and ventilation
Treating life-threatening thoracic injuries

What comprises adequate assessment of breathing?	Inspection—for air movement, respiratory rate, cyanosis, tracheal shift, jugular venous distention (JVD), asymmetric chest expansion, use of accessory muscles of respiration, open chest wounds Auscultation—for breath sounds Percussion—for hyperresonance or dullness over either lung field Palpation—for presence of subcutaneous emphysema, flail segments
What are the life-threatening conditions that MUST be diagnosed and treated during the breathing step?	Tension pneumothorax, open pneumothorax, massive hemothorax

Pneumothorax

What is it?	Injury to the lung, resulting in release of air into the pleural space between the normally apposed parietal and visceral pleura
How is it diagnosed?	**Tension pneumothorax is a clinical diagnosis:** dyspnea, JVD, tachypnea, anxiety, pleuritic chest pain, unilateral decreased or absent breath sounds, tracheal shift away from the affected side, hyperresonance on the affected side
What is the treatment of a tension pneumothorax?	Emergent digital thoracostomy (finger into pleural cavity) or **needle thoracostomy** followed by **tube thoracostomy** placed in the anterior/midaxillary line in the fourth intercostal space (level of the nipple in men)
What is the medical term for a "sucking chest wound"?	Open pneumothorax
What is a tube thoracostomy?	"Chest tube"
How is an open pneumothorax diagnosed and treated?	**Diagnosis:** usually obvious, with air movement through a chest wall defect and pneumothorax on CXR **Treatment in the ER:** tube thoracostomy (chest tube), occlusive dressing over chest wall defect or "three-sided" dressing

What does a pneumothorax look like on chest x-ray (CXR)?

Loss of lung markings (figure shows a right-sided pneumothorax; arrows point out edge of lung–air interface)

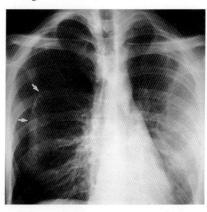

Flail Chest

What is it?

Two separate fractures in three or more consecutive ribs

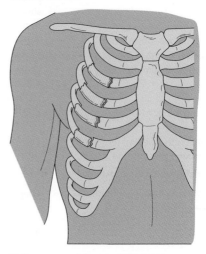

How is it diagnosed?

Flail segment of chest wall that moves **paradoxically** (sucks in with inspiration and pushes out with expiration opposite the rest of the chest wall)

What is the major cause of respiratory compromise with flail chest?

Underlying pulmonary contusion!

What is the treatment?	**Intubation** with positive pressure ventilation and PEEP PRN (let ribs heal on their own)

Cardiac Tamponade

What is it?	Bleeding into the pericardial sac, resulting in constriction of heart, decreasing inflow, and resulting in decreased cardiac output (the pericardium does not stretch!)
What are the signs and symptoms?	Tachycardia/shock with **Beck's triad**, pulsus paradoxus, Kussmaul's sign
Define the following:	
Beck's triad	1. Hypotension 2. Muffled heart sounds 3. JVD
Kussmaul's sign	JVD with inspiration
How is cardiac tamponade diagnosed?	Ultrasound (FAST exam)
What is the treatment?	Pericardial window—if blood returns then median sternotomy to rule out and treat cardiac injury

Massive Hemothorax

How is it diagnosed?	Unilaterally decreased or absent breath sounds; dullness to percussion; CXR, CT scan, chest tube output
What is the treatment?	Volume replacement **Tube thoracostomy** (chest tube) Removal of the blood (which will allow apposition of the parietal and visceral pleura, sealing the defect and slowing the bleeding)
What are indications for emergent thoracotomy for hemothorax?	Massive hemothorax = 1. >1,500 cc of blood on initial placement of chest tube 2. Persistent >200 cc of bleeding via chest tube per hour × 4 hours

Circulation

What are the goals in assessing circulation?	Securing adequate tissue perfusion; treatment of external bleeding
What is the initial test for adequate circulation?	Palpation of pulses: As a rough guide, if a radial pulse is palpable, then systolic pressure is at least 80 mm Hg; if a femoral or carotid pulse is palpable, then systolic pressure is at least 60 mm Hg

What comprises adequate assessment of circulation?	Heart rate, blood pressure, peripheral perfusion, urinary output, mental status, capillary refill (normal <2 seconds), exam of skin: cold, clammy = hypovolemia
Who can be hypovolemic with normal blood pressure?	Young patients; autonomic tone can maintain blood pressure until cardiovascular collapse is imminent
Which patients may not mount a tachycardic response to hypovolemic shock?	Those with concomitant spinal cord injuries Those on β-blockers Well-conditioned athletes
How are sites of external bleeding treated?	By direct pressure; ± tourniquets
What is the best and preferred intravenous (IV) access in the trauma patient?	"Two large-bore IVs" (14–16 gauge), IV catheters in the upper extremities (peripheral IV access)
For a femoral vein catheter, how can the anatomy of the right groin be remembered?	Lateral to medial **"NAVEL"**: Nerve Artery Vein Empty space Lymphatics Thus, the vein is medial to the femoral artery pulse (Or, Think: "venous close to penis")
What is the trauma resuscitation fluid of choice in the hypotensive trauma patient?	Blood and blood products
In the nonhypotensive trauma patient?	Lactated Ringer's (LR); most use NS for TBI patients
What types of decompression do trauma patients receive?	Gastric decompression with an NGT and Foley catheter bladder decompression after **normal rectal exam** and no indication of urethral injury
What are the contraindications to placement of a Foley?	Signs of urethral injury: Severe pelvic fracture in men Blood at the urethral meatus (penile opening) "High-riding," "ballotable" prostate (loss of urethral tethering) Scrotal/perineal injury/ecchymosis
What test should be obtained prior to placing a Foley catheter if urethral injury is suspected?	Retrograde UrethroGram **(RUG):** dye in penis retrograde to the bladder and x-ray looking for extravasation of dye
How is gastric decompression achieved with a maxillofacial fracture?	**Not** with an NGT because the tube may perforate through the cribriform plate into the brain; place an **oral**-gastric tube (OGT), not an NGT

Disability

What are the goals in assessing disability?

Determination of neurologic injury (Think: neurologic disability)

What comprises adequate assessment of disability?

Mental status—Glasgow Coma Scale (GCS)
Pupils—a blown pupil suggests ipsilateral brain mass (blood) as herniation of the brain compresses CN III
Motor/sensory—screening exam for lateralizing extremity movement, sensory deficits

Describe the GCS scoring system:

Eye opening (E)
    4—Opens spontaneously
    3—Opens to voice (command)
    2—Opens to pressure stimulus
    1—Does not open eyes
    (Think: Eyes = "four eyes")

Motor response (M)
    6—Obeys commands
    5—Localizes painful stimulus
    4—Withdraws from pressure
    3—Decorticate posture
    2—Decerebrate posture
    1—No movement
    (Think: Motor = "6-cylinder motor")

Verbal response (V)
    5—Appropriate and oriented
    4—Confused
    3—Inappropriate words
    2—Incomprehensible sounds
    1—No sounds
    (Verbal = Jackson 5)

What is a normal human GCS?

GCS 15

What is the GCS score for a dead man?

GCS 3

What is the GCS score for a patient in a "coma"?

GCS ≤8

GCS indication for intubation?

≤8

How does scoring differ if the patient is intubated?

Verbal evaluation is omitted and replaced with a "T"; thus, the highest score for an intubated patient is 10 T

Exposure and Environment

What are the goals in obtaining adequate exposure?

Complete disrobing to allow a thorough visual inspection and digital palpation of the patient during the secondary survey

| What is the "environment" of the E in ABCDEs? | Keep a warm environment (i.e., keep the patient warm; a hypothermic patient can become coagulopathic) |

SECONDARY SURVEY

What principle is followed in completing the secondary survey?	Complete physical exam, including all orifices: ears, nose, mouth, vagina, rectum
Why look in the ears?	Hemotympanum is a sign of basilar skull fracture; otorrhea is a sign of basilar skull fracture
Examination of what part of the trauma patient's body is often forgotten?	Patient's back (logroll the patient and examine!)
What are typical signs of basilar skull fracture?	Raccoon eyes, Battle's sign, clear otorrhea or rhinorrhea, hemotympanum
What diagnosis in the anterior chamber must not be missed on the eye exam?	Traumatic hyphema = blood in the anterior chamber of the eye
What potentially destructive lesion must not be missed on the nasal exam?	Nasal septal hematoma: Hematoma must be evacuated; if not, it can result in pressure necrosis of the septum!
What is the best indication of a mandibular fracture?	Dental malocclusion: Tell the patient to "bite down" and ask, "Does that feel normal to you?"
What signs of thoracic trauma are often found on the neck exam?	Crepitus or subcutaneous emphysema from tracheobronchial disruption/PTX; tracheal deviation from tension pneumothorax; JVD from cardiac tamponade; carotid bruit heard with seatbelt neck injury resulting in carotid artery injury
What is the best physical exam for broken ribs or sternum?	Lateral and anterior–posterior compression of the thorax to elicit pain/instability
What physical signs are diagnostic for thoracic great vessel injury?	None: Diagnosis of great vessel injury requires a high index of suspicion based on the mechanism of injury, associated injuries, and CXR/radiographic findings (e.g., widened mediastinum)
What is the best way to diagnose or rule out aortic injury?	CT angiogram (CTA)
What must be considered in every penetrating injury of the thorax at or below the level of the nipple?	Concomitant injury to the abdomen (Remember, the diaphragm extends to the level of the nipples in the male on full expiration)

What is the significance of subcutaneous air?

Indicates PTX, until proven otherwise

What is the physical exam technique for examining the thoracic and lumbar spine?

Logrolling the patient to allow complete visualization of the back and palpation of the spine to elicit pain over fractures, step off (spine deformity)

What conditions must exist to pronounce an abdominal physical exam negative?

Alert patient without any evidence of head/spinal cord injury or drug/EtOH intoxication (Even then, the abdominal exam is not 100% accurate)

What physical signs may indicate intra-abdominal injury?

Tenderness; guarding; peritoneal signs; progressive distention (always use a gastric tube for decompression of air); seatbelt sign

What is the seatbelt sign?

Ecchymosis on lower abdomen from wearing a seatbelt (≈10% of patients with this sign have a small bowel perforation!)

What must be documented from the rectal exam?

Sphincter tone (as an indication of spinal cord function); presence of blood (as an indication of colon or rectal injury); prostate position (as an indication of urethral injury)

What is the best physical exam technique to test for pelvic fractures?

Lateral compression of the iliac crests and greater trochanters and anterior–posterior compression of the symphysis pubis to elicit pain/instability

What is the "halo" sign?

Cerebrospinal fluid from nose/ear will form a clear "halo" around the blood on a cloth

What physical signs indicate possible urethral injury, thus contraindicating placement of a Foley catheter?

High-riding, ballotable prostate on rectal exam; presence of blood at the meatus; scrotal or perineal ecchymosis

What must be documented from the extremity exam?

Any fractures or joint injuries; any open wounds; motor and sensory exam, particularly distal to any fractures; distal pulses; peripheral perfusion

What complication after prolonged ischemia to the lower extremity must be treated immediately?

Compartment syndrome

What is the treatment for this condition?

Fasciotomy (four compartments below the knee)

What injuries must be suspected in a trauma patient with a progressive decline in mental status?

Epidural hematoma, subdural hematoma, brain swelling with rising intracranial pressure (ICP). But **hypoxia/hypotension must be ruled out!**

TRAUMA STUDIES

What are the classic blunt trauma ER x-rays?	1. AP (anterior–posterior) chest film 2. AP pelvis film
What are the common trauma labs?	Blood for complete blood count, chemistries, amylase, liver function tests (LFTs), lactic acid, coagulation studies, and **type and crossmatch;** urine for urinalysis
How can a C-spine be evaluated?	1. Clinically by physical exam 2. Radiographically
What patients can have their C-spines cleared by a physical exam?	No neck pain on palpation with full range of motion (FROM) with no neurologic injury (GCS 15), no EtOH/drugs, no distracting injury, no pain meds
How do you rule out a C-spine bony fracture?	With a CT scan of the C-spine
What do you do if no bony C-spine fracture is apparent on CT scan and you cannot obtain an MRI in a COMATOSE patient?	This is controversial, but most centers remove the c-collar
Which x-rays are used for evaluation of cervical spine LIGAMENTOUS injury?	MRI (lateral flexion and extension C-spine films also used but infrequently)
What study is used to rule out thoracic aortic injury?	CT scan of mediastinum looking for mediastinal hematoma with CTA
What is the most common site of thoracic aortic traumatic tear?	Just distal to the take-off of the left subclavian artery
What studies are available to evaluate for intra-abdominal injury?	FAST, CT scan, DPL
What is a FAST exam?	Ultrasound: **F**ocused **A**ssessment with **S**onography for **T**rauma = **FAST**
What does the FAST exam look for?	Blood in the peritoneal cavity looking at Morison's pouch, bladder, spleen, and pericardial sac
What does DPL stand for?	**D**iagnostic **P**eritoneal **L**avage
What diagnostic test is the test of choice for evaluation of the unstable patient with blunt abdominal trauma?	FAST
What is the indication for abdominal CT scan in blunt trauma?	Normal vital signs with abdominal pain/tenderness/mechanism

What is the indication for FAST in blunt trauma?	Unstable vital signs (hypotension)
What injuries does CT scan miss?	Small bowel injuries and diaphragm injuries
What study is used to evaluate the urethra in cases of possible disruption due to blunt trauma?	**R**etrograde **U**rethro**G**ram (**RUG**)
What are the most emergent orthopedic injuries?	1. Hip dislocation—must be reduced immediately 2. Exsanguinating pelvic fracture (binder or external fixator)
What is the treatment of a gunshot wound to the belly?	Exploratory laparotomy
What is the evaluation of a stab wound to the belly?	If there are peritoneal signs, heavy bleeding, shock, perform exploratory laparotomy; otherwise, many surgeons perform a CT scan and/or observe or laparoscopy

PENETRATING NECK INJURIES

What depth of neck injury must be further evaluated?	Penetrating injury through the platysma
Define the anatomy of the neck by trauma zones:	
Zone III	Angle of the mandible and up
Zone II	Angle of the mandible to the cricoid cartilage
Zone I	Below the cricoid cartilage

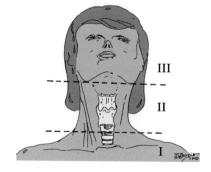

How do most surgeons treat penetrating neck injuries (those that penetrate the platysma) by neck zone:

Zone III — Selective exploration

Zone II — Surgical exploration versus selective exploration

Zone I — Selective exploration

What is selective exploration? — Selective exploration is based on diagnostic studies that include A-gram or CT A-gram, bronchoscopy, esophagoscopy

What are the indications for surgical exploration in all penetrating neck wounds (zones I, II, III)? — "**Hard** signs" of significant neck damage: **shock**, exsanguinating hemorrhage, expanding hematoma, pulsatile hematoma, neurologic injury, subQ emphysema

How can you remember the order of the neck trauma zones and Le Forte fractures? — In the direction of carotid blood flow

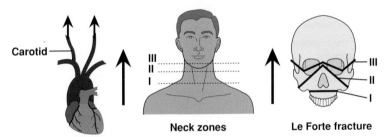

Neck zones   **Le Forte fracture**

MISCELLANEOUS TRAUMA FACTS

What is the minimal urine output for an adult trauma patient? — 50 mL/hr

How much blood can be lost into the thigh with a closed femur fracture? — Up to 1.5 L of blood

Can an adult lose enough blood in the "closed" skull from a brain injury to cause hypovolemic shock? — Absolutely not! But infants can lose enough blood from a brain injury to cause shock

Can a patient be hypotensive after an isolated head injury? — Yes, but rule out hemorrhagic shock!

What is the brief ATLS history?	**"AMPLE"** history: **A**llergies **M**edications **P**MH **L**ast meal (when) **E**vents (of injury, etc.)
In what population is a surgical cricothyroidotomy not recommended?	Any patient age <12 years; instead perform needle cricothyroidotomy
What are the signs of a laryngeal fracture?	Subcutaneous emphysema in neck Altered voice Palpable laryngeal fracture
What is the treatment of rectal penetrating injury?	**Diverting proximal colostomy;** closure of perforation (if easy, and definitely if intraperitoneal); and presacral drainage
What is the treatment of EXTRAperitoneal minor bladder rupture?	"Bladder catheter" (Foley) drainage and observation; intraperitoneal or large bladder rupture requires operative closure
What intra-abdominal injury is associated with seatbelt use?	Small bowel injuries (L2 fracture, pancreatic injury)
What is the treatment of a pelvic fracture?	± Pelvic binder until the external fixator is placed; IVF/blood; ± A-gram to embolize bleeding pelvic vessels
Bleeding from pelvic fractures is most commonly caused by arterial or venous bleeding?	Venous (≈85%)
If a patient has a laceration through an eyebrow, should you shave the eyebrow prior to suturing it closed?	No—20% of the time, the eyebrow will not grow back if shaved!
What is the treatment of extensive irreparable biliary, duodenal, and pancreatic head injury?	Trauma Whipple
What is the most common intra-abdominal organ injured with penetrating trauma?	Small bowel
How high up do the diaphragms go?	To the nipples (intercostal space #4); thus, intra-abdominal injury with penetrating injury below the nipples must be ruled out
Classic trauma question: "If you have only one vial of blood from a trauma victim to send to the lab, what test should be ordered?"	Type and cross (for blood transfusion)

What is the treatment of penetrating injury to the colon?

If the patient is in shock, resection and colostomy

If the patient is stable, the trend is primary anastomosis/repair

What is the treatment of small bowel injury?

Primary closure or resection and primary anastomosis

What is the treatment of minor pancreatic injury?

Drainage (e.g., JP drains)

What is the most commonly injured abdominal organ with blunt trauma?

Liver (in recent studies)

What is the treatment for significant duodenal injury?

Pyloric exclusion:
1. Close duodenal injury
2. Staple off pylorus
3. Gastrojejunostomy

What is the treatment for massive tail of pancreas injury?

Distal pancreatectomy (usually perform splenectomy also)

What is "damage control" surgery?

Stop major hemorrhage and GI soilage

Pack and get out of the O.R. ASAP to bring the patient to the ICU to warm, correct coags, and resuscitate

Return patient to O.R. when stable, warm, and not acidotic

What is the "lethal triad"?

"ACH":
1. **A**cidosis
2. **C**oagulopathy
3. **H**ypothermia

(Think: **ACH**e = **A**cidosis, **C**oagulopathy, **H**ypothermia)

What comprises the workup/ treatment of a stable parasternal chest gunshot/stab wound?

1. CXR
2. FAST, chest tube, ± O.R. for subxiphoid window; if blood returns, then sternotomy to assess for cardiac injury

What is the diagnosis with NGT in chest on CXR?

Ruptured diaphragm with stomach in pleural cavity (go to ex lap)

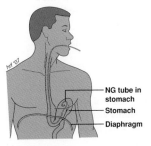

NG tube in stomach

Stomach

Diaphragm

What films are typically obtained to evaluate extremity fractures?

Complete views of the involved extremity, including the joints above and below the fracture

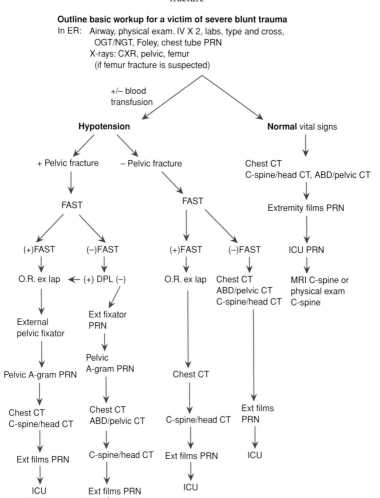

Outline basic workup for a victim of severe blunt trauma

In ER: Airway, physical exam. IV X 2, labs, type and cross, OGT/NGT, Foley, chest tube PRN

X-rays: CXR, pelvic, femur (if femur fracture is suspected)

+/− blood transfusion

Hypotension

Normal vital signs

+ Pelvic fracture

− Pelvic fracture

Chest CT
C-spine/head CT, ABD/pelvic CT

FAST

FAST

Extremity films PRN

(+)FAST   (−)FAST

(+)FAST   (−)FAST   ICU PRN

O.R. ex lap ← (+) DPL (−)

O.R. ex lap   Chest CT   MRI C-spine or
ABD/pelvic CT   physical exam
C-spine/head CT   C-spine

External pelvic fixator

Ext fixator PRN

Pelvic A-gram PRN

Pelvic A-gram PRN

Chest CT

Chest CT
C-spine/head CT

Chest CT
ABD/pelvic CT

Chest CT

Ext films PRN

Ext films PRN

C-spine/head CT

C-spine/head CT

ICU

ICU

Ext films PRN

Ext films PRN

ICU

ICU

Note: AP = anteroposterior; Ext = extremity; OGT = orogastric tube; FAST = Focused Assessment Sonogram for Trauma; lat = lateral; C = cervical.

What finding on ABD/pelvic CT scan requires ex lap in the blunt trauma patient with normal vital signs?

Free air; also strongly consider in the patient with no solid organ injury but lots of free fluid = both to rule out hollow viscus injury

Can you rely on a negative FAST in the unstable patient with a pelvic fracture?

No—perform DPL (above umbilicus)

Which lab tests are used to look for intra-abdominal injury in children?

LFTs = ↑ AST/ALT

What is the treatment for human and dog bites?

Leave wound open, irrigation, antibiotics

What percentage of pelvic fracture bleeding is exclusively venous?

85%

What is sympathetic ophthalmia?

Blindness in one eye that results in subsequent blindness in the contralateral eye (autoimmune)

What can present after blunt trauma with neurologic deficits and a normal brain CT scan?

Diffuse **A**xonal **I**njury (**DAI**), carotid artery injury

What is the usual presentation of an anterior hip dislocation?

Externally rotated with anterior hip fullness (Think: **A** for **Anterior**)

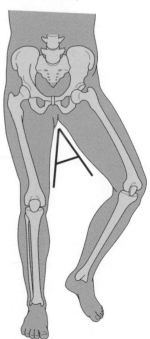

What is characteristic regarding the appearance of a brown recluse spider?

Brown with a "violin" shape on the thorax

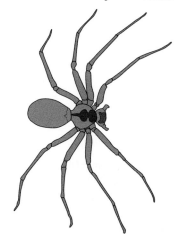

What does a brown recluse spider bite look and feel like?

Painful area of redness and blisters occasionally progressing to necrotic tissue

What drug is used to treat a brown recluse spider bite?

Dapsone

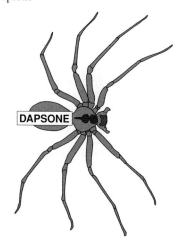

What do black widow spiders look like?

Black color with a red "hourglass" on their abdomens

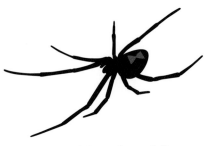

What are the symptoms of a black widow spider bite?

Muscle cramps, abdominal pain, chills, nausea, vomiting, weakness, sweating

How do you treat severe black widow spider bites?

Muscle relaxants and ANTIVENOM

RAPID-FIRE REVIEW

What is the correct diagnosis?

Coiled NGT in the left pleural cavity after blunt trauma	Diaphragm rupture
Blunt trauma patient with GCS <8 and otorrhea	Basilar fracture
20-year-old male s/p baseball bat to his head, arrives in a coma; CT scan reveals a lens shaped (lenticular) hematoma next to inner table of skull	Epidural hematoma
44-year-old male s/p fall from a ladder presents with GCS of 5; CT scan reveals a crescent-shaped hematoma next to inner table of the skull	Subdural hematoma
Trauma patient with increasing JVD with inspiration	Cardiac tamponade (Kussmaul's sign)
Trauma patient with hypertension and bradycardia	Cushing's response to increased ICP
Trauma patient with hypotension and bradycardia	Spinal cord injury

Name the most likely diagnosis:

28-year-old female involved in a high-speed, side-impact motor vehicle collision (MVC); stable vital signs; CXR reveals widened mediastinum

Thoracic aortic injury

21-year-old male involved in high-speed MVC with obvious unstable pelvis, gross blood from the urethral meatus, high-riding prostate on rectal exam

Urethral injury

45-year-old female involved in high-speed MVC complains of abdominal pain and shortness of breath; decreased breath sounds on the left; CXR reveals the NGT coiled up in the left chest

Ruptured left diaphragm

56-year-old involved in a high-speed motorcycle collision complains of severe shortness of breath; on exam, the left chest wall moves inwards not outwards on inhalation

Flail chest—"paradoxic respirations"

67-year-old involved in a high-speed MVC presents with a GCS of 5, bilateral periorbital ecchymosis, left mastoid ecchymosis, and clear fluid draining form the left ear

Basilar skull fracture—Battle's and raccoon signs

50-year-old female s/p high speed MVC with rib fractures and flail chest develops hypoxia 12 hours later in the ICU; CXR shows no pneumo- or hemothorax but reveals pulmonary infiltrates/congestion

Pulmonary contusion

29-year-old s/p a MVC arrives with hypotension, sats of 83%, JVD, decreased breath sounds on left

Tension pneumothorax

55-year-old male s/p 3-story fall reveals the NGT coiled up in chest on CXR

Diaphragm injury

22-year-old male s/p MVC with transection of right optic nerve; progresses to blindness in the contralateral left eye 3 weeks later	Sympathetic ophthalmia
8-year-old male s/p bicycle accident with handlebar to abdomen with duodenal hematoma	NGT, TPN, and observe; may take weeks to open up
30-year-old male involved in a skiing collision with a tree, arrives in the ER awake (GCS of 15) but then gets confused and next goes unresponsive (GCS of 3)	"Lucid interval" of an epidural hematoma

Name the diagnostic modality:

47-year-old female s/p MVC with a seatbelt sign (ecchymosis) on the left neck	CTA of cervical vessels
22-year-old male s/p gunshot wound to umbilicus; bullet is in the spine on x-rays	Exploratory laparotomy
27-year-old female with normal vital signs and stab to right flank	CT scan with triple contrast (rectal, PO, IV)

Chapter 38 | Burns

Define:

TBSA	Total Body Surface Area
STSG	Split-Thickness Skin Graft
Are acid or alkali chemical burns more serious?	In general, **ALKALI** burns are more serious because the body cannot buffer the alkali, thus allowing them to burn for much longer
How is myoglobinuria treated?	To avoid renal injury, think **"HAM"**: **H**ydration with IV fluids **A**lkalization of urine with IV bicarbonate **M**annitol diuresis

Define level of burn injury:

Superficial (previously known as first-degree) burns	Epidermis only
Partial-thickness (previously known as second-degree) burns	Epidermis and varying levels of dermis

Full-thickness (previously known as third-degree) burns	All layers of the skin including the entire dermis
How do superficial burns present?	Painful, dry, red areas that do not form blisters (think of sunburn)
How do partial-thickness burns present?	Painful, hypersensitive, swollen, mottled areas with **blisters** and open weeping surfaces
How do full-thickness burns present?	Painless, insensate, swollen, dry, mottled white, and charred areas; often described as dried leather
What is the major clinical difference between partial- and full-thickness burns?	Full-thickness burns are painless, and partial-thickness burns are painful
By which measure is burn severity determined?	Depth of burn and TBSA affected by partial- and full-thickness burns TBSA is calculated by the "rule of nines" in adults and by a modified rule in children to account for the disproportionate size of the head and trunk
What is the "rule of nines"?	In an adult, the total body surface area that is burned can be estimated by the following: Each upper limb = 9% Each lower limb = 18% Anterior and posterior trunk = 18% each Head and neck = 9% Perineum and genitalia = 1%

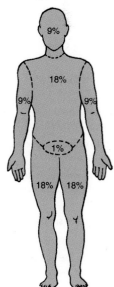

What is the "rule of the palm"?

Surface area of the patient's palm is ≈1% of the TBSA used for estimating size of small burns

What is the burn center referral criteria for the following?

   Partial-thickness burns

>20% TBSA

   Full-thickness burns

>5% TBSA

Partial thickness >10% TBSA in children and the elderly

Any burns involving the face, hands, feet, or perineum

Any burns with inhalation injury

Any burns with associated trauma

Any electrical burns

What is the treatment of superficial burns?

Keep clean, ± Neosporin®, pain meds

What is the treatment of partial-thickness burns?

Remove blisters; apply antibiotic ointment (usually Silvadene®) and dressing; pain meds; some use silver bandages

Most partial-thickness burns do not require skin grafting (epidermis grows from hair follicles and from margins)

What is the treatment of full-thickness burns?

Early excision of eschar (within first week postburn) and STSG

How can you decrease bleeding during excision?

Tourniquets as possible, topical epinephrine, topical thrombin

What is an autograft STSG?

STSG from the patient's own skin

What is an allograft STSG?

STSG from a deceased donor (temporary coverage)

What thickness is the STSG?

10/1,000 to 15/1,000 of an inch (down to the dermal layer)

What prophylaxis should the burn patient get in the ER?

Tetanus

What is used to evaluate the eyes after a full-thickness burn?

Fluorescein

What principles guide the initial assessment and resuscitation of the burn patient?

ABCDEs, then urine output; check for eschar and compartment syndromes

What are the signs of smoke inhalation?

Smoke and soot in sputum/mouth/nose, nasal/facial hair burns, throat/mouth erythema, history of loss of consciousness/explosion/fire in small enclosed area, dyspnea, low O_2 saturation, confusion, headache, coma

What diagnostic imaging is used for smoke inhalation?	Bronchoscopy
What lab value assesses smoke inhalation?	**Carboxyhemoglobin** level (carboxyhemoglobin level >60% is associated with a 50% mortality); treat with 100% O_2 and time
How should the airway be managed in the burn patient with an inhalational injury?	With a low threshold for **intubation;** oropharyngeal swelling may occlude the airway so that intubation is impossible; 100% oxygen should be administered immediately and continued until significant carboxyhemoglobin is ruled out
What is "burn shock"?	**Burn shock** describes the loss of fluid from the intravascular space as a result of burn injury, which causes "leaking capillaries" that require crystalloid infusion
What is the "Parkland formula"?	V = TBSA Burn (%) × Weight (kg) × 4 Formula widely used to estimate the volume (V) of crystalloid necessary for the initial resuscitation of the burn patient; half of the calculated volume is given in the **first 8 hours**, the rest in the next 16 hours
What burns qualify for the Parkland formula?	≥20% TBSA partial- and full-thickness burns only
What is the Brooke formula for burn resuscitation?	Replace 2 cc for the 4 cc in the Parkland formula
What is the rule of 10s?	For determining hourly IVF rate: TBSA × 10 (patients 40–80 kg)
How is the crystalloid given?	Through two large-bore peripheral venous catheters
Can you place an IV or central line through burned skin?	YES
What is the adult urine output goal?	30 to 50 cc (titrate IVF)
Why is glucose-containing IVF contraindicated in burn patients in the first 24 hours post burn?	Patient's serum glucose will be elevated on its own because of the stress response
What fluid is used after the first 24 hours post burn?	Colloid; use D5W **and** 5% albumin at 0.5 cc/kg/% burn surface area
Why should D5W IV be administered after 24 hours post burn?	Because of the massive sodium load in the first 24 hours of LR infusion and because of the massive evaporation of H_2O from the burn injury, the patient will need free water; after 24 hours, the capillaries begin to work and then the patient can usually benefit from **albumin** and D5W

What is the minimal urine output for burn patients?

Adults 30 cc; children 1 to 2 cc/kg/hr

What is most important for volume status monitoring in the burn patient?

Urine output

Why do most severely burned patients require nasogastric decompression?

Patients with >20% TBSA burns usually develop a paralytic ileus → vomiting → aspiration risk → pneumonia

What stress prophylaxis must be given to the burn patient?

PPI to prevent burn stress ulcer (Curling's ulcer)

What are the signs of burn wound infection?

Increased WBC with left shift, **discoloration of burn eschar** (most common sign), green pigment, necrotic skin lesion in unburned skin, edema, ecchymosis tissue below eschar, partial-thickness burns that turn into full-thickness burns, hypotension

Is fever a good sign of infection in burn patients?

NO

What are the common organisms found in burn wound infections?

Staphylococcus aureus, Pseudomonas, Streptococcus, Candida albicans

How is a burn wound infection diagnosed?

Send burned tissue in question to the laboratory for quantitative burn wound bacterial count; if the count is >105/g, infection is present and IV antibiotics should be administered

Why are systemic IV antibiotics contraindicated in fresh burns?

Bacteria live in the eschar, which is avascular (the systemic antibiotic will not be delivered to the eschar); thus, apply topical antimicrobial agents

Note some advantages and disadvantages of the following topical antibiotic agents:

Silver sulfadiazine (Silvadene®)

Painless, but little eschar penetration, misses *Pseudomonas,* and has idiosyncratic **neutropenia;** sulfa allergy is a contraindication

Mafenide acetate (Sulfamylon®)

Penetrates eschars, broad spectrum (but misses *Staphylococcus*), causes pain on application; triggers allergic reaction in 7% of patients; may cause **acid–base imbalances** (Think: **M**afenide **AC**etate = **M**etabolic **AC**idosis); agent of choice for ear burns

Polysporin®	Polymyxin B sulfate; painless, clear, used for facial burns; does not have a wide antimicrobial spectrum
Are prophylactic systemic antibiotics administered to burn patients?	No—prophylactic antibiotics have not been shown to reduce the incidence of sepsis, but rather have been shown to select for resistant organisms; IV antibiotics are reserved for established wound infections, pneumonia, urinary tract infections, etc.
Circumferential, full-thickness burns to the extremities are at risk for what complication?	Distal neurovascular impairment
How is it treated?	Escharotomy: full-thickness longitudinal incision through the eschar with scalpel or electrocautery
Is tetanus prophylaxis required in the burn patient?	Yes, it is mandatory in all patients except those actively immunized within the past 12 months (with incomplete immunization: toxoid × 3)
Can infection convert a partial-thickness injury into a full-thickness injury?	Yes!
How is carbon monoxide inhalation overdose treated?	100% O_2 (± hyperbaric O_2)
Which electrolyte must be closely followed acutely after a burn?	Na^+ (sodium)
What is the name of the gastric/duodenal ulcer associated with burn injury?	Curling's ulcer (Think: **CURLING** iron burn = **CURLING**'s burn ulcer)
How are STSGs nourished in the first 24 hours?	IMBIBITION (fed from wound bed exudate)

RAPID-FIRE REVIEW

What is the treatment?	
30-year-old female involved in a house fire with circumferential burns to both upper extremities with no palpable distal pulses	Escharotomies (cut burn scar releasing tourniquet effect)
55-year-old female s/p house fire with elevated carboxyhemoglobin	100% oxygen

Chapter 39 | Upper GI Bleeding

What is it?	Bleeding into the lumen of the proximal GI tract, proximal to the ligament of Treitz
What are the signs/symptoms?	Hematemesis, melena, syncope, shock, fatigue, coffee-ground emesis, hematochezia, epigastric discomfort, epigastric tenderness, signs of hypovolemia, guaiac-positive stools
Why is it possible to have hematochezia?	Blood is a cathartic, and hematochezia usually indicates a vigorous rate of bleeding from the UGI source
Are stools melenic or melanotic?	Melenic (melanotic is incorrect)
What is the most common cause of significant UGI bleeding?	PUD—duodenal and gastric ulcers (50%)
What is the *common* differential diagnosis of UGI bleeding?	1. Acute gastritis 2. Duodenal ulcer 3. Esophageal varices 4. Gastric ulcer 5. Esophageal 6. Mallory–Weiss tear
What is the diagnostic test of choice with UGI bleeding?	EGD (>95% diagnosis rate)
What are the treatment options with the endoscope during an EGD?	Coagulation, injection of epinephrine (for vasoconstriction), injection of sclerosing agents (varices), variceal ligation (banding)
Which lab tests should be performed?	Chem-7, bilirubin, LFTs, CBC, **type and cross**, PT/PTT, amylase
Why is BUN elevated?	Because of absorption of blood by the GI tract
What is the initial treatment?	1. **IVFs** (16 G or larger peripheral IVS × 2), **Foley** catheter (monitor fluid status) 2. **NGT** suction (determine rate and amount of blood) 3. Water lavage (use warm H_2O—will remove clots) 4. **EGD:** endoscopy (determine etiology/location of bleeding and possible treatment—coagulate bleeders)
Why irrigate in an upper GI (UGI) bleed?	To remove the blood clot so you can see the mucosa

What test may help identify the site of MASSIVE UGI bleeding when EGD fails to diagnose cause and blood continues per NGT?	Selective mesenteric angiography
What are the indications for surgical intervention in UGI bleeding?	Refractory or recurrent bleeding and site known, >3 unit PRBCs to stabilize or >6 unit PRBCs overall
What percentage of patients requires surgery?	≈10%
What percentage of patients spontaneously stops bleeding?	≈80% to 85%
What is the mortality of acute UGI bleeding?	Overall 10%, age 60 to 80 years 15%, age >80 years 25%
What are the risk factors for death following UGI bleed?	Age >60 years Shock >5 units of PRBC transfusion Concomitant health problems

PEPTIC ULCER DISEASE (PUD)

What is it?	Gastric and duodenal ulcers
What is the incidence in the United States?	≈10% of the population will suffer from PUD during their lifetime!
What are the possible consequences of PUD?	Pain, hemorrhage, perforation, obstruction
What percentage of patients with PUD develops bleeding from the ulcer?	≈20%
Which bacteria are associated with PUD?	*Helicobacter pylori*
What is the treatment for *H. pylori*?	1. Clarithromycin, amoxicillin, proton-pump inhibitor (PPI), ± bismuth or 2. Bismuth, metronidazole, tetracycline, PPI
What is the name of the sign with RLQ pain/peritonitis as a result of succus collecting from a perforated peptic ulcer?	Valentino's sign

DUODENAL ULCERS

In which age group are these ulcers most common?	40 to 65 years of age (younger than patients with gastric ulcer)
What is the ratio of male-to-female patients?	Men > women (3:1)
What is the most common location?	Most are within 2 cm of the pylorus in the duodenal bulb
What is the classic pain response to food intake?	Food classically relieves duodenal ulcer pain (Think: **D**uodenum = **D**ecreased with food)
What is the cause?	Increased production of gastric acid
What syndrome must you always think of with a duodenal ulcer?	Zollinger–Ellison syndrome (ZES)
What are the major symptoms?	Epigastric pain Bleeding
What are the signs?	Tenderness in epigastric area (possibly), guaiac-positive stool, melena, hematochezia, hematemesis
What is the differential diagnosis?	Acute abdomen, pancreatitis, cholecystitis, **all causes of UGI bleeding**, ZES, gastritis, MI, gastric ulcer, reflux
How is the diagnosis made?	History, PE, EGD, UGI series (if patient is not actively bleeding)
When is surgery indicated with a bleeding duodenal ulcer?	Most surgeons use: >6 unit PRBC transfusions, >3 unit PRBCs needed to stabilize, or for significant rebleed
What is the medical treatment?	PPIs or H_2 receptor antagonists—heals ulcers in 4 to 6 weeks in most cases Treatment for *H. pylori*
When is surgery indicated?	The acronym **"I HOP":** **I**ntractability **H**emorrhage (massive or relentless) **O**bstruction (gastric outlet obstruction) **P**erforation
How is a bleeding duodenal ulcer surgically corrected?	Opening of the duodenum through the pylorus Oversewing of the bleeding vessel
What artery is involved with bleeding duodenal ulcers?	Gastroduodenal artery

What are the common surgical options for the following conditions:

Truncal vagotomy	Pyloroplasty
Duodenal perforation	Graham patch (most common) Truncal vagotomy and pyloroplasty incorporating ulcer Graham patch and highly selective vagotomy Truncal vagotomy and antrectomy (higher mortality rate, but lowest recurrence rate)
Duodenal ulcer intractability	PGV (highly selective vagotomy) Vagotomy and pyloroplasty

GASTRIC ULCERS

In which age group are these ulcers most common?	40 to 70 years old (older than the duodenal ulcer population) Rare in patients age <40 years
How does the incidence in men compare with that of women?	Men > women
Which is more common overall: gastric or duodenal ulcers?	Duodenal ulcers are more than twice as common as gastric ulcers (Think: **D**uodenal = **D**ouble rate)
What is the classic pain response to food?	Food classically increases gastric ulcer pain
What is the cause?	**Decreased cytoprotection** or gastric protection (i.e., decreased bicarbonate/mucous production)
Is gastric acid production high or low?	Gastric acid production is normal or low!
What are the associated risk factors?	Smoking, alcohol, burns, trauma, CNS tumor/trauma, NSAIDs, steroids, shock, severe illness, male gender, advanced age
What are the symptoms?	Epigastric pain ± Vomiting, anorexia, and nausea
How is the diagnosis made?	History, PE, EGD with multiple biopsies (looking for gastric cancer)
What is the most common location?	≈70% are on the lesser curvature; 5% are on the greater curvature

When and why should biopsy be performed?	With all gastric ulcers, to rule out gastric cancer If the ulcer does not heal in 6 weeks after medical treatment, **rebiopsy** (always biopsy in O.R. also) must be performed
What is the medical treatment?	Similar to that of duodenal ulcer—PPIs or H_2 blockers, *H. pylori* treatment
When do patients with gastric ulcers need to have an EGD?	1. For diagnosis with biopsies 2. 6 weeks post diagnosis to confirm healing and rule out gastric cancer!
What are the indications for surgery?	The acronym **"I CHOP"**: **I**ntractability **C**ancer (rule out) **H**emorrhage (massive or relentless) **O**bstruction (gastric outlet obstruction) **P**erforation (*Note:* Surgery is indicated if gastric cancer cannot be ruled out)
What is the common operation for hemorrhage, obstruction, and a mass with perforation?	Distal gastrectomy with excision of the ulcer **without** vagotomy unless there is duodenal disease (i.e., BI or BII)
What is a common option for a perforated gastric ulcer?	Graham patch
What must be performed in every operation for gastric ulcers?	Biopsy looking for gastric cancer

PERFORATED PEPTIC ULCER

What are the symptoms?	**Acute** onset of upper abdominal pain
What is the differential diagnosis?	Acute pancreatitis, acute cholecystitis, perforated acute appendicitis, colonic diverticulitis, MI, any perforated viscus
Which diagnostic tests are indicated?	X-ray: free air under diaphragm or in lesser sac in an upright CXR
What is the initial treatment?	NPO: NGT (↓ contamination of the peritoneal cavity) IVF/Foley catheter Antibiotics/PPIs Surgery
What is a Graham patch?	Piece of omentum incorporated into the suture closure of perforation
What type of perforated ulcer may present just like acute pancreatitis?	Posterior perforated duodenal ulcer into the pancreas (i.e., epigastric pain radiating to the back; high serum amylase)

What is the classic difference between duodenal and gastric ulcer symptoms as related to food ingestion?	Duodenal = decreased pain Gastric = increased pain (Think: **D**uodenal = **D**ecreased pain)

TYPES OF SURGERIES

Define the following terms:

Graham patch	Place viable omentum over perforation and tack into place with sutures

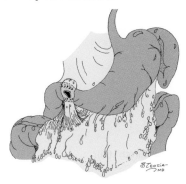

Truncal vagotomy	Resection of a 1- to 2-cm segment of each vagal **trunk** as it enters the abdomen on the distal esophagus, decreasing gastric acid secretion
What other procedure must be performed along with a truncal vagotomy?	"Drainage procedure" (pyloroplasty, antrectomy, or gastrojejunostomy), because vagal fibers provide relaxation of the pylorus, and, if you cut them, the pylorus will not open

Define the following terms:

Vagotomy and pyloroplasty	Pyloroplasty performed with vagotomy to compensate for decreased gastric emptying

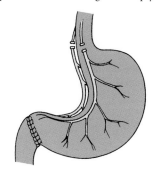

Vagotomy and antrectomy

Remove antrum and pylorus in addition to vagotomy; reconstruct as a Billroth I or II

What is the advantage of proximal gastric vagotomy (highly selective vagotomy)?

No drainage procedure is needed; vagal fibers to the pylorus are preserved; rate of dumping syndrome is low

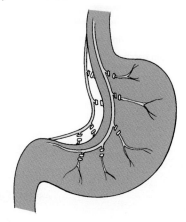

What is a Billroth I (BI)?

Truncal vagotomy, antrectomy, and gastroduodenostomy (Think: B**I** = **ONE** limb off of the stomach remnant)

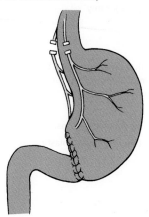

What are the contraindications for a Billroth I?

Gastric cancer or suspicion of gastric cancer

What is a Billroth II (BII)?	Truncal vagotomy, antrectomy, and gastrojejunostomy (Think: B**II** = **TWO** limbs off of the stomach remnant)

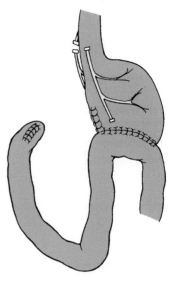

STRESS GASTRITIS

What is it?	**Superficial** mucosal erosions in the stressed patient
What are the risk factors?	Sepsis, intubation, trauma, shock, burn, brain injury
What is the prophylactic treatment?	H_2 blockers, PPIs, antacids, sucralfate
What are the signs/symptoms?	NGT blood (usually), painless (usually)
How is it diagnosed?	EGD, if bleeding is significant
What is the treatment for gastritis?	LAVAGE out blood clots, give a maximum dose of PPI in a 24-hour IV drip

MALLORY–WEISS SYNDROME

What is it?	Postretching, postemesis longitudinal tear (submucosa and mucosa) of the stomach near the GE junction; approximately three fourths are in the stomach

For what percentage of all UGI bleeds does this syndrome account?	≈10%
What are the causes of a tear?	Increased gastric pressure, often aggravated by hiatal hernia
What are the risk factors?	Retching, alcoholism (50%), >50% of patients have hiatal hernia
What are the symptoms?	Epigastric pain, thoracic substernal pain, emesis, hematemesis
What percentage of patients will have hematemesis?	85%
How is the diagnosis made?	EGD
What is the "classic" history?	Alcoholic patient after binge drinking—first, vomit food and gastric contents, followed by forceful retching and bloody vomitus
What is the treatment?	Room temperature water lavage (90% of patients stop bleeding), electrocautery, arterial embolization, or surgery for refractory bleeding
When is surgery indicated?	When medical/endoscopic treatment fails

ESOPHAGEAL VARICEAL BLEEDING

What is it?	Bleeding from formation of esophageal varices from backup of portal pressure via the coronary vein to the submucosal esophageal venous plexuses secondary to portal hypertension from liver cirrhosis
What is the "rule of two thirds" of esophageal variceal hemorrhage?	Two thirds of patients with portal hypertension develop esophageal varices Two thirds of patients with esophageal varices bleed
What are the signs/symptoms?	Liver disease, portal hypertension, hematemesis, caput medusa, ascites
How is the diagnosis made?	EGD (very important because only 50% of UGI bleeding in patients with known esophageal varices are bleeding from the varices; the other 50% have bleeding from ulcers, etc.)
What is the acute medical treatment?	Lower portal pressure with octreotide or vasopressin
What are the treatment options?	Sclerotherapy or band ligation via endoscope, TIPS, liver transplant

What is the problem with shunts?	Decreased portal pressure, but increased encephalopathy

BOERHAAVE'S SYNDROME

What is it?	Postemetic esophageal rupture
Who was Dr. Boerhaave?	Dutch physician who first described the syndrome in the Dutch Grand Admiral Van Wassenaer in 1724
Why is the esophagus susceptible to perforation and more likely to break down an anastomosis?	No serosa
What is the most common location?	Posterolateral aspect of the esophagus to the left, 3 to 5 cm above the GE junction
What is the cause of rupture?	Increased intraluminal pressure, usually caused by violent retching and vomiting
What is the associated risk factor?	Esophageal reflux disease (50%)
What are the symptoms?	Pain postemesis (may radiate to the back, dysphagia) (Think Boerhaave's = Boer HEAVES)
What are the signs?	Left pneumothorax, Hamman's sign, left pleural effusion, subcutaneous/mediastinal emphysema, fever, tachypnea, tachycardia, signs of infection by 24 hours, neck crepitus, widened mediastinum on CXR
What is Mackler's triad?	1. Emesis 2. Lower chest pain 3. Cervical emphysema (subQ air)
What is Hamman's sign?	"Mediastinal crunch or clicking" produced by the heart beating against air-filled tissues
How is the diagnosis made?	History, physical examination, CXR, esophagram with water-soluble contrast
What is the treatment?	Surgery within 24 hours to drain the mediastinum and surgically close the perforation and placement of pleural patch; broad-spectrum antibiotics
What is the mortality rate if >24 hours until surgery for perforated esophagus?	≈33%
Overall, what is the most common cause of esophageal perforation?	Iatrogenic (most commonly cervical esophagus)

RAPID-FIRE REVIEW

Name the diagnostic modality:

45-year-old male with dark blood per rectum, NGT returns clear fluid and no bile	EGD to rule out UGI source

Chapter 40 | Stomach

GASTRIC PHYSIOLOGY

Define the products of the following stomach cells:

Gastric parietal cells	HCl Intrinsic factor
Chief cells	**PEP**sinogen (Think: "a **PEP**py chief")
Mucous neck cells	Bicarbonate Mucus
G cells	Gastrin (Think: **G** cells = **G**astrin)
Where are G cells located?	Antrum
What is pepsin?	Proteolytic enzyme that hydrolyzes peptide bonds
What is intrinsic factor?	Protein secreted by the parietal cells that combines with vitamin B12 and allows for absorption in the terminal ileum

GASTROESOPHAGEAL REFLUX DISEASE (GERD)

What is it?	Excessive reflux of gastric contents into the esophagus, "heartburn"
What are the causes?	Decreased lower esophageal sphincter (LES) tone (>50% of cases) Decreased esophageal motility to clear refluxed fluid Gastric outlet obstruction Hiatal hernia in ≈50% of patients

What are the signs/symptoms?	Heartburn, regurgitation, respiratory problems/pneumonia from aspiration of refluxed gastric contents; substernal pain
What tests are included in the workup?	EGD UGI contrast study with esophagogram 24-hour acid analysis (pH probe in esophagus) Manometry, EKG, CXR
What is the medical treatment?	Small meals PPIs (proton-pump inhibitors) or H_2 blockers Elevation of head at night and no meals prior to sleeping
What are the indications for surgery?	Intractability (failure of medical treatment) Respiratory problems as a result of reflux and aspiration of gastric contents (e.g., pneumonia) Severe esophageal injury (e.g., ulcers, hemorrhage, stricture, ± Barrett's esophagus)
What is Barrett's esophagus?	Columnar metaplasia from the normal squamous epithelium as a result of chronic irritation from reflux
What is the major concern with Barrett's esophagus?	Developing cancer
What type of cancer develops in Barrett's esophagus?	Adenocarcinoma
What percentage of patients with GERD develops Barrett's esophagus?	10%
What percentage of patients with Barrett's esophagus will develop adenocarcinoma?	7% lifetime (5%–10%)
What is the treatment of Barrett's esophagus with dysplasia?	Nonsurgical: endoscopic mucosal resection and photodynamic therapy; other options include radiofrequency ablation, cryoablation (these methods are also often used for mucosal adenocarcinoma)

Define the following surgical options for severe GERD:

Laparoscopic Nissen fundoplication

360° fundoplication—2 cm long (laparoscopically)

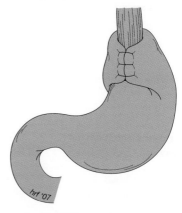

Toupet

Incomplete (≈200°) posterior wrap (laparoscopic) often used with severe decreased esophageal motility

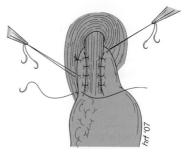

How does the Nissen wrap work?

Thought to work by improving the LES:
1. Increasing LES tone
2. Elongating LES ≈3 cm
3. Returning LES into abdominal cavity

In what percentage of patients does lap Nissen work?

85% (70%–95%)

What are the postoperative complications of lap Nissen?

1. Gas bloat syndrome
2. Stricture
3. Dysphagia
4. Spleen injury requiring splenectomy
5. Esophageal perforation
6. Pneumothorax

What is gas bloat syndrome?

Inability to burp or vomit

GASTRIC CANCER

What are the associated risk factors?	Diet—smoked meats, high nitrates, low fruits and vegetables, alcohol, tobacco Environment—raised in high-risk area, poor socioeconomic status, atrophic gastritis, male gender, blood type A, previous partial gastrectomy, pernicious anemia, polyps, *Helicobacter pylori*
Which blood type is associated with gastric cancer?	Blood type A (Think: there is an "**A**" in gastric but no "O" or "B" = g**A**stric = type "**A**")
What are the symptoms?	The acronym **"WEAPON"**: **W**eight loss **E**mesis **A**norexia **P**ain/epigastric discomfort **O**bstruction **N**ausea
What is a Blumer's shelf?	Solid peritoneal deposit anterior to the rectum, forming a "shelf," palpated on **rectal examination**
What is a Virchow's node?	Metastatic gastric cancer to the nodes in the left supraclavicular fossa
What is a surveillance laboratory finding?	CEA elevated in 30% of cases (if +, useful for postoperative surveillance)
What is the initial workup?	EGD with biopsy, endoscopic U/S to evaluate the level of invasion, CT scan of abdomen/pelvis for metastasis, CXR, labs
What is the histology?	Adenocarcinoma
What is the differential diagnosis for gastric tumors?	Adenocarcinoma, leiomyoma, leiomyosarcoma, lymphoma, carcinoid, ectopic pancreatic tissue, gastrinoma, benign gastric ulcer, polyp
Which morphologic type is named after a "leather bottle"?	Linitis plastica—the entire stomach is involved and looks thickened (10% of cancers)
Which patients with gastric cancer are NONoperative?	1. Distant metastasis (e.g., liver metastasis) 2. Peritoneal implants
What is the role of laparoscopy?	To rule out peritoneal implants and to evaluate for liver metastasis
What is the genetic alteration seen in >50% of patients with gastric cancer?	P53

How can you remember P53 for gastric cancer?	**G**astric **C**ancer = **GC** = P53; or, think: "GCP...53"—it sings!
What is the treatment?	Surgical resection with wide (>5 cm checked by frozen section) margins and lymph node dissection
What operation is performed for tumor in the:	
Antrum	Distal subtotal gastrectomy
Midbody	Total gastrectomy
Proximal	Total gastrectomy
What is a subtotal gastrectomy?	Subtotal gastrectomy = 75% of stomach removed

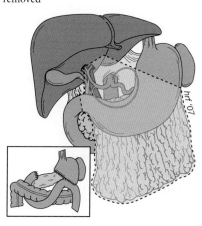

What is a total gastrectomy?	Stomach is removed and a Roux-en-Y limb is sewn to the esophagus

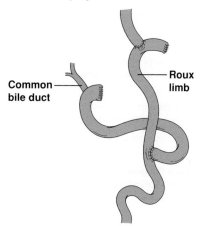

| When should splenectomy be performed? | When the tumor directly invades the spleen/splenic hilum or with splenic hilar adenopathy |
| What is the adjuvant treatment? | Stages II and III: postoperative chemotherapy and radiation |

GIST

What is it?	GastroIntestinal Stromal Tumor
What was it previously known as?	Leiomyosarcoma
What is the cell of origin?	CAJAL, interstitial cells of Cajal
Where is it found?	GI tract—"esophagus to rectum"—most commonly found in **stomach** (60%), small bowel (30%), duodenum (5%), rectum (3%), colon (2%), esophagus (1%)
What are the symptoms?	GI bleed, occult GI bleed, abdominal pain, abdominal mass, nausea, distention
How is it diagnosed?	CT scan, EGD, colonoscopy
How are distant metastases diagnosed?	PET scan
What is the tumor marker?	C-KIT (CD117 antigen)
What is the prognosis?	Local spread, distant metastases Poor long-term prognosis: size >5 cm, mitotic rate >5 per 50 hpf (high-power field)
What is the treatment?	Resect with negative margins, ± chemotherapy
Is there a need for lymph node dissection?	NO
What is the chemotherapy for metastatic or advanced disease?	Imatinib—tyrosine kinase inhibitor

MALTOMA

What is it?	Mucosal-Associated Lymphoproliferative Tissue
What is the most common site?	Stomach (70%)
What is the causative agent?	*H. pylori*
What is the medical treatment?	Nonsurgical—treat for *H. pylori* with triple therapy and chemotherapy/XRT in refractory cases

GASTRIC VOLVULUS

What is it?	Twisting of the stomach
What are the symptoms?	Borchardt's triad: 1. Distention of epigastrium 2. Cannot pass an NGT 3. Emesis followed by inability to vomit
What is the treatment?	Exploratory laparotomy to untwist, and gastropexy

RAPID-FIRE REVIEW

Name the most likely diagnosis:

54-year-old female with reflux disease and columnar epithelium on distal esophageal biopsy	Barrett's esophagus

Chapter 41 | Bariatric Surgery

What is it?	Weight reduction surgery for the morbidly obese
Define morbid obesity:	1. BMI >40 (basically, >100 lb above ideal body weight) or 2. BMI >35 with a medical problem related to morbid obesity
What is BMI?	Body Mass Index
What medical conditions are associated with morbid obesity?	Sleep apnea, coronary artery disease, pulmonary disease, diabetes mellitus, venous stasis ulcers, arthritis, infections, sex-hormone abnormalities, hypertension, breast cancer, colon cancer
What are the current best options for surgery?	1. Sleeve gastrectomy 2. Gastric bypass (malabsorptive) 3. Vertical-banded gastroplasty

Define sleeve gastrectomy:

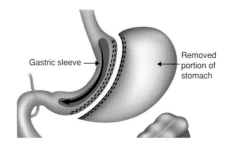

Gastric sleeve

Removed portion of stomach

Define gastric bypass:

Stapling off of small gastric pouch (restrictive)

Roux-en-Y limb to gastric pouch (bypass)

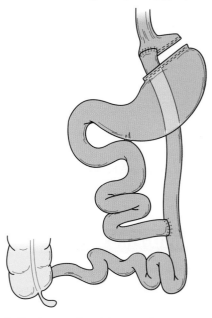

How does gastric bypass work?

1. Creates a small gastric reservoir
2. Causes dumping symptoms when a patient eats too much food or high-calorie foods; the food is "dumped" into the Roux-en-Y limb
3. Bypass of small bowel by Roux-en-Y limb

What is the most common sign of an anastomotic leak after a gastric bypass?

Tachycardia

What is a LAP-BAND®?

Laparoscopically placed **band** around stomach with a subcutaneous port to adjust constriction; results in smaller gastric reservoir

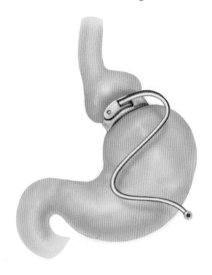

What is a Petersen's hernia?

Seen after bariatric gastric bypass—internal herniation of small bowel through the mesenteric defect from the Roux-en-Y limb

RAPID-FIRE REVIEW

Name the most likely diagnosis:

34-year-old female POD #2 gastric bypass with tachycardia and vague abdominal discomfort

Anastomotic leak

What is the correct diagnosis?

POD #2 s/p open gastric bypass for morbid obesity, patient becomes tachypneic and short of breath; sats = 86%, ABG $PO_2 = 52$, $CO_2 = 30$, EKG normal, chest x-ray normal

Pulmonary embolus

Chapter 42 | Ostomies

Define the following terms:

Ostomy	Operation that connects the GI tract to abdominal wall skin or the lumen of another hollow organ; a man-made fistula
Stoma	Opening of the ostomy (Greek *mouth*)
Gastrostomy	G-tube through the abdominal wall to the stomach for drainage or feeding
Jejunostomy	J-tube through the abdominal wall to the jejunum for feeding
Colostomy	Connection of colon mucosa to the abdominal wall skin for stool drainage
End colostomy	Proximal end of colon brought to the skin for stool drainage
Mucous fistula	Distal end of transected colon brought to the skin for decompression; the mucosa produces mucus, an ostomy is a fistula, and, hence, the term **mucous fistula** (proximal colon brought up as a colostomy or, if the proximal colon is removed, an ileostomy)
Hartmann's pouch	Distal end of transected colon stapled and dropped back into the peritoneal cavity, resulting in a blind pouch; mucus is decompressed through the anus (proximal colon is brought up as an end colostomy or, if proximal colon is removed, an end ileostomy)
Double-barrel colostomy	End colostomy and a mucous fistula (i.e., two barrels brought up to the skin)

Loop colostomy

Loop of large bowel is brought up to the abdominal wall skin and a plastic rod is placed underneath the loop; the colon is then opened and sewn to the abdominal wall skin as a colostomy

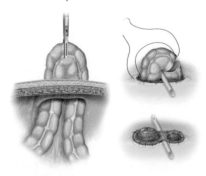

Brooke ileostomy

Ileostomy folded over itself to provide clearance from skin

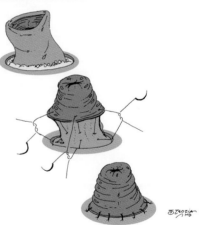

Why doesn't an ileostomy or colostomy close?

Epithelialization (mucosa to skin) from the acronym **F**RIEND

Why doesn't a gastrostomy close?

Foreign body (the plastic tube) from the acronym **F**RIEND

If the plastic tube, G-tube, or J-tube is removed, how fast can the hole to the stomach or jejunum close?

In a matter of hours! (Therefore, if it comes out inadvertently from a well-established tract, it must be replaced immediately)

What is a "tube check"?	Gastrografin contrast study to confirm that a G-tube or J-tube is within the lumen of the stomach or jejunum, respectively

RAPID-FIRE REVIEW

Name the most likely diagnosis:

S/P gastrojejunostomy with postprandial tachycardia, diarrhea, and abdominal pain	Dumping syndrome

Chapter 43 | Small Intestine

SMALL BOWEL

Anatomy

What comprises the small bowel?	Duodenum, jejunum, and ileum
How long is the duodenum?	≈12 inches—thus the name: duodenum!
What marks the end of the duodenum and the start of the jejunum?	Ligament of Treitz
What is the length of the entire small bowel?	≈6 meters (20 feet)
What are the plicae circulares?	*Plicae* means "folds," *circulares* means "circular"; thus, circular folds of mucosa (a.k.a. "valvulae conniventes") in small bowel lumen
What does the terminal ileum absorb?	B12, fatty acids, bile salts

Small Bowel Obstruction

What is small bowel obstruction (SBO)?	Mechanical obstruction to the passage of intraluminal contents
What are the signs/symptoms?	Abdominal discomfort, cramping, nausea, abdominal distention, emesis, high-pitched bowel sounds
What lab tests are performed with SBO?	Electrolytes, CBC, type and screen, urinalysis

What are classic electrolyte/ acid–base findings with proximal obstruction?	Hypovolemia, hypochloremia, hypokalemia, alkalosis
What must be ruled out on physical exam in patients with SBO?	Incarcerated hernia (also look for surgical scars)
What major AXR findings are associated with SBO?	Distended loops of small bowel air–fluid levels on upright film

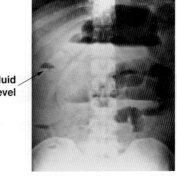

Air–fluid level

Define complete SBO:	Complete obstruction of the lumen
What is the danger of complete SBO?	Closed loop strangulation of the bowel leading to bowel necrosis
Define partial SBO	Incomplete SBO
What is initial management of all patients with SBO?	NPO, NGT, IVF, Foley
What tests can differentiate partial from complete bowel obstruction?	CT scan with oral contrast
What are the ABCs of SBO?	Causes of SBO: 1. **A**dhesions 2. **B**ulge (hernias) 3. **C**ancer and tumors
What is superior mesenteric artery (SMA) syndrome?	Seen with weight loss—SMA compresses duodenum, causing obstruction
What is the treatment of complete SBO?	Laparotomy and lysis of adhesions
What is the treatment of incomplete SBO?	Initially, conservative treatment with close observation plus NGT decompression
Intraoperatively, how can the level of obstruction be determined in patients with SBO?	Transition from dilated bowel proximal to the decompressed bowel distal to the obstruction

What is the most common indication for abdominal surgery in patients with Crohn's disease?

SBO due to strictures

Can a patient have complete SBO and bowel movements and flatus?

Yes; the bowel distal to the obstruction can clear out gas and stool

After a small bowel resection, why should the mesenteric defect always be closed?

To prevent an internal hernia

What may cause SBO if patient is on Coumadin®?

Bowel wall hematoma

What is the #1 cause of SBO in adults (industrialized nations)?

Postoperative adhesions

What is the #1 cause of SBO around the world?

Hernias

What is the #1 cause of SBO in children?

Hernias

What are the signs of strangulated bowel with SBO?

Fever, severe/continuous pain, hematemesis, **shock**, gas in the bowel wall or portal vein, abdominal free air, **peritoneal signs, acidosis** (increased lactic acid)

What are the clinical parameters that will lower the threshold to operate on a partial SBO?

Increasing **WBC**
Fever
Tachycardia/tachypnea
Abdominal pain

What is an absolute indication for operation with partial SBO?

Peritoneal signs, free air on AXR

What classic saying is associated with complete SBO?

"Never let the sun set or rise on complete SBO"

What condition commonly mimics SBO?

Paralytic ileus (AXR reveals gas distention throughout, including the colon)

What is the differential diagnosis of paralytic (nonobstructive) ileus?

Postoperative ileus after abdominal surgery (normally resolves in 3–5 days)
Electrolyte abnormalities (hypokalemia is most common)
Medications (anticholinergic, narcotics)
Inflammatory intra-abdominal process
Sepsis/shock
Spine injury/spinal cord injury
Retroperitoneal hemorrhage

What tumor classically causes SBO due to "mesenteric fibrosis"?

Carcinoid tumor

Small Bowel Tumors

What is the differential diagnosis of benign tumors of the small intestine?

Leiomyoma, lipoma, lymphangioma, fibroma, adenomas, hemangiomas

What are the signs and symptoms of small bowel tumors?

Abdominal pain, weight loss, obstruction (SBO), and perforation

What is the most common benign small bowel tumor?

Leiomyoma

What is the most common malignant small bowel tumor?

Adenocarcinoma

What is the differential diagnosis of malignant tumors of the small intestine?

1. Adenocarcinoma (50%)
2. Carcinoid (25%)
3. Lymphoma (20%)
4. Sarcomas (<5%)

What is the workup of a small bowel tumor?

UGI with small bowel follow-through, enteroclysis, CT scan, enteroscopy

What is the treatment for malignant small bowel tumor?

Resection and removal of mesenteric draining lymph nodes

What malignancy is classically associated with metastasis to the small bowel?

Melanoma

Meckel's Diverticulum

What is it?

Remnant of the omphalomesenteric duct/vitelline duct, which connects the yolk sac with the primitive midgut in the embryo

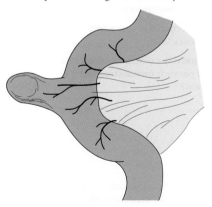

What is the usual location?

Within ≈2 feet of the ileocecal valve on the **antimesenteric** border of the bowel

What is the major differential diagnosis?	Appendicitis
Is it a true diverticulum?	**Yes**; all layers of the intestine are found in the wall
What is the incidence?	≈2% of the population at autopsy
What is the gender ratio?	Twice as common in **men**
What is the average age at onset of symptoms?	Most frequently in the first **2 years of life,** but can occur at any age
What are the possible complications?	**Intestinal hemorrhage** (painless)—50%; accounts for half of all lower GI bleeding in patients younger than 2 years Bleeding results from ectopic gastric mucosa secreting acid → ulcer → bleeding **Intestinal obstruction**—25%; most common complication in adults; includes volvulus and intussusception **Inflammation** (± perforations)—20%
What are the signs/symptoms?	Lower GI bleeding, abdominal pain, SBO
What is the most common complication of Meckel's diverticulum in adults?	Intestinal obstruction
In what percentage of cases is heterotopic tissue found in the diverticulum?	>50%
What heterotopic tissue type is most often found?	**Gastric mucosa** (60%), but duodenal, pancreatic, and colonic mucosa are also found
What is the "rule of 2s"?	**2**% of patients are **symptomatic** Found ≈**2** feet from the ileocecal valve Found in **2**% of the population Most symptoms occur before age **2** years Ectopic tissue found in 1 of **2** patients Most diverticula are ≈**2** inches long **2**:1 male-to-female ratio

What is the role of incidental Meckel's diverticulectomy (surgical removal upon finding asymptomatic diverticulum)?	1. Most would remove in all children
	2. Adults:
	  Ectopic tissue (fullness) or
	  Mesodiverticular band

What is a Meckel's scan?	Scan for ectopic gastric mucosa in Meckel's diverticulum; uses **technetium pertechnetate** IV, which is preferentially taken up by gastric mucosa
What is the treatment of a Meckel's diverticulum that is causing bleeding and obstruction?	Surgical resection, with small bowel resection as the actual ulcer is usually on the mesenteric wall opposite the diverticulum!

RAPID-FIRE REVIEW

Name the diagnostic modality:

25-year-old female with history of several abdominal surgeries now with 2-day history of abdominal distention, vomiting, and no gas or bowel movements	Abd/pelvis CT scan with oral contrast to rule out SBO
52-year-old male alcoholic with history of blood in vomit	EGD

What is the treatment?

67-year-old female with history of several abdominal surgeries presents with several days of crampy abdominal pain and vomiting, and x-ray reveals air–fluid levels; normal WBC afebrile, normal lactic acid level, pH is normal, mild tenderness on exam	CT scan with oral contrast and NGT decompression, IVF, serial and exams for SBO (oral contrast is thought to be therapeutic!)

What is the correct diagnosis?

Jejunal ulcers	Zollinger–Ellison syndrome
17-year-old s/p MVC with abdominal pain, seatbelt sign across abd, free fluid without solid organ injury on abd CT scan	Small bowel injury

Name the radiographic test for localizing the following:

Meckel's diverticulum	Technetium-99m sodium pertechnetate scan

Chapter 44 | Appendix

What vessel provides blood supply to the appendix?	Appendiceal artery—branch of the ileocolic artery
Name the mesentery of the appendix:	Mesoappendix (contains the appendiceal artery)
How can the appendix be located if the cecum has been identified?	Follow the teniae coli down to the appendix; the teniae converge on the appendix

APPENDICITIS

What is it?	Inflammation of the appendix caused by **obstruction** of the appendiceal lumen, producing a closed loop with resultant inflammation that can lead to necrosis and perforation
What are the causes?	Lymphoid hyperplasia, fecalith (a.k.a. "appendicolith")
What is the lifetime incidence of acute appendicitis in the United States?	$\approx 7\%$!
What is the most common cause of emergent abdominal surgery in the United States?	Acute appendicitis
How does appendicitis classically present?	Classic chronologic order: 1. Periumbilical pain (intermittent and crampy) 2. Nausea/vomiting 3. Anorexia 4. Pain migrates to RLQ (constant and intense pain), usually in <24 hours
Why does periumbilical pain occur?	Referred pain
Why does RLQ pain occur?	Peritoneal irritation
What are the signs/symptoms?	Signs of peritoneal irritation may be present: guarding, muscle spasm, rebound tenderness, obturator and psoas signs, low-grade fever (high grade if perforation occurs), RLQ hyperesthesia
Define the following terms:	
Obturator sign	Pain upon internal rotation of the leg with the hip and knee flexed; seen in patients with pelvic appendicitis
Psoas sign	Pain elicited by extending the hip with the knee in full extension or by flexing the hip against resistance; seen classically in retrocecal appendicitis
Rovsing's sign	Palpation or rebound pressure of the LLQ results in pain in the RLQ; seen in appendicitis

McBurney's point

Point 1/3 from the anterior superior iliac spine to the umbilicus (often the point of maximal tenderness)

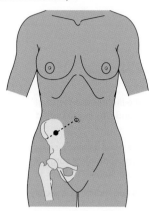

What is the differential diagnosis for:

Everyone

Meckel's diverticulum, Crohn's disease, perforated ulcer, pancreatitis, mesenteric lymphadenitis, constipation, gastroenteritis, intussusception, volvulus, tumors, UTI (e.g., cystitis), pyelonephritis, torsed epiploicae, cholecystitis, cecal tumor, diverticulitis (floppy sigmoid)

Females

Ovarian cyst, ovarian torsion, tuboovarian abscess, mittelschmerz, pelvic inflammatory disease (PID), ectopic pregnancy, ruptured pregnancy

What lab tests should be performed?

CBC: increased WBC (>10,000 per mm^3 in >90% of cases), most often with a "left shift"

Urinalysis: to evaluate for pyelonephritis or renal calculus

Can you have an abnormal urinalysis with appendicitis?

Yes; mild hematuria and pyuria are common in appendicitis with pelvic inflammation, resulting in inflammation of the ureter

What additional tests can be performed if the diagnosis is not clear?

Spiral CT scan, U/S (may see a large, noncompressible appendix or fecalith)

In acute appendicitis, what classically precedes vomiting?

Pain (in gastroenteritis, the pain classically follows vomiting)

What radiographic studies are often performed?	CXR: to rule out RML or RLL pneumonia, free air
	AXR: abdominal films are usually nonspecific, but calcified fecalith present in ≈5% of cases
What are the CT scan findings with acute appendicitis?	Periappendiceal fat stranding, appendiceal diameter >6 mm, periappendiceal fluid, fecalith
What are the preoperative medications/preparation?	1. Rehydration with **IV fluids** (LR)
	2. Preoperative **antibiotics** with anaerobic coverage (appendix is considered part of the colon)
What is a lap appy?	Laparoscopic appendectomy
What is the treatment for *non*perforated acute appendicitis?	Nonperforated—prompt appendectomy (prevents perforation), 24 hours of antibiotics, discharge home usually on POD #1
What is the treatment for *perforated* acute appendicitis?	Perforated—IV fluid resuscitation and prompt appendectomy; all pus is drained with postoperative antibiotics continued for 3 to 7 days; wound is left open in most cases of perforation after closing the fascia (heals by secondary intention or delayed primary closure), ± drain
How is an appendiceal abscess that is diagnosed preoperatively treated?	**Percutaneous** drainage of the abscess, antibiotic administration, and elective appendectomy ≈6 weeks later (a.k.a. "interval appendectomy")
If a normal appendix is found upon exploration, should you take out the normal appendix?	Yes
How long after removal of a NONRUPTURED appendix should antibiotics continue postoperatively?	For 24 hours
Which antibiotic is used for NONPERFORATED appendicitis?	Anaerobic coverage: Cefoxitin®, Cefotetan®, Unasyn®, Cipro®, and Flagyl®
What antibiotic is used for a PERFORATED appendix?	**Broad-spectrum antibiotics** (e.g., amp/Cipro®/clinda or a penicillin such as Zosyn®)
How long do you give antibiotics for perforated appendicitis?	Until the patient has a normal WBC count and is afebrile, ambulating, and eating a regular diet (usually 3 to 7 days)
What is the risk of perforation?	≈25% by 24 hours from onset of symptoms, ≈50% by 36 hours, and ≈75% by 48 hours

What is the most common general surgical abdominal emergency in pregnancy?

Appendicitis (about 1/1,750; **appendix may be in the RUQ** because of the enlarged uterus)

What are the possible complications of appendicitis?

Pelvic abscess, liver abscess, free perforation, portal pylethrombophlebitis (very rare)

What percentage of negative appendectomies is acceptable?

Up to 20%; taking out some normal appendixes is better than missing a case of acute appendicitis that eventually ruptures

Who is at risk of dying from acute appendicitis?

Very old and very young patients

What bacteria are associated with "mesenteric adenitis" that can closely mimic acute appendicitis?

Yersinia enterocolitica

CLASSIC INTRAOPERATIVE QUESTIONS

What are the layers of the abdominal wall during a McBurney incision?

1. Skin
2. Subcutaneous fat
3. Scarpa's fascia
4. External oblique
5. Internal oblique
6. Transversus muscle
7. Transversalis fascia
8. Preperitoneal fat
9. Peritoneum

How can you find the appendix after identifying the cecum?

Follow the teniae down to where they converge on the appendix

If you find Crohn's disease in the terminal ileum, will you remove the appendix?

Yes, if the cecal/appendiceal base is not involved

If the appendix is normal what do you inspect intraoperatively?

Terminal ileum: Meckel's diverticulum, Crohn's disease, intussusception
Gynecologic: Cysts, torsion, etc.
Groin: hernia, rectus sheath hematoma, adenopathy (adenitis)

APPENDICEAL TUMORS

What is the most common appendiceal tumor?

Carcinoid tumor

What is the treatment of appendiceal carcinoid <1.5 cm?

Appendectomy (if not through the bowel wall)

What is the treatment of appendiceal carcinoid >1.5 cm?

Right hemicolectomy

What percentage of appendiceal carcinoids is malignant?	<5%
What is the differential diagnosis of appendiceal tumor?	Carcinoid, adenocarcinoma, malignant mucoid adenocarcinoma
What type of appendiceal tumor can cause the dreaded pseudomyxoma peritonei if the appendix ruptures?	Malignant mucoid adenocarcinoma

RAPID-FIRE REVIEW

Name the diagnostic modality:

8-year-old with history of RLQ pain, s/p appendectomy	Technetium-99m pertechnetate Meckel's scan looking for a Meckel's diverticulum

Chapter 45 | Carcinoid Tumors

What is a carcinoid tumor?	Tumor arising from neuroendocrine cells (APUDomas), a.k.a. "**Kulchitsky cells**"; basically, a tumor that secretes **serotonin**
Why is it called "carcinoid"?	Suffix "-oid" means "resembling"; thus, carcinoid resembles a carcinoma but is clinically and histologically less aggressive than most GI carcinomas
How can you remember that Kulchitsky cells are found in carcinoid tumors?	Think: "COOL CAR" or KULchitsky CARcinoid
What are the common sites of occurrence?	Think "**AIR**": 1. **A**ppendix (most common) 2. **I**leum 3. **R**ectum 4. Bronchus Other sites: jejunum, stomach, duodenum, colon, ovary, testicle, pancreas, thymus
What are the signs/symptoms?	Depends on location; most cases are asymptomatic; also SBO, abdominal pain, bleeding, weight loss, diaphoresis, **pellagra skin changes**, intussusception, carcinoid syndrome, wheezing
Why SBO with carcinoid?	Classically = severe mesenteric fibrosis

What are the pellagra-like symptoms?	Think "**3D**": 1. **D**ermatitis 2. **D**iarrhea 3. **D**ementia
What causes pellagra in carcinoid patients?	Decreased **niacin** production
What is carcinoid syndrome?	Syndrome of symptoms caused by release of substances from a carcinoid tumor
What are the symptoms of carcinoid syndrome?	Remember the acronym "**B FDR**": **B**ronchospasm **F**lushing (skin) **D**iarrhea **R**ight-sided heart failure (from valve failure)
What is a complete memory aid for carcinoid?	Think: "**Be FDR** in a **cool CAR**" (COOL = **KUL**chitsky cells): FDR = Flush Diarrhea Right-sided heart failure; CAR = CARcinoid

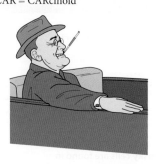

Why does right-sided heart failure develop but not left-sided heart failure?	Lungs act as a filter (just like the liver); thus, the left heart doesn't see all the vasoactive compounds
Classic cardiac complication with carcinoid syndrome:	**Tips**: **T**ricuspid **I**nsufficiency **P**ulmonary **S**tenosis
What is the incidence of carcinoid SYNDROME in patients who have a carcinoid TUMOR?	≈10%
What released substances cause carcinoid syndrome?	**Serotonin** and vasoactive peptides
What is the medical treatment for carcinoid syndrome?	Octreotide IV
What is the medical treatment of diarrhea alone?	Ondansetron (Zofran®)—serotonin **antagonist**

How does the liver prevent carcinoid syndrome?	By degradation of serotonin and the other vasoactive peptides when the **tumor drains into the portal vein**
Why does carcinoid syndrome occur in some tumors and not in others?	Occurs when **venous drainage from the tumor gains access to the systemic circulation** by avoiding hepatic degradation of the vasoactive substances
What tumors can produce carcinoid syndrome?	**Liver metastases** Retroperitoneal disease draining into paravertebral veins Primary tumor outside the GI tract, portal venous drainage (e.g., ovary, **testicular**, bronchus)
What does the liver break down serotonin into?	5-Hydroxyindoleacetic acid (**5-HIAA**)
What percentage of patients with a carcinoid has an elevated urine 5-HIAA level?	50%
What are the associated diagnostic lab findings?	**Elevated urine 5-HIAA** as well as elevated urine and blood **serotonin** levels
How do you remember 5-HIAA for carcinoid?	Think of a **5-HIGH CAR** pileup = **5-HI**AA **CAR**cinoid

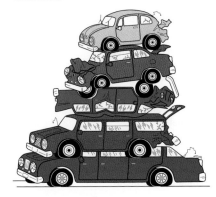

What stimulation test can often elevate serotonin levels and cause symptoms of carcinoid syndrome?	Pentagastrin stimulation
How do you localize a GI carcinoid?	Barium enema, upper GI series with small bowel follow-through, colonoscopy, enteroscopy, enteroclysis, EGD, radiology tests
What are the special radiologic (scintigraphy) localization tests?	^{131}I-MIBG (^{131}I metaiodobenzylguanidine) ^{111}In-octreotide PET scan utilizing ^{11}C-labeled HTP

What is the surgical treatment?	Excision of the primary tumor and single or feasible metastasis in the liver (liver transplant is an option with unresectable liver metastasis); chemotherapy for advanced disease
What is the medical treatment?	Medical therapy for palliation of the carcinoid syndrome (serotonin antagonists, somatostatin analogue [**octreotide**])
How effective is octreotide?	It relieves diarrhea and flushing in more than 85% of cases and may shrink tumor in 10% to 20% of cases
What is a common antiserotonin drug?	**Cyproheptadine**
What is the overall prognosis?	Two thirds of patients are alive at 5 years
What is the prognosis of patients with liver metastasis or carcinoid syndrome?	50% are alive at 3 years
What does carcinoid tumor look like?	Usually intramural bowel mass; appears as **yellowish** tumor upon incision
For appendiceal carcinoid, when is a right hemicolectomy indicated versus an appendectomy?	If the tumor is >**1.5 cm,** right **hemicolectomy** is indicated; if there are no signs of serosal or cecal involvement and tumor is <**1.5 cm, appendectomy** should be performed
Which primary site has the highest rate of metastasis?	Ileal primary tumor
Can a carcinoid tumor be confirmed malignant by looking at the histology?	No, metastasis must be present to diagnose malignancy
What is the correlation between tumor size and malignancy potential?	Vast majority of tumors <2 cm are benign; in tumors >2 cm, malignancy potential is significant
What treatments might you use for the patient with unresectable liver metastasis that is refractory to medical treatment?	Chemoembolization or radiofrequency ablation

RAPID-FIRE REVIEW

Name the diagnostic modality:

50-year-old male with history of flushing, diarrhea, JVD with echo revealing right-sided heart failure	24-hour urinary 5-HIAA (5-hydroxyindoleacetic acid) level to workup carcinoid syndrome

Chapter 46 | Fistulas

What is a fistula?
Abnormal **communication** between two hollow organs or a hollow organ and the skin (i.e., two epithelial cell layers)

What are the predisposing factors and conditions that maintain patency of a fistula?
The acronym **"HIS FRIEND"**:
High-output fistula (>500 cc/day)
Intestinal destruction (>50% of circumference)
Short-segment fistula <2.5 cm

Foreign body (e.g., G-tube)
Radiation
Infection
Epithelialization (e.g., colostomy)
Neoplasm
Distal obstruction

SPECIFIC TYPES OF FISTULAS

Enterocutaneous

What is it?
Fistula from GI tract to skin (enterocutaneous = **bowel to skin**)

What are the causes?
Anastomotic leak, trauma/injury to the bowel/colon, Crohn's disease, abscess, diverticulitis, inflammation/infection, inadvertent suture through bowel

What is the workup?
1. CT scan to rule out abscess/inflammatory process
2. Fistulagram

What are the possible complications?
High-output fistulas, malnutrition, skin breakdown

What is the treatment?
NPO; TPN; drain abscesses, rule out and correct underlying causes; may feed distally (or if fistula is distal, feed elemental diet proximally); half will close spontaneously, but the other half require operation and resection of the involved bowel segment

Which enterocutaneous fistula closes faster: short or long?
Long fistula (may be counterintuitive—but true)

Colonic Fistulas

What are they?

Include colovesical, colocutaneous, colovaginal, and coloenteric fistulas

What are the most common causes?

Diverticulitis (most common cause), cancer, IBD, foreign body, and irradiation

What is the most common type?

Colovesical fistula, which often presents with recurrent urinary tract infections; other signs include pneumaturia, dysuria, and fecaluria

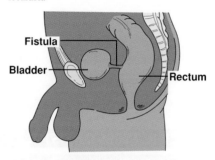

How is the diagnosis made?

Via barium enema (BE) and cystoscopy

What is the treatment?

Surgery: segmental colon resection and primary anastomosis; repair/resection of the involved organ

External Pancreatic Fistula

What is it?

Pancreaticocutaneous fistula; drainage of pancreatic exocrine secretions through to abdominal skin (usually through drain tract/wound)

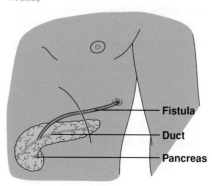

What is the treatment?	NPO, TPN, skin protection, **octreotide**
What is a "refractory" pancreatic fistula?	Pancreaticocutaneous fistula that does not resolve with conservative medical management (minority of cases)
What is the diagnostic test for "refractory" pancreatic fistulas?	ERCP to define site of fistula tract (i.e., tail versus head of pancreas)
How is refractory tail of a pancreas fistula treated?	Resection of the tail of the pancreas and the fistula
How is refractory head of a pancreas fistula treated?	Pancreaticojejunostomy

RAPID-FIRE REVIEW

Name the diagnostic modality:

40-year-old male with history of passing air with his urine	CT scan looking for colocystic fistula usually from diverticulitis

What is the correct diagnosis?

21-year-old s/p GSW to abdomen with small bowel resections develops tachycardia, fever, and green bilious wound drainage	Anastomotic leak and enterocutaneous fistula

Chapter 47 | Colon and Rectum

ANATOMY

Identify the arterial blood supply to the colon:

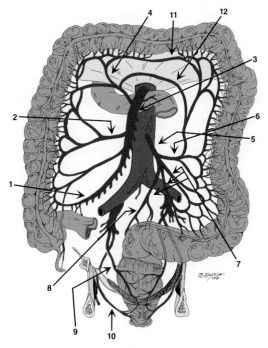

1. Ileocolic artery
2. Right colic artery
3. Superior mesenteric artery (SMA)
4. Middle colic artery
5. Inferior mesenteric artery (IMA)
6. Left colic artery
7. Sigmoidal artery
8. Superior hemorrhoidal artery (superior rectal)
9. Middle hemorrhoidal artery
10. Inferior hemorrhoidal artery
11. Marginal artery of Drummond
12. Meandering artery of Gonzalez

What are the white lines of Toldt?   Lateral peritoneal reflections of the ascending and descending colon

What parts of the GI tract do not have a serosa?	Esophagus, middle and distal **rectum**
What are the major anatomic differences between the colon and the small bowel?	Colon has teniae coli, haustra, and appendices epiploicae (fat appendages), whereas the small intestine is smooth
What is the blood supply to the rectum?	
Proximal	Superior hemorrhoidal (or superior rectal) from the IMA
Middle	Middle hemorrhoidal (or middle rectal) from the hypogastric (internal iliac)
Distal	Inferior hemorrhoidal (or inferior rectal) from the pudendal artery (a branch of the hypogastric artery)
What is the venous drainage of the rectum?	
Proximal	Via the IMV to the splenic vein, then **to the portal vein**
Middle	Via the iliac vein to the **IVC**
Distal	Via the iliac vein to the **IVC**

COLORECTAL CARCINOMA

What is it?	Adenocarcinoma of the colon or rectum
What is the incidence?	Most common GI cancer Second most common cancer in the United States Incidence increases with age starting at 40 and peaks at 70 to 80 years
How common is it as a cause of cancer deaths?	Second most common cause of cancer deaths
What is the lifetime risk of colorectal cancer?	6%
What is the male-to-female ratio?	≈1:1
What are the risk factors?	**Dietary:** Low-fiber, high-fat diets correlate with increased rates **Genetic:** Family history is important when taking history FAP, Lynch's syndrome **IBD:** Ulcerative colitis > Crohn's disease, age, previous colon cancer

What is Lynch's syndrome?

HNPCC = **H**ereditary **N**on**P**olyposis **C**olon **C**ancer—autosomal-dominant inheritance of high risk for development of colon cancer

What are current ACS recommendations for polyp/colorectal screening in asymptomatic patients without family (first-degree) history of colorectal cancer?

Starting at age 50, at least one of the following test regimens is recommended:
Colonoscopy q10 yrs
Double-contrast barium enema (DCBE) q5 yrs
Flex sigmoidoscopy q5 yrs
CT colonography q5 yrs

What are the current recommendations for colorectal cancer screening if there is a history of colorectal cancer in a first-degree relative <60 years old?

Colonoscopy at age 40, or 10 years before the age at diagnosis of the youngest first-degree relative, and every 5 years thereafter

What signs/symptoms are associated with the following conditions?

Right-sided lesions

Right side of bowel has a large luminal diameter, so a tumor may attain a large size before causing problems
Microcytic anemia, occult/melena more than hematochezia PR, postprandial discomfort, fatigue

Left-sided lesions

Left side of bowel has smaller lumen and semisolid contents
Change in bowel habits (small-caliber stools), colicky pain, signs of obstruction, abdominal mass, heme(+), or gross red blood
Nausea, vomiting, constipation

What is the incidence of rectal cancer?

Comprises 20% to 30% of all colorectal cancer

What are the signs/symptoms of rectal cancer?

Most common symptom is hematochezia (passage of red blood ± stool) or mucus; also tenesmus, feeling of incomplete evacuation of stool (because of the mass), and rectal mass

What is the differential diagnosis of a colon tumor/mass?

Adenocarcinoma, carcinoid tumor, lipoma, liposarcoma, leiomyoma, leiomyosarcoma, lymphoma, diverticular disease, ulcerative colitis, Crohn's disease, polyps

Which diagnostic tests are helpful?

History and physical exam (**Note: ≈10% of cancers are palpable on rectal exam**), heme occult, CBC, barium enema, colonoscopy

What disease does microcytic anemia signify until proven otherwise in a man or postmenopausal woman?	Colon cancer
What tests help find metastases?	CXR (lung metastases), LFTs (liver metastases), abdominal CT scan (liver metastases), other tests based on history and physical exam (e.g., head CT scan for left arm weakness looking for brain metastasis)
What is the preoperative workup for colorectal cancer?	History, physical exam, LFTs, CEA, CBC, Chem-10, PT/PTT, type and cross 2 units PRBCs, CXR, U/A, abdominopelvic CT scan
By what means does the cancer spread?	Direct extension: circumferentially and then through bowel wall to later invade other abdominoperineal organs Hematogenous: portal circulation to liver; lumbar/vertebral veins to lungs Lymphogenous: regional lymph nodes (LNs) Transperitoneal
Is CEA useful?	Not for initial screening but for baseline and recurrence surveillance (but offers no proven survival benefit)
What unique diagnostic test is helpful in patients with rectal cancer?	Endorectal ultrasound (probe is placed transanally and depth of invasion and nodes are evaluated)
How are tumors staged?	TNM staging system
Explain the TNM stages:	
Stage I	Invades submucosa or muscularis propria (T1–2, N0, M0)
Stage II	Invades through muscularis propria or surrounding structures but with negative nodes (T3–4, N0, M0)
Stage III	**Positive nodes**, no distant metastasis (any T, N1–3, M0)
Stage IV	Positive **distant metastasis** (any T, any N, M1)
What is the approximate 5-year survival by stage?	
Stage I	**90%**
Stage II	**70%**
Stage III	**50%**
Stage IV	**10%**

What percentage of patients with colorectal cancer has liver metastases on diagnosis?	≈20%
What are the common preoperative IV antibiotics?	Cefoxitin (Mefoxin®), carbapenem
If the patient is allergic (hives, swelling), what antibiotics should be prescribed?	IV ciprofloxacin (Cipro®) and metronidazole (Flagyl®)
What are the treatment options?	Resection: wide surgical resection of lesion and its regional lymphatic drainage
What decides low anterior resection (LAR) versus abdominal perineal resection (APR)?	Distance from the anal verge, pelvis size
What do all rectal cancer operations include?	Total mesorectal excision—remove the rectal mesentery, including the LNs
What is the minimal surgical margin for rectal cancer?	2 cm
How many LNs should be resected with a colon cancer mass?	12 LNs minimum = for staging, and may improve prognosis
What is the adjuvant treatment of stage III colon cancer?	5-FU and leucovorin (or levamisole) chemotherapy (if postoperative nodal metastasis)
What is the adjuvant treatment for T3–4 rectal cancer?	**Preoperative radiation therapy** and 5-FU chemotherapy as a "radiosensitizer"
What is the most common site of distant (hematogenous) metastasis from colorectal cancer?	Liver
What is the treatment of liver metastases from colorectal cancer?	Resect with ≥1 cm margins and administer chemotherapy if feasible
What is the surveillance regimen?	Physical exam, stool guaiac, CBC, CEA, LFTs (every 3 months for 3 years, then every 6 months for 2 years), CXR every 6 months for 2 years and then yearly, colonoscopy at years 1 and 3 postoperatively, CT scans directed by exam
Why is follow-up so important in the first 3 postoperative years?	≈90% of colorectal recurrences are within 3 years of surgery
What are the most common causes of colonic obstruction in the adult population?	Colon cancer, diverticular disease, colonic volvulus

What is the 5-year survival rate after liver resection with clean margins for colon cancer liver metastasis?	≈33% (28%–50%)
What is the 5-year survival rate after diagnosis of unresectable colon cancer liver metastasis?	0%

COLONIC AND RECTAL POLYPS

What are they?	Tissue growth into bowel lumen, usually consisting of mucosa, submucosa, or both
How are they anatomically classified?	Sessile (flat) Pedunculated (on a stalk)
What are the histologic classifications of the following types?	
Inflammatory (pseudopolyp)	As in Crohn's disease or ulcerative colitis
Hamartomatous	Normal tissue in abnormal configuration
Hyperplastic	Benign—normal cells—no malignant potential
Neoplastic	Proliferation of undifferentiated cells; premalignant or malignant cells
What are the subtypes of neoplastic polyps?	Tubular adenomas (usually pedunculated) Tubulovillous adenomas Villous adenomas (usually sessile and look like broccoli heads)
What determines malignant potential of an adenomatous polyp?	Size Histologic type Atypia of cells
What is the correlation between size and malignancy?	Polyps >2 cm have a high risk of carcinoma (33%–55%)
What about histology and cancer potential of an adenomatous polyp?	Villous > tubovillous > tubular (Think: **VILL**ous = **VILL**ain)
What is the approximate percentage of carcinomas found in the following polyps overall?	
Tubular adenoma	5%
Tubulovillous adenoma	20%
Villous adenoma	40%

Where are most polyps found?	Rectosigmoid (30%)
What are the signs/symptoms?	Bleeding (red or dark blood), change in bowel habits, mucus per rectum, electrolyte loss, totally asymptomatic
What are the diagnostic tests?	Colonoscopy
What is the treatment?	Endoscopic resection (snared) if polyps; large sessile villous adenomas should be removed with bowel resection and LN resection

POLYPOSIS SYNDROMES

Familial Polyposis

What is another name for this condition?	Familial Adenomatous Polyposis (**FAP**)
What are the characteristics?	Hundreds of adenomatous polyps within the rectum and colon that begin developing at puberty; all undiagnosed; untreated patients develop cancer by ages 40 to 50
What is the inheritance pattern?	Autosomal dominant (i.e., 50% of offspring)
What is the genetic defect?	Adenomatous Polyposis Coli (APC) gene
What is the treatment?	Total proctocolectomy and ileostomy Total colectomy and rectal mucosal removal (mucosal proctectomy) and ileoanal anastomosis
With FAP, what other tumor must be looked for?	Duodenal tumors

Gardner's Syndrome

What are the characteristics?	Neoplastic polyps of the **small bowel** and **colon;** cancer by age 40 in 100% of undiagnosed patients, as in FAP
What are the other associated findings?	**Desmoid** tumors (in abdominal wall or cavity), **osteomas** of skull (seen on x-ray), **sebaceous** cysts, adrenal and thyroid tumors, retroperitoneal fibrosis, duodenal and periampullary tumors

How can the findings associated with Gardner's syndrome be remembered?	Think of a gardener planting **"SOD"**: **S**ebaceous cysts **O**steomas **D**esmoid tumors

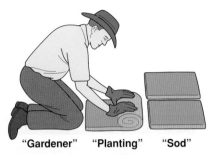

"Gardener"   "Planting"   "Sod"

What is a desmoid tumor?	Tumor of the musculoaponeurotic sheath, usually of the abdominal wall; benign, but grows locally; treated by wide resection
What medications may slow the growth of a desmoid tumor?	Tamoxifen, sulindac, steroids
What is the inheritance pattern?	Varying degree of penetrance from an autosomal-dominant gene
What is the treatment of colon polyps in patients with Gardner's syndrome?	Total proctocolectomy and ileostomy Total colectomy and rectal mucosal removal (mucosal proctectomy) and ileoanal anastomosis

Peutz–Jeghers' Syndrome

What are the characteristics?	Hamartomas throughout the GI tract (jejunum/ileum > colon > stomach)
What is the associated cancer risk from polyps?	Increased
What is the associated cancer risk for women with Peutz–Jeghers'?	Ovarian cancer (granulosa cell tumor is most common)
What is the inheritance pattern?	Autosomal dominant
What are the other signs?	Melanotic pigmentation (black/brown) of buccal mucosa (mouth), lips, digits, palms, feet (soles) (Think: **P**eutz = **P**igmented)
What is the treatment?	Removal of polyps, if symptomatic (i.e., bleeding, intussusception, or obstruction) or large (>1.5 cm)

What are juvenile polyps?	Benign hamartomas in the small bowel and colon; not premalignant (a.k.a. "retention polyps")
What is Cronkhite–Canada syndrome?	Diffuse GI hamartoma polyps (i.e., no cancer potential) associated with malabsorption/ weight loss, diarrhea, and **loss of electrolytes/proteins;** signs include alopecia, nail atrophy, skin pigmentation
What is Turcot's syndrome?	Colon polyps with malignant **CNS tumors** (glioblastoma multiforme)

DIVERTICULAR DISEASE OF THE COLON

Diverticulosis

What is diverticulosis?	Condition in which diverticula can be found within the colon, especially the sigmoid; diverticula are actually **false diverticula** in that only mucosa and submucosa herniate through the bowel musculature; true diverticula involve all layers of the bowel wall and are rare in the colon

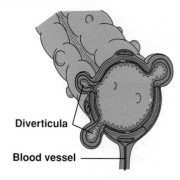

Diverticula

Blood vessel

Describe the pathophysiology:	**Weakness** in the bowel wall develops at points where nutrient **blood vessels** enter between antimesenteric and mesenteric teniae; increase intraluminal pressures then cause herniation through these areas
What is the incidence?	≈50% to 60% in the United States by age 60, with only 10% to 20% becoming symptomatic
What is the most common site?	95% of people with diverticulosis have **sigmoid** colon involvement

Who is at risk?	People with **low-fiber diets**, chronic constipation, and a positive family history; incidence increases with age
What are the symptoms/complications?	**Bleeding:** may be massive Diverticulitis, asymptomatic (80% of cases)
What is the diagnostic approach?	
Bleeding	Without signs of inflammation: colonoscopy
Pain and signs of inflammation	Abdominal/pelvic CT scan
What is the treatment of diverticulosis?	High-fiber diet is recommended
What are the indications for operation with diverticulosis?	Complications of diverticulitis (e.g., fistula, obstruction, stricture); recurrent episodes; hemorrhage; suspected carcinoma; prolonged symptoms; abscess not drainable by percutaneous approach
When is it safe to get a colonoscopy or barium enema/sigmoidoscopy?	Due to risk of perforation, this is performed 6 weeks after inflammation resolves to rule out colon cancer

Diverticulitis

What is it?	Infection or perforation of a diverticulum
What is the pathophysiology?	**Obstruction** of diverticulum by a fecalith leading to inflammation and microperforation
What are the signs/symptoms?	LLQ pain (cramping or steady), change in bowel habits (**diarrhea**), fever, chills, anorexia, LLQ mass, nausea/vomiting, dysuria
What are the associated lab findings?	Increased WBCs
What are the associated radiographic findings?	On x-ray: ileus, partially obstructed colon, air–fluid levels, free air if perforated On abdominal/pelvic CT scan: swollen, edematous bowel wall; particularly helpful in diagnosing an abscess
What are the associated barium enema findings?	Barium enema should be avoided in acute cases
Is colonoscopy safe in an acute setting?	No, there is increased risk of perforation
What are the possible complications?	Abscess, diffuse peritonitis, fistula, obstruction, perforation, stricture
What is the most common fistula with diverticulitis?	Colovesical fistula (to bladder)

What is the best test for diverticulitis?	CT scan
What is the initial therapy?	IV fluids, NPO, broad-spectrum antibiotics with anaerobic coverage, NG suction (as needed for emesis/ileus)
When is surgery warranted?	Obstruction, fistula, free perforation, abscess not amenable to percutaneous drainage, sepsis, deterioration with initial conservative treatment
What is the lifelong risk of recurrence after:	
First episode?	33%
Second episode?	50%
What are the indications for elective resection?	Case-by-case decisions, but usually after two episodes of diverticulitis; should be considered after the **first** episode in a young, diabetic, or immunosuppressed patient or to rule out cancer
What surgery is usually performed ELECTIVELY for recurrent bouts?	One-stage operation: resection of involved segment and primary anastomosis (with preoperative bowel prep)
What type of surgery is usually performed for an acute case of diverticulitis with a complication?	1. **Hartmann's procedure:** resection of involved segment with an end colostomy and stapled rectal stump 2. Resection, primary anastomosis loop ileostomy
What is the treatment of diverticular abscess?	Percutaneous drainage; if abscess is not amenable to percutaneous drainage, then surgical approach for drainage is necessary
How common is massive lower GI bleeding with diverticulitis?	Very **rare**! Massive lower GI bleeding is seen with divercu**losis**, not diverticulitis
What are the most common causes of massive lower GI bleeding in adults?	Diverticulosis (especially right sided), vascular ectasia
What must you rule out in any patient with diverticulitis/diverticulosis?	Colon cancer

Colonic Volvulus

What is it?	**Twisting of colon on itself** about its mesentery, resulting in obstruction and, if complete, vascular compromise with potential necrosis, perforation, or both

What is the most common type of colonic volvulus?	Sigmoid volvulus (makes sense because the sigmoid is a redundant/"floppy" structure!)

Sigmoid Volvulus

What is it?	Volvulus or "twist" in the sigmoid colon

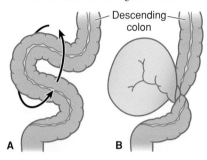

What is the incidence?	≈75% of colonic volvulus cases (Think: **S**igmoid = **S**uperior)
What are the etiologic factors?	High-residue diet resulting in bulky stools and tortuous, elongated colon; chronic constipation; laxative abuse; pregnancy; seen most commonly in bedridden elderly or institutionalized patients, many of whom have history of prior abdominal surgery or distal colonic obstruction
What are the signs/symptoms?	Acute abdominal pain, progressive abdominal distention, anorexia, obstipation, cramps, nausea/vomiting
What findings are evident on abdominal plain film?	Distended loop of sigmoid colon, often in the classic "bent inner tube" or "omega" sign with the loop aiming toward the RUQ
What are the signs of necrotic bowel in colonic volvulus?	Free air, pneumatosis (air in bowel wall)
How is the diagnosis made?	CT scan, sigmoidoscopy, or radiographic exam with Gastrografin® enema
Under what conditions is Gastrografin® enema useful?	If sigmoidoscopy and plain films fail to confirm the diagnosis; **"bird's beak"** is pathognomonic seen on enema contrast study as the contrast comes to a sharp end
What are the signs of strangulation?	Discolored or hemorrhagic mucosa on sigmoidoscopy, bloody fluid in the rectum, frank ulceration or necrosis at the point of the twist, peritoneal signs, fever, hypotension, ↑ WBCs

What is the initial treatment?	**Nonoperative:** If there is no strangulation, sigmoidoscopic reduction is successful in ≈85% of cases; enema study will occasionally reduce (5%)
What is the percentage of recurrence after nonoperative reduction of a sigmoid volvulus?	≈40%!
What are the indications for surgery?	Emergently if strangulation is suspected or nonoperative reduction unsuccessful (Hartmann's procedure); most patients should undergo resection during same hospitalization of redundant sigmoid after successful nonoperative reduction because of high recurrence rate (40%)

Cecal Volvulus

What is it?	Twisting of the cecum upon itself and the mesentery

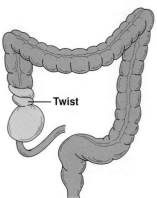

What is a cecal "bascule" volvulus?	Instead of the more common axial twist, the cecum folds upward (lies on the ascending colon)
What is the incidence?	≈25% of colonic volvulus (i.e., much less common than sigmoid volvulus)
What is the etiology?	Idiopathic, poor fixation of the right colon, many patients have history of abdominal surgery

What are the signs/symptoms?	Acute onset of abdominal or colicky pain beginning in the RLQ and progressing to a constant pain, vomiting, obstipation, abdominal distention, and SBO; many patients will have had previous similar episodes
How is the diagnosis made?	Abdominal plain film; dilated, ovoid colon with large air/fluid level in the RLQ often forming the classic **"coffee bean"** sign with the apex aiming toward the epigastrium or LUQ (must rule out gastric dilation with NG aspiration)
What diagnostic studies should be performed?	Water-soluble contrast study (Gastrografin®), if diagnosis cannot be made by AXR, CT scan
What is the treatment?	Emergent surgery, right colectomy with primary anastomosis or ileostomy and mucous fistula (primary anastomosis may be performed in stable patients)
What are the major differences in the EMERGENT management of cecal volvulus versus sigmoid?	Patients with cecal volvulus require **surgical** reduction, whereas the vast majority of patients with sigmoid volvulus undergo initial **endoscopic** reduction of the twist

RAPID-FIRE REVIEW

Name the most likely diagnosis:

67-year-old male smoker on Coumadin® for chronic DVT notices LLQ pain after a strenuous coughing spell; LLQ mass detected on physical exam	Rectus sheath hematoma

What is the treatment?

60-year-old male with LLQ pain and "parrot's beak" on x-ray c/w sigmoid volvulus	Proctosigmoidoscopy to decompress initially
78-year-old male with RLQ and "coffee bean" colonic dilation on x-ray c/w cecal volvulus	Ex lap with resection with primary anastomosis or ileostomy

Chapter 48 │ Anus

ANATOMY

Identify the following:

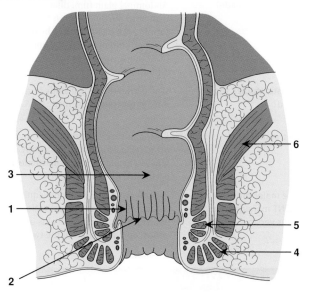

1. Anal columns
2. Dentate line
3. Rectum
4. External sphincter
5. Internal sphincter
6. Levator ani muscle

ANAL CANCER

What is the most common carcinoma of the anus?

Squamous cell carcinoma (80%)
(Think: **ASS** = **A**nal **S**quamous **S**uperior)

What cell types are found in carcinomas of the anus?

1. Squamous cell carcinoma (80%)
2. Cloacogenic (transitional cell)
3. Adenocarcinoma/melanoma/
   basal cell carcinoma

What is the incidence of anal carcinoma?

Rare (1% of colon cancers incidence)

What is anal Bowen's disease?	Squamous cell carcinoma in situ (Think: **B.S.** = **B**owen **S**quamous)
How is Bowen's disease treated?	With local wide excision
What is Paget's disease of the anus?	Adenocarcinoma in situ of the anus (Think: **P.A.** = **P**aget's **A**denocarcinoma)
How is Paget's disease treated?	With local wide excision
What are the risk factors for anal cancer?	Human papillomavirus, condyloma, herpes, HIV, chronic inflammation (fistulae/Crohn's disease), immunosuppression, homosexuality in males, cervical/vaginal cancer, STDs, smoking
What is the most common symptom of anal carcinoma?	Anal bleeding
What are the other signs/ symptoms of anal carcinoma?	Pain, mass, mucus per rectum, pruritus
What percentage of patients with anal cancer is asymptomatic?	≈25%
To what locations do anal canal cancers metastasize?	Lymph nodes, liver, bone, lung
What is the lymphatic drainage below the dentate line?	Below to inguinal lymph nodes (above to pelvic chains)
Are most patients with anal cancer diagnosed early or late?	Late (diagnosis is often missed)
What is the workup of a patient with suspected anal carcinoma?	History Physical exam: digital rectal exam, proctoscopic exam, and colonoscopy Biopsy of mass Abdominal/pelvic CT scan, transanal U/S CXR LFTs
Define:	
Margin cancer	Anal verge out 5 cm onto the perianal skin
Canal cancer	Proximal to anal verge up to the border of the internal sphincter
How is an anal canal epidermal carcinoma treated?	NIGRO protocol: 1. Chemotherapy (5-FU and mitomycin C) 2. Radiation 3. Postradiation therapy scar biopsy (6–8 weeks postradiation therapy [XRT])
What percentage of patients have a "complete" response with the NIGRO protocol?	90%

What is the 5-year survival with the NIGRO protocol?	5%
What is the treatment for local recurrence of anal cancer after the NIGRO protocol?	May repeat chemotherapy/XRT or salvage abdominoperineal resection (APR)
How is a small (<5 cm) anal margin cancer treated?	Surgical excision with 1-cm margins
How is a large (>5 cm) anal margin cancer treated?	Chemoradiation
What is the treatment of anal melanoma?	Wide excision or APR (especially if tumor is large) ± XRT, chemotherapy, postoperatively
What is the 5-year survival rate with anal melanoma?	<10%
How many patients with anal melanoma have an amelanotic anal tumor?	Approximately 1/3, thus making diagnosis difficult without pathology
What is the prognosis of anal melanoma?	<5% 5-year survival rate

Fistula-in-Ano

What is it?	Anal fistula, from rectum to perianal skin
What are the causes?	Usually anal crypt/gland infection (usually perianal abscess)
What are the signs/symptoms?	Perianal drainage, perirectal abscess, recurrent perirectal abscess, "diaper rash," itching
What disease should be considered with fistula–in-ano?	Crohn's disease
How is the diagnosis made?	Exam, proctoscope
What is Goodsall's rule?	Fistulas originating **anterior** to a transverse line through the anus will course **straight** ahead and exit anteriorly, whereas those exiting **posteriorly** have a **curved** tract

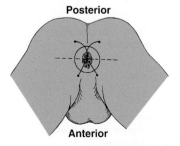

How can Goodsall's rule be remembered?

Think of a dog with a **straight** nose (anterior) and **curved** tail (posterior)

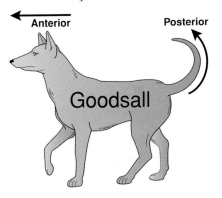

What is the management of anorectal fistulas?

1. Define the anatomy
2. Marsupialization of fistula tract (i.e., fillet tract open)
3. Wound care: routine sitz baths and dressing changes
4. Seton placement if fistula is through the sphincter muscle

What is a seton?

Thick suture placed through fistula tract to allow slow transection of sphincter muscle; scar tissue formed will hold the sphincter muscle in place and allow for continence after transection

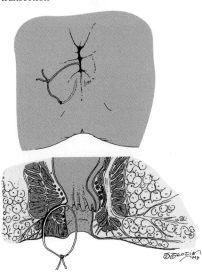

What percentage of patients with a perirectal abscess develops a fistula in ano after drainage?	$\approx 50\%$
How do you find the internal rectal opening of an anorectal fistula in the O.R.?	Inject H_2O_2 (or methylene blue) in external opening—then look for bubbles (or blue dye) coming out of internal opening!
What is a sitz bath?	Sitting in a warm bath (usually done after bowel movement and TID)

Perirectal Abscess

What is it?	Abscess formation around the anus/rectum
What are the signs/symptoms?	Rectal pain, drainage of pus, fever, perianal mass
How is the diagnosis made?	Physical/digital exam reveals perianal/rectal submucosal mass/fluctuance
What is the cause?	Crypt abscess in dentate line with spread
What is the treatment?	As with all abscesses (except simple liver amebic abscess) **drainage**, sitz bath, anal hygiene, stool softeners
What is the indication for postoperative IV antibiotics for drainage?	Cellulitis, immunosuppression, diabetes, heart valve abnormality
What percentage of patients develops a fistula in ano during the 6 months after surgery?	$\approx 50\%$

Anal Fissure

What is it?	Tear or fissure in the anal epithelium
What is the most common site?	Posterior midline (comparatively low blood flow)
What is the cause?	Hard stool passage (constipation), hyperactive sphincter, disease process (e.g., Crohn's disease)
What are the signs/symptoms?	Pain in the anus, painful (can be excruciating) bowel movement, rectal bleeding, blood on toilet tissue after bowel movement, sentinel tag, tear in the anal skin, extremely painful rectal exam, sentinel pile, hypertrophied papilla
What is a sentinel pile?	Thickened mucosa/skin at the distal end of an anal fissure that is often confused with a small hemorrhoid

What is the anal fissure triad for a chronic fissure?

1. Fissure
2. Sentinel pile
3. Hypertrophied anal papilla

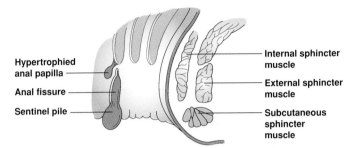

What is the conservative treatment?

Sitz baths, stool softeners, high-fiber diet, excellent anal hygiene, topical nifedipine, Botox®

What disease processes must be considered with a chronic anal fissure?

Crohn's disease, anal cancer, sexually transmitted disease, ulcerative colitis, AIDS

What are the indications for surgery?

Chronic fissure refractory to conservative treatment

What is one surgical option?

Lateral internal sphincterotomy (LIS)—cut the internal sphincter to release it from spasm

What is the "rule of 90%" for anal fissures?

90% occur posteriorly
90% heal with medical treatment alone
90% of patients who undergo LIS heal successfully

Perianal Warts

What are they?

Warts around the anus/perineum

What is the cause?

Condyloma acuminatum (human papillomavirus)

What is the major risk?

Squamous cell carcinoma

What is the treatment if warts are small?

Topical podophyllin, imiquimod (Aldara®)

What is the treatment if warts are large?

Surgical resection or laser ablation

Hemorrhoids

What are they?

Engorgement of the venous plexuses of the rectum, anus, or both; with protrusion of the mucosa, anal margin, or both

Why do we have "healthy" hemorrhoidal tissue?	It is thought to be involved with fluid/air continence
What are the signs/symptoms?	Anal mass/prolapse, bleeding, itching, pain
Which type, internal or external, is painful?	External, below the dentate line
If a patient has excruciating anal pain and history of hemorrhoids, what is the likely diagnosis?	Thrombosed external hemorrhoid (treat by excision)
What are the causes of hemorrhoids?	Constipation/straining, portal hypertension, pregnancy
What is an internal hemorrhoid?	Hemorrhoid above the (proximal) dentate line
What is an external hemorrhoid?	Hemorrhoid below the dentate line
What are the three "hemorrhoid quadrants"?	1. Left lateral 2. Right posterior 3. Right anterior

Classification by Degrees

Define the following terms for internal hemorrhoids:

First-degree hemorrhoid

Hemorrhoid that does not prolapse

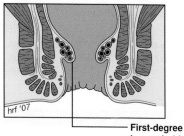

First-degree hemorrhoid

Second-degree hemorrhoid

Prolapses with defecation, but returns on its own

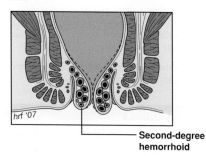

Second-degree hemorrhoid

Third-degree hemorrhoid	Prolapses with defecation or any type of Valsalva maneuver and requires active manual reduction (eat fiber!)

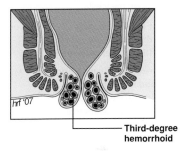

Third-degree hemorrhoid

Fourth-degree hemorrhoid	Prolapsed hemorrhoid that cannot be reduced
What is the treatment?	High-fiber diet, anal hygiene, topical steroids, sitz baths Rubber band ligation (in most cases anesthetic is not necessary for internal hemorrhoids) Surgical resection for large refractory hemorrhoids, infrared coagulation, harmonic scalpel
What is a "closed" versus an "open" hemorrhoidectomy?	Closed (Ferguson) "closes" the mucosa with sutures after hemorrhoid tissue removal Open (Milligan-Morgan) leaves mucosa "open"
What are the dreaded complications of hemorrhoidectomy?	Exsanguination (bleeding may pool proximally in lumen of colon without any signs of external bleeding) Pelvic infection (may be extensive and potentially fatal) Incontinence (injury to sphincter complex) Anal stricture
What condition is a contraindication for hemorrhoidectomy?	Crohn's disease
Classically, what must be ruled out with lower GI bleeding believed to be caused by hemorrhoids?	Colon cancer (colonoscopy)

RAPID-FIRE REVIEW

Name the most likely diagnosis:

56-year-old female with hemorrhoids that prolapse with defecation but then retract by themselves	Second-degree internal hemorrhoids

34-year-old female with hemorrhoids that prolapse after defecation and that she has to "push back in"	Third-degree internal hemorrhoids
56-year-old female with hemorrhoids that are "stuck out" after a bowel movement	Fourth-degree internal hemorrhoid
22-year-old female with bright red blood from her rectum with history of extremely painful bowel movements	Anal fissure

Chapter 49 | Lower GI Bleeding

What is the definition of lower GI bleeding?	Bleeding distal to the ligament of Treitz; vast majority occurs in the colon
What are the symptoms?	**Hematochezia (bright red blood per rectum [BRBPR])**, with or without abdominal pain, melena, anorexia, fatigue, syncope, shortness of breath, shock
What are the signs?	BRBPR, positive hemoccult, abdominal tenderness, hypovolemic shock, orthostasis
What are the causes?	Diverticulosis (usually **right** sided in severe hemorrhage), vascular ectasia, colon cancer, hemorrhoids, trauma, hereditary hemorrhagic telangiectasia, intussusception, volvulus, ischemic colitis, IBD (especially ulcerative colitis), anticoagulation, rectal cancer, Meckel's diverticulum (with ectopic gastric mucosa), stercoral ulcer (ulcer from hard stool), infectious colitis, aortoenteric fistula, chemotherapy, irradiation injury, infarcted bowel, strangulated hernia, anal fissure
What medicines should be looked for causally with a lower GI bleed?	Coumadin®, aspirin, Plavix®
What are the most common causes of massive lower GI bleeding?	1. Diverticulosis 2. Vascular ectasia
What lab tests should be performed?	CBC, Chem-7, PT/PTT, type and cross
What is the initial treatment?	IVFs: Lactated Ringer's; packed red blood cells as needed, IV × 2, Foley catheter to follow urine output, discontinue aspirin, NGT

What diagnostic tests should be performed for all lower GI bleeds?

History, physical exam, NGT aspiration (to rule out UGI bleeding; bile or blood must be seen; otherwise, perform EGD), anoscopy/proctoscopic exam

What must be ruled out in patients with lower GI bleeding?

Upper GI bleeding! Remember, NGT aspiration is not 100% accurate (even if you get bile without blood)

How can you have a UGI bleed with only clear succus back in the NGT?

Duodenal bleeding ulcer can bleed distal to the pylorus with the NGT sucking normal nonbloody gastric secretions! **If there is any question, perform EGD**

What would an algorithm for diagnosing and treating lower GI bleeding look like?

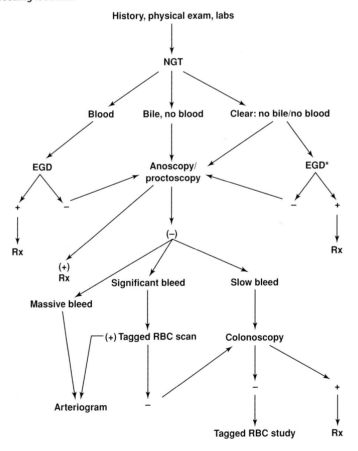

*Based on clinical suspicion

What is the diagnostic test of choice for localizing a slow to moderate lower GI bleeding source?	Colonoscopy
What test is performed to localize bleeding if there is too much active bleeding to see the source with a colonoscope?	A-gram (mesenteric angiography)
What is more sensitive for a slow, intermittent amount of blood loss: A-gram or tagged RBC study?	Radiolabeled RBC scan is more sensitive for blood loss at a rate of ≥0.5 mL/min or intermittent blood loss because it has a longer half-life (for arteriography, bleeding rate must be ≥1.0 mL/min)
What is the treatment if bleeding site is KNOWN and massive or recurrent lower GI bleeding continues?	Segmental resection of the bowel
What is the surgical treatment of massive lower GI bleeding WITHOUT localization?	Exploratory laparotomy with intraoperative enteroscopy and total abdominal colectomy as last resort
What percentage of cases spontaneously stops bleeding?	80% to 90% stop bleeding with resuscitative measures only (at least temporarily)
What percentage of patients requires emergent surgery for lower GI bleeding?	Only ≈10%
Does melena always signify active colonic bleeding?	NO—the colon is very good at storing material and often will store melena/maroon stools and pass them days later (follow patient, UO, HCT, and vital signs)
What is the therapeutic advantage of doing a colonoscopy?	Options of injecting substance (epinephrine) or coagulating vessels is an advantage with C-scope to control bleeding
What is the therapeutic advantage of doing an A-gram?	Ability to inject vasopressin and/or embolization, with at least temporary control of bleeding in >85%

RAPID-FIRE REVIEW

Name the diagnostic modality:

45-year-old male with dark blood per rectum	NGT aspiration to evaluate for upper GI bleed (if blood, then EGD; if bile and no blood, then workup for lower GI bleed)
45-year-old male with significant massive blood per rectum; NGT reveals bile and no blood	Angiography to find lower GI source

Chapter 50 | Inflammatory Bowel Disease: Crohn's Disease and Ulcerative Colitis

What is IBD?	Inflammatory Bowel Disease, inflammatory disease of the GI tract
What are the two inflammatory bowel diseases?	Crohn's disease and ulcerative colitis
How can the extraintestinal manifestations be remembered?	Think of the acronym **"A PIE SACK"**: Aphthous ulcers Pyoderma gangrenosum Iritis Erythema nodosum Sclerosing cholangitis Arthritis, Ankylosing spondylitis Clubbing of fingers Kidney (amyloid deposits, nephrotic syndrome)

COMPARISON OF CROHN'S DISEASE AND ULCERATIVE COLITIS

Incidence

Crohn's disease:

Incidence	3–6/100,000
At-risk population	High in the Jewish population, low in the African American population, similar rates between African American and US White populations
Sex	Female > male
Distribution	Bimodal distribution (i.e., two peaks in incidence): peak incidence at 25 to 40 years of age; second bimodal distribution peak at 50 to 65 years of age

Ulcerative colitis:

Incidence	10/100,000
At-risk population	High in the Jewish population, low in the African American population Positive family history in 20% of cases
Sex	Male > female

Distribution	Bimodal distribution at 20 to 35 and 50 to 65 years of age

Initial Symptoms

Crohn's disease?	**Abdominal pain**, **diarrhea**, fever, weight loss, anal disease
Ulcerative colitis?	**Bloody diarrhea** (hallmark), fever, weight loss

Anatomic Distribution

Crohn's disease?	Classic phrasing **"mouth to anus"** Small bowel only (20%) Small bowel and colon (40%) Colon only (30%)
Ulcerative colitis?	Colon only (Think: ulcerative **COL**itis = **COL**on alone)

Route of Spread

Crohn's disease?	Small bowel, colon, or both with **"skip areas"** of normal bowel; hence, the name "regional enteritis"
Ulcerative colitis?	Almost always involves the rectum and spreads proximally always in a continuous route without "skip areas"
What is "backwash" ileitis?	Mild inflammation of the terminal ileum in ulcerative colitis; thought to be "backwash" of inflammatory mediators from the colon into the terminal ileum

Bowel Wall Involvement

Crohn's disease?	Full thickness (transmural involvement)
Ulcerative colitis?	Mucosa/submucosa only

Anal Involvement

Crohn's disease?	Common (fistulae, abscesses, fissures, ulcers)
Ulcerative colitis?	Uncommon

Rectal Involvement

Crohn's disease?	Rare
Ulcerative colitis?	100%

Mucosal Findings

Crohn's disease (6)?	1. Aphthoid ulcers 2. Granulomas 3. Linear ulcers 4. Transverse fissures 5. Swollen mucosa 6. **Full-thickness wall involvement**
Ulcerative colitis (5)?	1. Granular, flat mucosa 2. Ulcers 3. **Crypt abscess** 4. Dilated mucosal vessels 5. **Pseudopolyps**
How can ulcerative colitis and Crohn's anal and wall involvement be remembered?	"CAT URP": Crohn's = **A**nal—**T**ransmural UC = **R**ectum—**P**artial wall thickness

Diagnostic Tests

Crohn's disease?	Colonoscopy with biopsy, barium enema, UGI with small bowel follow-through, stool cultures
Ulcerative colitis?	Colonoscopy, barium enema, UGI with small bowel follow-through (to look for Crohn's disease), stool cultures

Complications

Crohn's disease?	**Anal** fistula/abscess, **fistula**, stricture, perforation, **abscesses**, toxic megacolon, colovesical fistula, enterovaginal fistula, hemorrhage, **obstruction**, cancer
Ulcerative colitis?	**Cancer, toxic megacolon**, **colonic perforation**, **hemorrhage**, strictures, obstruction, complications of surgery

Cancer Risk

Crohn's disease?	Overall increased risk, but about half that of ulcerative colitis
Ulcerative colitis?	≈5% risk of developing colon cancer at 10 years; then, risk increases ≈1% per year; thus, an incidence of ≈20% after 20 years of the disease (30% at 30 years)

Incidence of Toxic Megacolon

Crohn's disease?	≈5%
Ulcerative colitis?	≈10%

Indications for Surgery

Crohn's disease?	Obstruction, massive bleeding, fistula, perforation, suspicion of cancer, abscess (refractory to medical treatment), toxic megacolon (refractory to medical treatment), strictures, dysplasia
Ulcerative colitis?	Toxic megacolon (refractory to medical treatment); cancer prophylaxis; massive bleeding; failure of child to mature because of disease and steroids; perforation; suspicion of or documented cancer; acute severe symptoms refractory to medical treatment; inability to wean off chronic steroids; obstruction; dysplasia; stricture
What are the common surgical options for ulcerative colitis?	1. Total proctocolectomy, distal rectal mucosectomy, and ileoanal pull through 2. Total proctocolectomy and Brooke ileostomy
What is "toxic megacolon"?	**Toxic** patient: sepsis, febrile, abdominal pain **Megacolon:** acutely and massively distended colon

Medical Treatment of IBD

What are the medication options for treating IBD?	**Sulfasalazine**, mesalamine (5-aminosalicylic acid) **Steroids,** metronidazole (Flagyl®), azathioprine, 6-mercaptopurine (6-mp), infliximab
Which medications are used for Crohn's Disease but not ulcerative colitis?	Methotrexate, Antibiotics (e.g., Flagyl®/Cipro®)
What are infliximab, adalimumab, certolizumab, natalizumab?	Monoclonal antibodies versus TNF-α (tumor necrosis factor-alpha)

RAPID-FIRE REVIEW

Name the most likely diagnosis:

24-year-old male with ulcerative colitis receives Lomotil® for excessive diarrhea and develops fever, abdominal pain and tenderness, and a massively dilated colon on abdominal x-ray	Toxic megacolon

28-year-old male with nonbloody diarrhea, low-grade fever, abdominal pain, perirectal abscesses, perianal fistulae

Crohn's disease

Chapter 51 | Liver

ANATOMY

Identify the arterial branches of the celiac trunk:

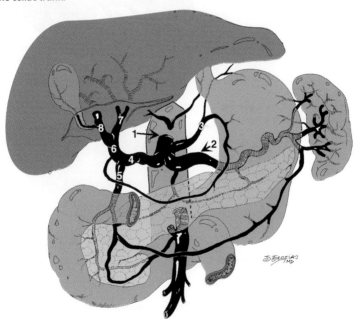

1. Celiac trunk
2. Splenic artery
3. Left gastric artery
4. Common hepatic artery
5. Gastroduodenal artery
6. Proper hepatic artery
7. Left hepatic artery
8. Right hepatic artery

What is the venous supply?	**Portal vein** (formed from the splenic vein and the superior mesenteric vein)
What is the hepatic venous drainage?	Via the hepatic veins, which drain into the IVC (three veins: left, middle, and right)
What sources provide oxygen to the liver?	Portal vein blood—50% Hepatic artery blood—50%
From what sources does the liver receive blood?	Portal system—75% Hepatic artery system—25%

Identify the segments of the liver (French system)

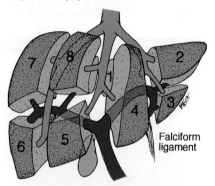

What is the overall arrangement of the segments in the liver?	Clockwise, starting at segment 1

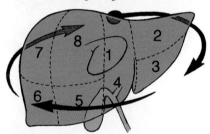

What is the maximum amount of liver that can be resected while retaining adequate liver function?	>80% (Remember Prometheus!)
What is Child's class? (Child–Turcotte–Pugh)	Classification system that estimates hepatic reserve in patients with hepatic failure and mortality
How can the criteria comprising the modified Child's classification be remembered?	Use the acronym: "**A BEAP**": **A**scites **B**ilirubin **E**ncephalopathy **A**lbumin **P**T (prothrombin time)

Define Child's classification:	Ascites	Bili	Enceph	ALB	PT INR
A	none	<2	none	>3.5	<1.7
B	controlled	2–3	minimal	2.8–3.5	1.7–2.2
C	uncontrolled	>3	severe	<2.8	>2.2

(Think: As in a letter grading system, A is better than B, B is better than C)

What is the operative mortality for a portacaval shunt versus overall intra-abdominal operations with cirrhosis in the following Child's classes?

A   <5% versus overall = 10%

B   <15% versus overall = 30%

C   ≈33% versus overall = 75%

What does the MELD score stand for?   Model for End-stage Liver Disease

What is measured in the MELD score?   INR, total bilirubin, serum creatinine (SCR); find good MELD calculators online

What is the mortality in cirrhotic patients for nonemergent nontransplant surgery?   Increase in mortality by 1% per 1 point in the MELD score until 20, then 2% for each MELD point

What is the mortality in cirrhotic patients for emergent nontransplant surgery?   14% increase in mortality per 1 point of the MELD score

TUMORS OF THE LIVER

What is the most common liver cancer?   **Metastatic disease** outnumbers primary tumors 20:1; primary site is usually the GI tract

What is the most common primary malignant liver tumor?   Hepatocellular carcinoma (hepatoma)

What is the most common primary benign liver tumor?   Hemangioma

What lab tests comprise the workup for liver metastasis?   LFTs (AST and alkaline phosphatase are most useful), CEA for suspected primary colon cancer

What are the associated imaging studies?   CT scan, U/S, A-gram

What is a right hepatic lobectomy?   Removal of the right lobe of the liver (i.e., all tissue to the right of Cantlie's line is removed)

What is a left hepatic lobectomy?	Removal of the left lobe of the liver (i.e., removal of all the liver tissue to the left of Cantlie's line)
What is a right trisegmentectomy?	Removal of all the liver tissue to the right of the falciform ligament
What chemical exposures are risk factors for angiosarcoma?	**Vinyl chloride**, arsenic, Thorotrast contrast

Hepatocellular Adenoma

What is it?	Benign liver tumor
Describe the histology:	Normal hepatocytes without bile ducts
What are the associated risk factors?	Women, birth control pills (Think: **ABC** = **A**denoma **B**irth **C**ontrol), anabolic steroids, glycogen storage disease
What is the average age of occurrence?	30 to 35 years of age
What are the signs/symptoms?	RUQ pain/mass, RUQ fullness, bleeding (rare)
What are the possible complications?	Rupture with bleeding (33%), necrosis, pain, risk of hepatocellular carcinoma
How is the diagnosis made?	CT scan, U/S, ± biopsy (rule out hemangioma with RBC-tagged scan!)
What is the treatment?	
Small	Stop birth control pills—it may regress; if not, surgical resection is necessary
Large (>5 cm), bleeding, painful, or ruptured	Surgical resection

Focal Nodular Hyperplasia (FNH)

What is it?	Benign liver tumor

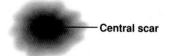

(Seen on CT and/or MRI)

Central scar

What is the histology?	Normal hepatocytes and bile ducts (adenoma has no bile ducts)
What is the average age of occurrence?	≈40 years

What are the associated risk factors?	Female gender
Are the tumors associated with birth control pills?	Yes, but not as clearly associated as with adenoma
How is the diagnosis made?	Nuclear technetium-99 study, U/S, CT scan, A-gram, biopsy
What is the classic CT scan finding?	Liver mass with **"central scar"** (Think: focal = central)
Is there a cancer risk with FNH?	No (there is a cancer risk with adenoma)
What is the treatment?	Resection or **embolization** if patient is symptomatic; otherwise, follow if diagnosis is confirmed; stop birth control pills

Hepatic Hemangioma

What is it?	Benign vascular tumor of the liver
What is its claim to fame?	Most common primary benign liver tumor (up to 7% of population)
What are the signs/symptoms?	RUQ pain/mass, bruits
What are the possible complications?	Pain, congestive heart failure, coagulopathy, obstructive jaundice, gastric outlet obstruction, Kasabach–Merritt syndrome, hemorrhage (rare)
What is Kasabach–Merritt syndrome?	Hemangioma **and** thrombocytopenia and fibrinogenopenia
How is the diagnosis made?	CT scan with IV contrast, tagged red blood scan, MRI, U/S
Should biopsy be performed?	No (risk of hemorrhage with biopsy)
What is the treatment?	**Observation** (>90%)
What are the indications for resection?	Symptoms, hemorrhage, cannot make a diagnosis

Hepatocellular Carcinoma

What is it?	Most common primary malignancy of the liver
By what name is it also known?	Hepatoma
What is its incidence?	Accounts for 80% of all primary malignant liver tumors
What are the associated risk factors?	Hepatitis B virus, cirrhosis, aflatoxin

What percentage of patients with cirrhosis will develop hepatocellular carcinoma?	≈5%
What are the signs/symptoms?	Dull RUQ pain, hepatomegaly (classic presentation: **painful hepatomegaly**)
What tests should be ordered?	U/S, CT scan, angiography, tumor marker elevation
What is the tumor marker?	Elevated α-fetoprotein
What is the most common way to get a tissue diagnosis?	Needle biopsy with CT scan, U/S, or laparoscopic guidance
What is the most common site of metastasis?	Lungs
What is the treatment of hepatocellular carcinoma?	Surgical resection, if possible (e.g., lobectomy); liver transplant
What are the treatment options if the patient is not a surgical candidate?	Percutaneous ethanol tumor injection, cryotherapy, and intra-arterial chemotherapy
What are the indications for liver transplantation?	Cirrhosis and NO resection candidacy as well as no distant or lymph node metastases and no vascular invasion; the tumor must be single, <5-cm tumor or have three nodules, with none >3 cm
What is the prognosis under the following conditions?	
Unresectable	Almost none survive 1 year
Resectable	≈35% are alive at 5 years
Which subtype has the best prognosis?	Fibrolamellar hepatoma (young adults)

ABSCESSES OF THE LIVER

What is a liver abscess?	Abscess (collection of pus) in the liver parenchyma
What are the types of liver abscess?	Pyogenic (bacterial), parasitic (amebic), fungal
What are the two most common types?	**Bacterial** (most common in the United States) and amebic (most common worldwide)

Bacterial Liver Abscess

What are the three most common bacterial organisms affecting the liver?	Gram negatives: *Escherichia coli*, *Klebsiella*, and *Proteus*

What are the most common sources/causes of bacterial liver abscesses?	Cholangitis, diverticulitis, liver cancer, liver metastasis
What are the signs/symptoms?	**Fever, chills, RUQ pain,** leukocytosis, increased liver function tests (LFTs), jaundice, sepsis, weight loss
What is the treatment?	IV antibiotics (triple antibiotics with metronidazole), percutaneous drainage with CT scan or U/S guidance
What are the indications for operative drainage?	Multiple/loculated abscesses or if multiple percutaneous attempts have failed

Amebic Liver Abscess

What is the etiology?	*Entamoeba histolytica* (typically reaches liver via portal vein from intestinal amebiasis)
How does it spread?	Fecal–oral transmission
What are the risk factors?	Patients from countries south of the United States–Mexican border, institutionalized patients, homosexual men, alcoholic patients
What are the signs/symptoms?	RUQ pain, fever, hepatomegaly, diarrhea
	Note: Chills are much less common with amebic abscesses than with pyogenic abscesses
What is the classic description of abscess contents?	"Anchovy paste" pus
How is the diagnosis made?	Lab tests, U/S, CT scan
What lab tests should be performed?	Indirect hemagglutination titers for *Entamoeba* antibodies elevated in >95% of cases, elevated LFTs
What is the treatment?	Metronidazole IV
What are the indications for percutaneous surgical drainage?	Refractory to metronidazole, bacterial coinfection, or peritoneal rupture

Hydatid Liver Cyst

What is it?	Usually a right lobe cyst filled with *Echinococcus granulosus*
What are the risk factors?	Travel; exposure to dogs, sheep, and cattle (carriers)
What are the signs/symptoms?	RUQ abdominal pain, jaundice, RUQ mass

How is the diagnosis made?	Indirect hemagglutination antibody test (serologic testing), Casoni skin test, U/S, CT scan, radiographic imaging
What are the findings on AXR?	Possible calcified outline of cyst
What are the major risks?	Erosion into the pleural cavity, pericardial sac, or biliary tree Rupture into the peritoneal cavity causing fatal anaphylaxis
What is the risk of surgical removal of echinococcal (hydatid) cysts?	Rupture or leakage of cyst contents into the abdomen may cause a fatal anaphylactic reaction
When should percutaneous drainage be performed?	Never; may cause leaking into the peritoneal cavity and anaphylaxis
What is the treatment?	Mebendazole, followed by surgical resection; large cysts can be drained and then injected with toxic irrigant (scoliocide) into the cyst unless aspirate is bilious (which means there is a biliary connection) followed by cyst removal
Which toxic irrigations are used?	Hypertonic saline, ethanol, or cetrimide

HEMOBILIA

What is it?	Blood draining via the common bile duct into the duodenum
What is the diagnostic triad?	Triad: 1. RUQ pain 2. Guaiac positive/upper GI bleeding 3. Jaundice
What are the causes?	Trauma with liver laceration, percutaneous transhepatic cholangiography (PTC), tumors
How is the diagnosis made?	EGD (blood out of the ampulla of Vater), A-gram
What is the treatment?	A-gram with embolization of the bleeding vessel
What is bilhemia?	Seen after trauma, connection of bile ducts and venous system, resulting in rapid and very elevated serum bilirubin

Chapter 52 | Portal Hypertension

Where does the portal vein begin?

At the confluence of the splenic vein and the SMV

What are the six potential routes of portal–systemic collateral blood flow (as seen with portal hypertension)?

1. Umbilical vein
2. Coronary vein to esophageal venous plexuses
3. Retroperitoneal veins (veins of Retzius)
4. Diaphragm veins (veins of Sappey)
5. Superior hemorrhoidal vein to middle and inferior hemorrhoidal veins and then to the iliac vein
6. Splenic veins to the short gastric veins

What is the pathophysiology of portal hypertension?

Elevated portal pressure resulting from resistance to portal flow

What is the etiology?

Prehepatic—Thrombosis of portal vein/ atresia of portal vein

Hepatic—**Cirrhosis** (distortion of normal parenchyma by regenerating hepatic nodules), hepatocellular carcinoma, fibrosis

Posthepatic—Budd–Chiari syndrome: thrombosis of hepatic veins

What is the most common cause of portal hypertension in the United States?

Cirrhosis (>90% of cases)

How many patients with alcoholism develop cirrhosis?

Surprisingly, <1 in 5

What percentage of patients with cirrhosis develops esophageal varices?

≈40%

How many patients with cirrhosis develop portal hypertension?

≈2/3

What is the most common physical finding in patients with portal hypertension?

Splenomegaly (spleen enlargement)

What are the four associated CLINICAL findings in portal hypertension?

1. Esophageal varices
2. Splenomegaly
3. Caput medusae (engorgement of periumbilical veins)
4. Hemorrhoids

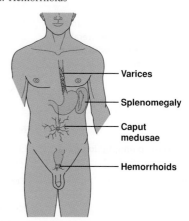

What other physical findings are associated with cirrhosis and portal hypertension?

Spider angioma, palmar erythema, ascites, truncal obesity and peripheral wasting, encephalopathy, asterixis (liver flap), gynecomastia, jaundice

What is the name of the periumbilical bruit heard with caput medusae?

Cruveilhier–Baumgarten bruit

What constitutes the portal–systemic collateral circulation in portal hypertension in the following conditions?

Esophageal varices

Coronary vein backing up into the azygos system

Caput medusae

Umbilical vein (via falciform ligament) draining into the epigastric veins

Retroperitoneal varices

Small mesenteric veins (veins of Retzius) draining retroperitoneally into lumbar veins

Hemorrhoids

Superior hemorrhoidal vein (which normally drains into the inferior mesenteric vein) backing up into the middle and inferior hemorrhoidal veins

What is the etiology?

Cirrhosis (90%), schistosomiasis, hepatitis, Budd–Chiari syndrome, hemochromatosis, Wilson's disease, portal vein thrombosis, tumors, splenic vein thrombosis

What is Budd–Chiari syndrome?	Thrombosis of the hepatic veins
What is the most feared complication of portal hypertension?	Bleeding from esophageal varices
What are esophageal varices?	Engorgement of the esophageal venous plexuses secondary to increased collateral blood flow from the portal system as a result of portal hypertension
What is the "rule of 2/3" of portal hypertension?	2/3 of patients with cirrhosis will develop portal hypertension 2/3 of patients with portal hypertension will develop esophageal varices 2/3 of patients with esophageal varices will bleed from the varices
In patients with cirrhosis and known varices who are suffering from upper GI bleeding, how often does that bleeding result from varices?	Only ≈50% of the time
What are the signs/symptoms?	Hematemesis, melena, hematochezia
What is the initial treatment of variceal bleeding?	As with all upper GI bleeding: large-bore IVs × 2, IV fluid, Foley catheter, type and cross blood, send labs, correct coagulopathy (vitamin K, fresh frozen plasma), ± intubation to protect from aspiration
What is the diagnostic test of choice?	**EGD (upper GI endoscopy)** Remember, **bleeding** is the result of varices only half the time; must rule out ulcers, gastritis, etc.
If esophageal varices cause bleeding, what are the EGD treatment options?	1. **Emergent endoscopic sclerotherapy:** a sclerosing substance is injected into the esophageal varices under direct endoscopic vision 2. **Endoscopic band ligation:** elastic band ligation of varices
What are the pharmacologic options?	**Somatostatin** (octreotide) or **IV vasopressin** (and nitroglycerin, to avoid MI) to achieve vasoconstriction of the mesenteric vessels; if bleeding continues, consider balloon (**Sengstaken–Blakemore tube**) tamponade of the varices, β-blocker
What is a Sengstaken–Blakemore tube?	Tube with a gastric and esophageal balloon for tamponading an esophageal bleed
What is the next therapy after the bleeding is controlled?	Repeat endoscopic sclerotherapy/banding

What are the options if sclerotherapy and conservative methods fail to stop the variceal bleeding or bleeding recurs?

Repeat sclerotherapy/banding and treat conservatively
TIPS
Surgical shunt (selective or partial)
Liver transplantation

What does the acronym TIPS stand for?

Transjugular **I**ntrahepatic **P**ortosystemic **S**hunt

What is a TIPS procedure?

Angiographic radiologist places a small tube stent intrahepatically between the hepatic vein and a branch of the portal vein via a percutaneous jugular vein route

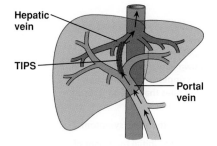

What is a Warren shunt?

Distal splenorenal shunt with ligation of the coronary vein—elective shunt procedure associated with low incidence of encephalopathy in patients postoperatively because only the splenic flow is diverted to decompress the varices

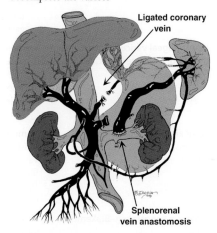

What is the most common perioperative cause of death following shunt procedure?

Hepatic failure, secondary to decreased blood flow (accounts for 2/3 of deaths)

What is the major postoperative morbidity after a shunt procedure?

Increased incidence of hepatic encephalopathy because of decreased portal blood flow to the liver and decreased clearance of toxins/metabolites from the blood

What medication is infused to counteract the coronary artery vasoconstriction of IV vasopressin?

Nitroglycerin IV drip

What lab value roughly correlates with degree of encephalopathy?

Serum ammonia level (*Note:* Thought to correlate with but not cause encephalopathy)

What medications are used to treat hepatic encephalopathy?

Lactulose PO, with or without neomycin PO

RAPID-FIRE REVIEW

Name the most likely diagnosis:

39-year-old male with caput medusae, hemorrhoids, and splenomegaly

Portal hypertension

Chapter 53 | Biliary Tract

ANATOMY

Name structures 1 through 8 of the biliary tract:

1. Intrahepatic ducts
2. Left hepatic duct
3. Right hepatic duct
4. Common hepatic duct
5. Gallbladder
6. Cystic duct
7. Common bile duct
8. Ampulla of Vater

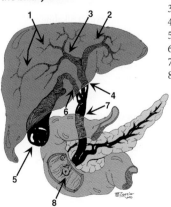

What is the name of the node in Calot's triangle?	Calot's node
What are the small ducts that drain bile directly into the gallbladder from the liver?	Ducts of Luschka
Which artery is susceptible to injury during cholecystectomy?	Right hepatic artery, because of its proximity to the cystic artery and Calot's triangle
Where is the infundibulum of the gallbladder?	Near the cystic duct
Where is the fundus of the gallbladder?	At the end of the gallbladder
What are the boundaries of the triangle of Calot?	**"Three Cs":** 1. **C**ystic duct 2. **C**ommon hepatic duct 3. **C**ystic artery

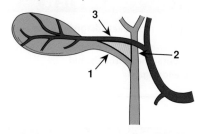

"Dr. Blackbourne, are you absolutely sure that the triangle of Calot includes the cystic artery and not the liver edge?"	Yes, look up *Gastroenterology* 2002;123(5): 1440

PHYSIOLOGY

What is the source of alkaline phosphatase?	Bile duct epithelium; expect alkaline phosphatase to be elevated in bile duct obstruction
What is in bile?	Cholesterol, lecithin (phospholipid), bile acids, and bilirubin
What does bile do?	Emulsifies fats
What is the enterohepatic circulation?	Circulation of bile acids from liver to gut and back to the liver
Where are most of the bile acids absorbed?	In the terminal ileum

What stimulates gallbladder emptying?	Cholecystokinin and vagal input
What is the source of cholecystokinin?	Duodenal mucosal cells
What are its actions?	Gallbladder emptying Opening of ampulla of Vater Slowing of gastric emptying Pancreas acinar cell growth and release of exocrine products

PATHOPHYSIOLOGY

At what level of serum total bilirubin does one start to get jaundiced?	2.5
Classically, what is thought to be the anatomic location where one first finds evidence of jaundice?	Under the tongue (ultraviolet light breaks down bilirubin at other sites!)
What are the signs and symptoms of obstructive jaundice?	Jaundice Dark urine Clay-colored stools (acholic stools) Pruritus (itching) Loss of appetite Nausea
What causes the itching in obstructive jaundice?	Bile salts in the dermis (not bilirubin!)
Define the following terms:	
Cholelithiasis	Gallstones in gallbladder

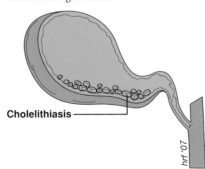

Cholelithiasis

hrf '07

Choledocholithiasis   Gallstone in common bile duct

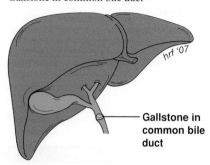

Gallstone in common bile duct

Cholecystitis   Inflammation of gallbladder

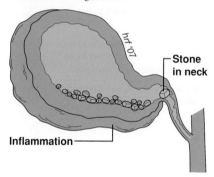

Stone in neck

Inflammation

Cholangitis	Infection of biliary tract
Cholangiocarcinoma	Adenocarcinoma of bile ducts
Klatskin's tumor	Cholangiocarcinoma of bile duct at the junction of the right and left hepatic ducts
Biliary colic	Pain from gallstones, usually from a stone at cystic duct Pain is located in the RUQ, epigastrium, or right subscapular region of the back Usually lasts minutes to hours but eventually goes away; it is often postprandial, especially after fatty foods
Biloma	Intraperitoneal bile fluid collection
Choledochojejunostomy	Anastomosis between common bile duct and jejunum
Hepaticojejunostomy	Anastomosis of hepatic ducts or common hepatic duct to jejunum

DIAGNOSTIC STUDIES

What is the initial diagnostic study of choice for evaluation of the biliary tract/gallbladder/cholelithiasis?

U/S!

Define the following diagnostic studies:

ERCP

Endoscopic Retrograde CholangioPancreatography

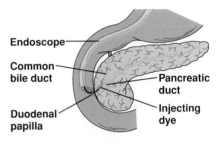

PTC

Percutaneous Transhepatic Cholangiogram

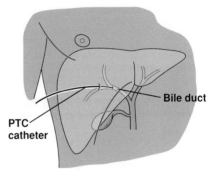

IOC

IntraOperative Cholangiogram (done laparoscopically or open to rule out choledocholithiasis)

HIDA/PRIDA scan

Radioisotope study; isotope concentrated in liver and secreted into bile; will demonstrate cholecystitis, bile leak, or CBD obstruction

How does the HIDA scan reveal cholecystitis?

Nonopacification of the gallbladder from obstruction of the cystic duct

BILIARY SURGERY

What is a cholecystectomy?

Removal of the gallbladder laparoscopically or through a standard Kocher incision

What is a "lap chole"?

LAParoscopic **CHOLE**cystectomy

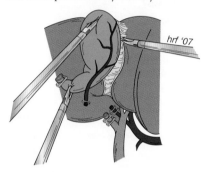

hrf '07

What is a sphincterotomy?

Cut through sphincter of Oddi to allow passage of gallstones from the common bile duct; most often done at ERCP; a.k.a. "papillotomy"

How should postoperative biloma be treated after a lap chole?

1. Percutaneous drain bile collection
2. ERCP with placement of biliary stent past leak (usually cystic duct remnant leak)

What is the treatment of major CBD injury after a lap chole?

Choledochojejunostomy

OBSTRUCTIVE JAUNDICE

What is it?

Jaundice (hyperbilirubinemia >2.5) from obstruction of bile flow to the duodenum

What is the differential diagnosis of *proximal* bile duct obstruction?

Cholangiocarcinoma
Lymphadenopathy
Metastatic tumor
Gallbladder carcinoma
Sclerosing cholangitis
Gallstones
Tumor embolus
Parasites
Postsurgical stricture
Hepatoma
Benign bile duct tumor

What is the differential diagnosis of DISTAL bile duct obstruction?	Choledocholithiasis (**gallstones**) Pancreatic carcinoma Pancreatitis Ampullary carcinoma Lymphadenopathy Pseudocyst Postsurgical stricture Ampulla of Vater dysfunction/stricture Lymphoma Benign bile duct tumor Parasites
What is the initial study of choice for obstructive jaundice?	U/S
What lab results are associated with obstructive jaundice?	Elevated alkaline phosphatase, elevated bilirubin with or without elevated LFTs

CHOLELITHIASIS

What is it?	Formation of gallstones
What is the incidence?	≈10% of US population will develop gallstones
What are the "Big 4" risk factors?	"**Four Fs**": **F**emale **F**at **F**orty **F**ertile (multiparity)
What are the types of stones?	Cholesterol stones (75%) Pigment stones (25%)
What are the types of pigmented stones?	Black stones (contain calcium bilirubinate) Brown stones (associated with biliary tract infection)
What are the causes of black-pigmented stones?	Cirrhosis, hemolysis
What is the pathogenesis of cholesterol stones?	Secretion of bile **supersaturated** with cholesterol (relatively decreased amounts of lecithin and bile salts); then, cholesterol precipitates out and forms solid crystals, then gallstones
What are the signs and symptoms?	Symptoms: biliary colic, cholangitis, choledocholithiasis, gallstone, pancreatitis
Is biliary colic pain really "colic"?	No, symptoms usually last for hours; therefore, colic is a misnomer!
What percentage of patients with gallstones is ASYMPTOMATIC?	80% of patients with cholelithiasis are asymptomatic!

What is thought to cause biliary colic?	Gallbladder contraction against a stone temporarily at the gallbladder/cystic duct junction; a stone in the cystic duct; or a stone passing through the cystic duct
What are the five major complications of gallstones?	1. Acute cholecystitis 2. Choledocholithiasis 3. Gallstone pancreatitis 4. Gallstone ileus 5. Cholangitis
How is cholelithiasis diagnosed?	History Physical examination **U/S**
How often does U/S detect choledocholithiasis?	≈33% of the time… not a very good study for choledocholithiasis!
How are symptomatic or complicated cases of cholelithiasis treated?	By cholecystectomy
What are the possible complications of a lap chole?	Common bile duct injury; right hepatic duct/artery injury; cystic duct leak; biloma (collection of bile)
What are the indications for cholecystectomy in the asymptomatic patient?	Sickle cell disease Calcified gallbladder (porcelain gallbladder) Patient is a child
What is choledocholithiasis?	Gallstones in the common bile duct
What is the management of choledocholithiasis?	1. ERCP with papillotomy and basket/balloon retrieval of stones (pre- or postoperatively) 2. Laparoscopic transcystic duct or trans common bile duct retrieval 3. Open common bile duct exploration
What medication may dissolve a cholesterol gallstone?	Chenodeoxycholic acid, ursodeoxycholic acid (Actigall®); but, if medication is stopped, gallstones often recur
What is the major feared complication of ERCP?	Pancreatitis

ACUTE CHOLECYSTITIS

What is the pathogenesis of acute cholecystitis?	Obstruction of cystic duct leads to inflammation of the gallbladder; ≈95% of cases result from calculi, and ≈5% from acalculous obstruction
What are the risk factors?	Gallstones

What are the signs and symptoms?	**Unrelenting** RUQ pain or tenderness **Fever** Nausea/vomiting Painful palpable gallbladder in 33% Positive Murphy's sign Right subscapular pain (referred) Epigastric discomfort (referred)
What is Murphy's sign?	Acute pain and **inspiratory arrest** elicited by palpation of the RUQ during inspiration
What are the complications of acute cholecystitis?	Abscess Perforation Choledocholithiasis Cholecystenteric fistula formation Gallstone ileus

What lab results are associated with acute cholecystitis?	Increased WBC; may have:
	    Slight elevation in alkaline phosphatase, LFTs
	    Slight elevation in amylase, total bilirubin

What is the diagnostic test of choice for acute cholecystitis?	U/S
What are the signs of acute cholecystitis on U/S?	Thickened gallbladder wall (>3 mm) Pericholecystic fluid Distended gallbladder Gallstones present/cystic duct stone Sonographic Murphy's sign (pain on inspiration after placement of U/S probe over gallbladder)
What is the difference between acute cholecystitis and biliary colic?	Biliary colic has temporary pain; acute cholecystitis has pain that does not resolve, usually with elevated WBCs, fever, and signs of acute inflammation on U/S
What is the treatment of acute cholecystitis?	IVFs, antibiotics, and early cholecystectomy

ACUTE ACALCULOUS CHOLECYSTITIS

What is it?	Acute cholecystitis without evidence of stones
What is the pathogenesis?	It is believed to result from sludge and gallbladder disuse and **biliary stasis**, perhaps secondary to absence of cholecystokinin stimulation (decreased contraction of gallbladder)

What are the risk factors?	Prolonged fasting TPN Trauma Multiple transfusions Dehydration Often occurs in prolonged postoperative or ICU setting
What are the diagnostic tests of choice?	U/S; sludge and inflammation usually present with acute acalculous cholecystitis HIDA scan
What are the findings on HIDA scan?	Nonfilling of the gallbladder
What is the management of acute acalculous cholecystitis?	Cholecystectomy or cholecystostomy tube if the patient is unstable (placed percutaneously by radiology or open surgery)

CHOLANGITIS

What is it?	Bacterial infection of the biliary tract from obstruction (either partial or complete); potentially life-threatening
What are the common causes?	Choledocholithiasis Stricture (usually postoperative) Neoplasm (usually ampullary carcinoma) Extrinsic compression (pancreatic pseudocyst/pancreatitis) Instrumentation of the bile ducts (e.g., PTC/ERCP) Biliary stent
What is the most common cause of cholangitis?	Gallstones in common bile duct (choledocholithiasis)
What are the signs and symptoms?	**Charcot's triad:** 1. Fever/chills 2. RUQ pain 3. Jaundice

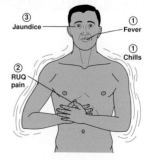

What is Reynold's pentad?	Charcot's triad PLUS: 4. Mental status changes 5. Shock
Which organisms are most commonly isolated with cholangitis?	Gram-negative organisms (*Escherichia coli, Klebsiella, Pseudomonas, Enterobacter, Proteus, Serratia*) are the most common
What are the diagnostic tests of choice?	U/S and contrast study (e.g., ERCP or IOC) after patient has "cooled off" with IV antibiotics
What is suppurative cholangitis?	Severe infection with sepsis—"pus under pressure"
What is the management of cholangitis?	**Nonsuppurative:** IVF and antibiotics, with definitive treatment later (e.g., lap chole ± ERCP) **Suppurative:** IVF, antibiotics, and decompression; decompression can be obtained by ERCP with papillotomy, PTC with catheter drainage, or laparotomy with T-tube placement

SCLEROSING CHOLANGITIS

What is it?	Multiple inflammatory fibrous thickenings of bile duct walls resulting in biliary strictures
What is its natural history?	Progressive obstruction possibly leading to cirrhosis and liver failure; 10% of patients will develop cholangiocarcinoma
What is the major risk factor?	Inflammatory bowel disease
What type of IBD is the most common risk factor?	Ulcerative colitis (≈66%)
What are the signs and symptoms of sclerosing cholangitis?	Same as those for obstructive jaundice: Jaundice Itching (pruritus) Dark urine Clay-colored stools Loss of energy Weight loss (Many patients are asymptomatic)
How is it diagnosed?	Elevated alkaline phosphatase, and PTC or ERCP revealing "beads on a string" appearance on contrast study

What are the management options?	Hepatoenteric anastomosis (if primarily extrahepatic ducts are involved) and resection of extrahepatic bile ducts because of the risk of cholangiocarcinoma Transplant (if primarily intrahepatic disease or cirrhosis) Endoscopic balloon dilations

GALLSTONE ILEUS

What is it?	Small bowel obstruction from a large gallstone (>2.5 cm) that has eroded through the gallbladder and into the duodenum/small bowel
What is the classic site of obstruction?	Ileocecal valve (but may cause obstruction in the duodenum, sigmoid colon)
What are the classic findings of gallstone ileus?	

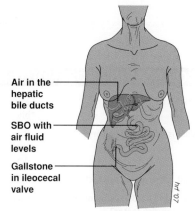

Air in the hepatic bile ducts

SBO with air fluid levels

Gallstone in ileocecal valve

What is the population at risk?	Gallstone ileus is most commonly seen in **women >70 years**
What are the signs/symptoms?	Symptoms of SBO: distention, vomiting, hypovolemia, RUQ pain
Gallstone ileus causes what percentage of cases of SBO?	<1%
What are the diagnostic tests of choice?	**Abdominal x-ray:** occasionally reveals radiopaque gallstone in the bowel; **40% of patients show air in the biliary tract**, small bowel distention, and air–fluid levels secondary to ileus UGI: used if diagnosis is in question; will show cholecystenteric fistula and the obstruction **Abdominal CT scan:** reveals air in biliary tract, SBO ± gallstone in intestine

What is the management?	Surgery: enterotomy with removal of the stone ± interval cholecystectomy (interval delayed)

CARCINOMA OF THE GALLBLADDER

What is it?	Malignant neoplasm arising in the gallbladder, vast majority are **adenocarcinoma (90%)**
What are the risk factors?	Gallstones, porcelain gallbladder, cholecystenteric fistula
What is a porcelain gallbladder?	Calcified gallbladder
What percentage of patients with a porcelain gallbladder will have gallbladder cancer?	≈50% (20%–60%)
What is the incidence?	≈1% of all gallbladder specimens
What are the symptoms?	Biliary colic, weight loss, anorexia; many patients are asymptomatic until late; may present as acute cholecystitis
What are the signs?	Jaundice (from invasion of the common duct or compression by involved pericholedochal lymph nodes), RUQ mass, palpable gallbladder (advanced disease)
What are the diagnostic tests of choice?	U/S, abdominal CT scan, ERCP
What is the route of spread?	Contiguous spread to the liver is most common
What is the management under the following conditions?	
Confined to mucosa	Cholecystectomy
Confined to muscularis/serosa	Radical cholecystectomy: cholecystectomy and wedge resection of overlying liver, and lymph node dissection ± chemotherapy/XRT
What is the main complication of a lap chole for gallbladder cancer?	Trocar site tumor implants (***Note:*** If known preoperatively, perform open cholecystectomy)
What is the prognosis for gallbladder cancer?	Dismal overall: <5% 5-year survival as most are unresectable at diagnosis T1 with cholecystectomy: 95% 5-year survival

CHOLANGIOCARCINOMA

What is it?	Malignancy of the extrahepatic or intrahepatic ducts—**primary bile duct cancer**
What is the histology?	Almost all are adenocarcinomas
Average age at diagnosis?	≈65 years, equally affects male/female
What are the signs and symptoms?	Those of biliary obstruction: jaundice, pruritus, dark urine, clay-colored stools, cholangitis
What is the most common location?	Proximal bile duct
What are the risk factors?	Choledochal cysts Ulcerative colitis Thorotrast contrast dye (used in 1950s) Sclerosing cholangitis Liver flukes (clonorchiasis) Toxin exposures (e.g., Agent Orange)
What is a Klatskin tumor?	Tumor that involves the junction of the right and left hepatic ducts

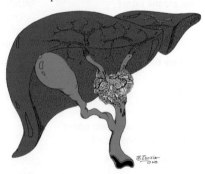

What are the diagnostic tests of choice?	U/S, CT scan, ERCP/PTC with biopsy/brushings for cytology, MRCP
What is an MRCP?	MRI with visualization of pancreatic and bile ducts
What is the management of proximal bile duct cholangiocarcinoma?	Resection with Roux-en-Y hepaticojejunostomy (anastomose bile ducts to jejunum) ± unilateral hepatic lobectomy
What is the management of distal common bile duct cholangiocarcinoma?	Whipple procedure

MISCELLANEOUS CONDITIONS

What is a porcelain gallbladder?	**Calcified gallbladder** seen on abdominal x-ray; results from chronic cholelithiasis/cholecystitis with calcified scar tissue in gallbladder wall; **cholecystectomy** required because of the strong association of **gallbladder carcinoma** with this condition
What is hydrops of the gallbladder?	Complete obstruction of the cystic duct by a gallstone, with filling of the gallbladder with fluid (not bile) from the gallbladder mucosa
What is Gilbert's syndrome?	Inborn error in liver bilirubin uptake and glucuronyl transferase resulting in hyperbilirubinemia (Think: **G**ilbert's = **G**lucuronyl)
What is Courvoisier's gallbladder?	Palpable, **nontender** gallbladder (unlike gallstone disease) associated with cancer of the head of the pancreas; able to distend because it has not been "scarred down" by gallstones
What is Mirizzi's syndrome?	Common hepatic duct obstruction as a result of **extrinsic** compression from a gallstone impacted in the cystic duct

RAPID-FIRE REVIEW

What is the correct diagnosis?

Elderly female with small bowel obstruction and air in the biliary tract	Gallstone ileus
38-year-old female with progressively worse RUQ pain and U/S reveals a thickened gallbladder wall, pericholecystic fluid, and a sonographic Murphy's sign	Acute cholecystitis
40-year-old s/p MVC with severe liver injury on hospital day 3 develops significant UGI bleed; EGD reveals no ulcer or gastritis	Hemobilia

Name the most likely diagnosis:

Lap chole POD #3, fever, RUQ fluid collection, no biliary dilation	Biloma (most common cause = cystic duct leak)

POD #7 following laparoscopic cholecystectomy—jaundice and dilated intrahepatic biliary ducts	Clipping or transection of common bile duct
33-year-old female with jaundice, fever, RUQ pain, hypotension, and confusion	Suppurative cholangitis
43-year-old female with RUQ pain and right subscapular pain for 2 hours intermittently over 4 months	Biliary colic
Name the diagnostic modality:	
22-year-old with RUQ pain with eating	U/S for cholelithiasis

Chapter 54 | Pancreas

Identify the regions of the pancreas:

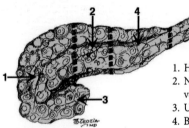

1. Head
2. Neck (in front of the superior mesenteric vein [SMV])
3. Uncinate process
4. Body
5. Tail

Why must the duodenum be removed if the head of the pancreas is removed?	They share the same blood supply (gastroduodenal artery)
What is the endocrine function of the pancreas?	Islets of Langerhans: α-cells: glucagon β-cells: insulin
What is the exocrine function of the pancreas?	Digestive enzymes: amylase, lipase, trypsin, chymotrypsin, carboxypeptidase
What maneuver is used to mobilize the duodenum and pancreas and evaluate the entire pancreas?	Kocher maneuver: Incise the lateral attachments of the duodenum and then lift the pancreas to examine the posterior surface

PANCREATITIS

Acute Pancreatitis

What is it?	Inflammation of the pancreas
What are the most common etiologies in the United States?	1. Alcohol abuse (50%) 2. Gallstones (30%) 3. Idiopathic (10%)
What is the acronym to remember all causes of pancreatitis?	"I GET SMASHED": 　Idiopathic 　Gallstones 　Ethanol 　Trauma 　Scorpion bite 　Mumps (viruses) 　Autoimmune 　Steroids 　Hyperlipidemia/Hypercalcemia 　ERCP 　Drugs
What are the symptoms?	Epigastric pain (frequently radiates to back); nausea and vomiting
What are the signs of pancreatitis?	Epigastric tenderness Diffuse abdominal tenderness Decreased bowel sounds (adynamic ileus) Fever Dehydration/shock
What lab tests should be ordered?	Amylase/lipase
What are the associated diagnostic findings?	Lab—High amylase, high lipase, high WBC AXR—Sentinel loop, colon cutoff, possibly gallstones (only 10% visible on x-ray) U/S—Phlegmon, cholelithiasis CT—Phlegmon, pancreatic necrosis
What is the most common sign of pancreatitis on AXR?	Sentinel loop(s)
What is the treatment?	NPO IVF NGT if vomiting Postpyloric tube feeds H2 blocker/PPI Analgesia (not morphine) Correction of coags/electrolytes ± Alcohol withdrawal prophylaxis "Tincture of time"

What are the possible complications?	Pseudocyst Abscess/infection Pancreatic necrosis Splenic/mesenteric/portal vessel rupture or thrombosis Pancreatic ascites/pancreatic pleural effusion Diabetes ARDS/sepsis/MOF Coagulopathy/DIC Encephalopathy Severe hypocalcemia
What is the prognosis?	Based on Ranson's criteria
Are postpyloric tube feeds safe in acute pancreatitis?	YES

What are Ranson's criteria for the following stages?

At presentation	1. Age >55 2. WBC >16,000 3. Glucose >200 4. AST >250 5. LDH >350
During the initial 48 hours	1. Base deficit >4 2. BUN increase >5 mg/dL 3. Fluid sequestration >6 L 4. Serum Ca^{2+} <8 5. Hct decrease >10% 6. PO_2 (ABG) <60 mm Hg (Amylase value is NOT one of Ranson's criteria!)

What is the mortality per positive criteria?

0 to 2	<5%
3 to 4	≈15%
5 to 6	≈40%
7 to 8	≈100%
How can the admission Ranson's criteria be remembered?	"**GA LAW** (Georgia law)": **G**lucose >200 **A**ge >55 **L**DH >350 **A**ST >250 **W**BC >16,000 ("Don't mess with the pancreas and don't mess with the Georgia law")

How can Ranson's criteria at less than 48 hours be remembered?

"C HOBBS (Calvin and Hobbes)":
Calcium <8 mg/dL

Hct drop of >10%
O_2 <60 (PaO_2)
Base deficit >4
BUN >5 increase
Sequestration >6 L

How can the AST versus LDH values in Ranson's criteria be remembered?

Alphabetically and numerically: A before L and 250 before 350
Therefore, AST >250 and LDH >350

What is the etiology of hypocalcemia with pancreatitis?

Fat saponification: fat necrosis binds to calcium

What complication is associated with splenic vein thrombosis?

Gastric varices (treatment with splenectomy)

Can TPN with lipids be given to a patient with pancreatitis?

Yes, if the patient does not suffer from hyperlipidemia (triglycerides >300)

What is the least common cause of acute pancreatitis (and possibly the most commonly asked cause on rounds!)?

Scorpion bite (found on the island of Trinidad)

Chronic Pancreatitis

What is it?

Chronic inflammation of the pancreas region causing destruction of the parenchyma, fibrosis, and calcification, resulting in loss of endocrine and exocrine tissue

What are the subtypes?

1. Chronic calcific pancreatitis
2. Chronic obstructive pancreatitis (5%)

What are the causes?

Alcohol abuse (most common; 70% of cases)
Idiopathic (15%)
Hypercalcemia (hyperparathyroidism)
Hyperlipidemia
Familial (found in families without any other risk factors)
Trauma
Iatrogenic
Gallstones

What are the symptoms?

Epigastric and/or back pain, weight loss, steatorrhea

What are the associated signs?

Type 1 diabetes mellitus (up to 1/3)
Steatorrhea (up to 1/4), weight loss

What are the signs of pancreatic exocrine insufficiency?

Steatorrhea (fat malabsorption from lipase insufficiency—stools float in water)
Malnutrition

What are the signs of pancreatic endocrine insufficiency?

Diabetes (glucose intolerance)

What are the common pain patterns?

Unrelenting pain
Recurrent pain

What is the differential diagnosis?

PUD, biliary tract disease, AAA, pancreatic cancer, angina

What percentage of patients with chronic pancreatitis has or will develop pancreatic cancer?

≈2%

What are the appropriate lab tests?

Amylase/lipase
72-hour fecal fat analysis
Glucose tolerance test (IDDM)

Why may amylase/lipase be normal in a patient with chronic pancreatitis?

Because of extensive pancreatic tissue loss ("burned-out pancreas")

What radiographic tests should be performed?

CT scan—has greatest sensitivity for gland enlargement/atrophy, calcifications, masses, pseudocysts
KUB—calcification in the pancreas
ERCP—ductal irregularities with dilation and stenosis ("chain of lakes"), pseudocysts

What is the medical treatment?

Discontinuation of alcohol use—can reduce attacks, though parenchymal damage continues secondary to ductal obstruction and fibrosis
Insulin for type 1 diabetes mellitus
Pancreatic enzyme replacement
Narcotics for pain

What is the surgical treatment?

Puestow—longitudinal pancreaticojejunostomy (pancreatic duct **must be dilated**)
Duval—distal pancreaticojejunostomy
Near-total pancreatectomy

What is the Frey's procedure?

Longitudinal pancreaticojejunostomy with core resection of the pancreatic head

What is the indication for surgical treatment of chronic pancreatitis?

Severe, prolonged/refractory pain

What are the possible complications of chronic pancreatitis?	Insulin-dependent diabetes mellitus Steatorrhea Malnutrition Biliary obstruction Splenic vein thrombosis Gastric varices Pancreatic pseudocyst/abscess Narcotic addiction Pancreatic ascites/pleural effusion Splenic artery aneurysm

Gallstone Pancreatitis

What is it?	Acute pancreatitis from a gallstone in or passing through the ampulla of Vater (the exact mechanism is unknown)
How is the diagnosis made?	Acute pancreatitis and cholelithiasis and/or choledocholithiasis and no other cause of pancreatitis (e.g., no history of alcohol abuse)
What radiologic tests should be performed?	U/S to look for gallstones CT scan to look at the pancreas, if symptoms are severe
What is the treatment?	Conservative measures and early interval cholecystectomy (laparoscopic cholecystectomy or open cholecystectomy) and intraoperative cholangiogram (IOC) in 3 to 5 days (after pancreatic inflammation resolves)
Why should early interval cholecystectomy be performed on patients with gallstone pancreatitis?	Pancreatitis will recur in ≈33% of patients within 8 weeks (so always perform early interval cholecystectomy and IOC in 3–5 days when pancreatitis resolves)
What is the role of ERCP?	1. Cholangitis 2. Refractory choledocholithiasis

Hemorrhagic Pancreatitis

What is it?	Bleeding into the parenchyma and retroperitoneal structures with extensive pancreatic necrosis
What are the signs?	Abdominal pain, shock/ARDS, Cullen's sign, Grey Turner's sign, Fox's sign
Define the following terms:	
Cullen's sign	**Bluish discoloration of the periumbilical area** from retroperitoneal hemorrhage tracking around to the anterior abdominal wall through fascial planes

Grey Turner's sign	**Ecchymosis or discoloration of the flank** in patients with retroperitoneal hemorrhage from dissecting blood from the retroperitoneum (Think: Grey **TURN**er = **TURN** side to side = flank [side] hematoma)
Fox's sign	**Ecchymosis of the inguinal ligament** from blood tracking from the retroperitoneum and collecting at the inguinal ligament
What are the significant lab values?	Increased amylase/lipase Decreased Hct Decreased calcium levels
What radiologic test should be performed?	CT scan with IV contrast

PANCREATIC ABSCESS

What is it?	Infected peripancreatic purulent fluid collection
What are the signs/symptoms?	Fever, unresolving pancreatitis, epigastric mass
What radiographic tests should be performed?	Abdominal CT scan with needle aspiration → send for Gram stain/culture
What are the associated lab findings?	Positive Gram stain and culture of bacteria
Which organisms are found in pancreatic abscesses?	Gram negative (most common): *Escherichia coli, Pseudomonas, Klebsiella* Gram positive: *Staphylococcus aureus, Candida*
What is the treatment?	Antibiotics and percutaneous drain placement or operative débridement and placement of drains

PANCREATIC NECROSIS

What is it?	Dead pancreatic tissue, usually following acute pancreatitis
How is the diagnosis made?	Abdominal CT scan with IV contrast; dead pancreatic tissue does not take up IV contrast and is not enhanced on CT scan (i.e., doesn't "light up")
What is the treatment?	
Sterile	Medical management
Suspicious of infection	CT-guided FNA
Toxic, hypotensive	Operative débridement

PANCREATIC PSEUDOCYST

What is it?	Encapsulated collection of pancreatic fluid

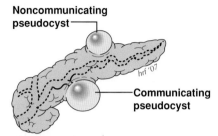

Noncommunicating pseudocyst

hrt '07

Communicating pseudocyst

What makes it a "pseudo" cyst?	Wall is formed by inflammatory fibrosis, NOT epithelial cell lining
What is the incidence?	≈1 in 10 after alcoholic pancreatitis
What are the associated risk factors?	Acute pancreatitis < chronic pancreatitis from alcohol
What is the most common cause of pancreatic pseudocyst in the United States?	Chronic alcoholic pancreatitis
What are the symptoms?	Epigastric pain/mass Emesis Mild fever Weight loss ***Note:*** Should be suspected when a patient with acute pancreatitis fails to resolve pain
What are the signs?	Palpable epigastric mass, tender epigastrium, ileus
What is the differential diagnosis of a pseudocyst?	Cystadenocarcinoma, cystadenoma
What are the possible complications of a pancreatic pseudocyst?	Infection, bleeding into the cyst, fistula, pancreatic ascites, gastric outlet obstruction, SBO, biliary obstruction
What is the treatment?	Drainage of the cyst or observation
What is the waiting period before a pseudocyst should be drained?	It takes 6 weeks for pseudocyst walls to "mature" or become firm enough to hold sutures, and most will resolve during this period if they are going to
What percentage of pseudocysts resolves spontaneously?	≈50%
What is the treatment for pseudocyst with bleeding into cyst?	Angiogram and embolization

What is the treatment for pseudocyst with infection?	Percutaneous external drainage/IV antibiotics

What size pseudocyst should be drained?	Most experts say:
	    Pseudocysts >5 cm have a small chance of resolving and have a higher chance of complications
	    Calcified cyst wall
	    Thick cyst wall

What are three treatment options for pancreatic pseudocyst?	1. Percutaneous aspiration/drain 2. Operative drainage 3. Transpapillary stent via ERCP (pseudocyst must communicate with pancreatic duct)
What is an endoscopic option for drainage of a pseudocyst?	**Endoscopic** cystogastrostomy
What must be done during a surgical drainage procedure for a pancreatic pseudocyst?	**Biopsy** of the cyst wall to rule out a cystic carcinoma (e.g., cystadenocarcinoma)
What is the most common cause of death due to pancreatic pseudocyst?	Massive hemorrhage into the pseudocyst

PANCREATIC CARCINOMA

What is it?	Adenocarcinoma of the pancreas arising from duct cells

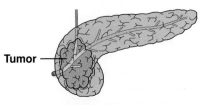

Tumor

What are the associated risk factors?	**Smoking 3× risk**, diabetes mellitus, heavy alcohol use, chronic pancreatitis, diet high in fried meats, previous gastrectomy
What is the average age?	>60 years
What are the different types?	>80% are duct cell adenocarcinomas; other types include cystadenocarcinoma and acinar cell carcinoma
What percentage arises in the pancreatic head?	**66%** arise in the pancreatic **head; 33%** arise in the **body and tail**
Why are most pancreatic cancers in the tail nonresectable?	These tumors grow without symptoms until it is too late and they have already spread—head of the pancreas tumors draw attention earlier because of biliary obstruction

What are the signs/symptoms of tumors based on locations?

Head of the pancreas

Painless jaundice from obstruction of common bile duct; weight loss; abdominal pain; back pain; weakness; **pruritus** from bile salts in skin; anorexia; **Courvoisier's sign**; acholic stools; dark urine; diabetes

Body or tail

Weight loss and pain (90%); migratory thrombophlebitis (10%); jaundice (<10%); nausea and vomiting; fatigue

What are the most common symptoms of cancer of the pancreatic HEAD?

1. Weight loss (90%)
2. Pain (75%)
3. Jaundice (70%)

What is "Courvoisier's sign"?

Palpable, nontender, distended gallbladder

What is the classic presentation of pancreatic cancer in the head of the pancreas?

Painless jaundice

What are the associated lab findings?

Increased direct bilirubin and alkaline phosphatase (as a result of biliary obstruction)
Increased LFTs
Elevated pancreatic tumor markers

Which tumor markers are associated with pancreatic cancer?

CA 19-9

What does CA 19-9 stand for?

Carbohydrate Antigen 19-9

What diagnostic studies are performed?

Abdominal CT scan, U/S, cholangiography (ERCP to rule out choledocholithiasis and cell brushings), endoscopic U/S with biopsy

What is the treatment based on location?

Head of the pancreas

Whipple procedure (pancreaticoduodenectomy)

Body or tail

Distal resection

What factors signify inoperability?

Vascular encasement (SMA, hepatic artery)
Liver metastasis
Peritoneal implants
Distant lymph node metastasis (periaortic/celiac nodes)
Distant metastasis
Malignant ascites

Is portal vein or SMV involvement an absolute contraindication for resection?

No—can be resected and reconstructed with vein interposition graft at some centers

What is the Whipple procedure (pancreaticoduodenectomy)?	Cholecystectomy Truncal vagotomy Antrectomy Pancreaticoduodenectomy—removal of head of pancreas and duodenum Choledochojejunostomy—anastomosis of common bile duct to jejunum Pancreaticojejunostomy—anastomosis of distal pancreas remnant to jejunum Gastrojejunostomy—anastomosis of stomach to jejunum
What mortality rate is associated with a Whipple procedure?	<5% at busy high-volume centers
What is the "pylorus-preserving Whipple"?	No antrectomy; anastomose duodenum to jejunum
What are the possible post-Whipple complications?	Delayed gastric emptying (if antrectomy is performed); **anastomotic leak** (from the bile duct or pancreatic anastomosis), causing pancreatic/biliary fistula; wound infection; postgastrectomy syndromes; sepsis; pancreatitis
Why must the duodenum be removed if the head of the pancreas is resected?	They share the same blood supply
What is the postoperative adjuvant therapy?	Chemotherapy ± XRT
What is the palliative treatment if the tumor is inoperable and biliary obstruction is present?	Percutaneous transhepatic cholangiography (PTC) or ERCP and placement of stent across obstruction
What is the prognosis at 1 year after diagnosis?	Dismal; 90% of patients die within 1 year of diagnosis
What is the survival rate at 5 years after resection?	20%

MISCELLANEOUS

What is an annular pancreas?	Pancreas encircling the duodenum; if obstruction is present, bypass, **do not resect**
What is pancreatic divisum?	Failure of the two pancreatic ducts to fuse; the normally small duct (**S**mall = **S**antorini) of Santorini acts as the main duct in pancreatic divisum (Think: the two pancreatic ducts are **D**ivided = **D**ivisum)
What is heterotopic pancreatic tissue?	Heterotopic pancreatic tissue usually found in the stomach, intestine, duodenum

What is a Puestow procedure?	Longitudinal filleting of the pancreas/pancreatic duct with a side-to-side anastomosis with the small bowel
What medication decreases output from a pancreatic fistula?	Somatostatin (GI-inhibitory hormone)
Which has a longer half-life: amylase or lipase?	Lipase; therefore, amylase may be normal and lipase will remain elevated longer

What is the WDHA syndrome?	Pancreatic **VIP**oma (**V**asoactive **I**ntestinal **P**olypeptide tumor)
	Tumor secretes VIP, which causes:
	    Watery
	    Diarrhea
	    Hypokalemia
	    Achlorhydria (inhibits gastric acid secretion)

What is the Whipple triad of pancreatic insulinoma?	1. Hypoglycemia (glucose <50) 2. Symptoms of hypoglycemia: mental status changes/vasomotor instability 3. Relief of symptoms with administration of glucose
What is the most common islet cell tumor?	Insulinoma
What pancreatic tumor is associated with gallstone formation?	Somatostatinoma (inhibits gallbladder contraction)
What is the triad found with pancreatic somatostatinoma tumor?	1. Gallstones 2. Diabetes 3. Steatorrhea
What are the two classic findings with pancreatic glucagonoma tumors?	1. Diabetes 2. Dermatitis/rash (necrotizing migratory erythema)

RAPID-FIRE REVIEW

Name the diagnostic modality:

40-year-old female with "migratory necrolytic dermatitis," diabetes	Glucagon assay (glucagon level), CT scan for glucagonoma
What is the treatment?	
2-year-old with annular pancreas	Bypass obstruction

40-year-old alcoholic with dead pancreatic tissue on CT scan develops hypotension and fever	Operative pancreatic débridement

What is the correct diagnosis?

28-year-old male with diarrhea, diabetes, and gallstones	Somatostatinoma
80-year-old with new-onset jaundice has a palpable, distended, nontender gallbladder on exam	Courvoisier's sign for head of the pancreas cancer mass

Chapter 55 | Breast

ANATOMY OF THE BREAST AND AXILLA

What four nerves must the surgeon be aware of during an axillary dissection?

1. **Long thoracic nerve**
2. **Thoracodorsal nerve**
3. Medial pectoral nerve
4. Lateral pectoral nerve

Describe the location of these nerves and the muscle each innervates:

Long thoracic nerve	Courses along the lateral chest wall in midaxillary line on serratus anterior muscle; innervates serratus anterior muscle
Thoracodorsal nerve	Courses lateral to long thoracic nerve on latissimus dorsi muscle; innervates latissimus dorsi muscle
Medial pectoral nerve	Runs **lateral** to or through the pectoral minor muscle, actually **lateral** to the lateral pectoral nerve; innervates the pectoral minor and pectoral major muscles
Lateral pectoral nerve	Runs **medial** to the medial pectoral nerve (names describe orientation from the brachial plexus!); innervates the pectoral major

Identify the nerves in the axilla:

1. Thoracodorsal nerve
2. Long thoracic nerve
3. Medial pectoral nerve
4. Lateral pectoral nerve
5. Axillary vein

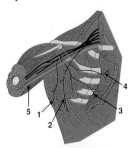

What is the name of the deformity if you cut the long thoracic nerve in this area?

"Winged scapula"

What is the name of the CUTANEOUS nerve that crosses the axilla in a transverse fashion? (Many surgeons try to preserve this nerve.)

Intercostobrachial nerve

What is the name of the large vein that marks the upper limit of the axilla?

Axillary vein

What is the lymphatic drainage of the breast?

Lateral: axillary LNs
Medial: parasternal nodes that run with
   internal mammary artery

What are the levels of axillary LNs?

Level I (low): lateral to pectoral minor
Level II (middle): deep to pectoral minor
Level III (high): medial to pectoral minor
In breast cancer, a higher level of
   involvement has a worse prognosis, but
   the level of involvement is less important
   than the number of positive nodes
   (Think: Levels I, II, and III are in the
   same inferior–superior anatomic order
   as the Le Fort facial fractures and the
   trauma neck zones; *I dare you to forget!*)

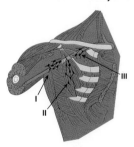

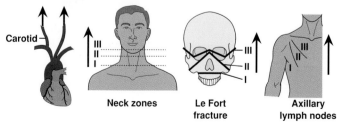

Neck zones   Le Fort   Axillary
                  fracture   lymph nodes

Carotid

What are Rotter's nodes?	Nodes between the pectoralis major and minor muscles; not usually removed unless they are enlarged or feel suspicious intraoperatively
What are the suspensory breast ligaments called?	Cooper's ligaments
Which hormone is mainly responsible for breast milk production?	Prolactin

BREAST CANCER

What is the incidence of breast cancer?	**12% lifetime risk**
What percentage of women with breast cancer has no known risk factor?	75%!
What percentage of all breast cancers occurs in women younger than 30 years?	≈2%
What are the major breast cancer susceptibility genes?	*BRCA1* and *BRCA2* (easily remembered: **BR** = **BR**east and **CA** = **CA**ncer)
What option exists to decrease the risk of breast cancer in women with BRCA?	Prophylactic bilateral mastectomy
What is the most common motivation for medicolegal cases involving the breast?	Failure to diagnose a breast carcinoma
What is the "TRIAD OF ERROR" for misdiagnosed breast cancer?	1. Age <45 years 2. Self-diagnosed mass 3. Negative mammogram *Note:* >75% of cases of **MISDIAGNOSED** breast cancer have these three characteristics

What are the history risk factors for breast cancer?	"NAACP":
	    Nulliparity
	    Age at menarche (<13 years)
	    Age at menopause (>55 years)
	    Cancer of the breast (in self or family)
	    Pregnancy with first child (>30 years)

What are physical/anatomic risk factors for breast cancer?	**"CHAFED LIPS":**
	Cancer in the breast (3% synchronous contralateral cancer)
	Hyperplasia (moderate/florid) (2× risk)
	Atypical hyperplasia (4× risk)
	Female (100× male risk)
	Elderly
	DCIS
	LCIS
	Inherited genes (BRCA I and II)
	Papilloma (1.5×)
	Sclerosing adenosis (1.5×)
Is "run of the mill" fibrocystic disease a risk factor for breast cancer?	No
What are the possible symptoms of breast cancer?	No symptoms
	Mass in the breast
	Pain (**most are painless**)
	Nipple discharge
	Local edema
	Nipple retraction
	Dimple
	Nipple rash
Why does skin retraction occur?	Tumor involvement of Cooper's ligaments and subsequent traction on ligaments pull skin inward
What are the signs of breast cancer?	Mass (1 cm is usually the smallest lesion that can be palpated on examination)
	Dimple
	Nipple rash
	Edema
	Axillary/supraclavicular nodes
What is the most common site of breast cancer?	≈50% of cancers develop in the upper outer quadrants
What are the different types of invasive breast cancer?	Infiltrating ductal carcinoma (≈75%)
	Medullary carcinoma (≈15%)
	Infiltrating lobular carcinoma (≈5%)
	Tubular carcinoma (≈2%)
	Mucinous carcinoma (colloid) (≈1%)
	Inflammatory breast cancer (≈1%)
What is the most common type of breast cancer?	Infiltrating ductal carcinoma

What is the differential diagnosis?	Fibrocystic disease of the breast Fibroadenoma Intraductal papilloma Duct ectasia Fat necrosis Abscess Radial scar Simple cyst
Describe the appearance of the edema of the dermis in inflammatory carcinoma of the breast:	Peau d'orange (orange peel)
What are the screening recommendations for breast cancer?	
Breast exam recommendations	Self-exam of breasts monthly Ages 20 to 40 years: breast exam every 2 to 3 years by a physician >40 years: annual breast exam by physician
Mammograms	Mammogram every year or every other year after age 40
When is the best time for breast self-exams?	1 week after menstrual period
Why is mammography a more useful diagnostic tool in older women than in younger?	Breast tissue undergoes fatty replacement with age, making masses more visible; younger women have more fibrous tissue, which makes mammograms harder to interpret
What are the radiographic tests for breast cancer?	Mammography and breast U/S, MRI
What is the classic picture of breast cancer on mammogram?	Spiculated mass

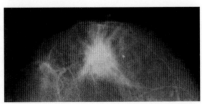

Which option is the best initial test to evaluate a breast mass in a female <30 years?	Breast U/S

What are the methods for obtaining tissue for pathologic examination?

Fine-needle aspiration (FNA), core biopsy (larger needle core sample), mammotome stereotactic biopsy, and open biopsy, which can be incisional (cutting a **piece** of the mass) or excisional (cutting out the **entire** mass)

What are the indications for biopsy?

Persistent mass after aspiration
Solid mass
Blood in cyst aspirate
Suspicious lesion by mammography/U/S/MRI
Bloody nipple discharge
Ulcer or dermatitis of nipple
Patient's concern of persistent breast abnormality

What is the process for performing a biopsy when a nonpalpable mass is seen on mammogram?

Stereotactic (mammotome) biopsy or needle localization biopsy

What is a needle localization biopsy (NLB)?

Needle localization by radiologist, followed by biopsy; removed breast tissue must be checked by mammogram to ensure all of the suspicious lesion has been excised

What is a mammotome biopsy?

Mammogram-guided computerized stereotactic core biopsies

What is obtained first, the mammogram or the biopsy?

Mammogram is obtained first; otherwise, tissue extraction (core or open) may alter the mammographic findings (FNA may be done prior to the mammogram because the fine needle usually will not affect the mammographic findings)

What would be suspicious mammographic findings?

Mass, microcalcifications, stellate/spiculated mass

What is a "radial scar" seen on mammogram?

Spiculated mass with central lucency, ± microcalcifications

What tumor is associated with a radial scar?

Tubular carcinoma; thus, biopsy is indicated

What is the "workup" for a breast mass?

1. Clinical breast exam
2. Mammogram or breast U/S
3. FNA, core biopsy, or open biopsy

How do you proceed if the mass appears to be a cyst?

Aspirate it with a needle

Is the fluid from a breast cyst sent for cytology?

Not routinely; bloody fluid should be sent for cytology

When do you proceed to open biopsy for a breast cyst?	1. In the case of a second cyst recurrence 2. Bloody fluid in the cyst 3. Palpable mass after aspiration
What is the preoperative staging workup in a patient with breast cancer?	Bilateral mammogram (cancer in one breast is a risk factor for cancer in the contralateral breast!) CXR (to check for lung metastasis) LFTs (to check for liver metastasis) Serum calcium level, alkaline phosphatase (if these tests indicate bone metastasis/"bone pain," proceed to bone scan) Other tests, depending on signs/symptoms (e.g., head CT scan if patient has focal neurologic deficit, to look for brain metastasis)
What hormone receptors must be checked for in the biopsy specimen?	**Estrogen and progesterone receptors**—this is **key for determining adjuvant treatment;** this information must be obtained on all specimens (including fine-needle aspirates)
What staging system is used for breast cancer?	**TMN:** T**umor/M**etastases/N**odes (AJCC)

Describe the staging (simplified):

Stage I	Tumor ≤2 cm in diameter without metastases, **no nodes**
Stage IIA	Tumor ≤2 cm in diameter with mobile axillary nodes **or** Tumor 2 to 5 cm in diameter, no nodes
Stage IIB	Tumor 2 to 5 cm in diameter with mobile axillary nodes **or** Tumor >5 cm with no nodes
Stage IIIA	Tumor >5 cm with mobile axillary nodes **or** Any size tumor with **fixed** axillary nodes, no metastases
Stage IIIB	Peau d'orange (skin edema) or Chest wall invasion/fixation or Inflammatory cancer or Breast skin ulceration or Breast skin satellite metastases or Any tumor and + ipsilateral **internal mammary** LNs
Stage IIIC	Any size tumor, no distant metastases POSITIVE: supraclavicular, infraclavicular, or internal mammary LNs

Stage IV	**Distant metastases** (including ipsilateral supraclavicular nodes)
What are the sites of metastases?	LNs (most common) Lung/pleura Liver Bones Brain
What are the major treatments of breast cancer?	Modified radical mastectomy Lumpectomy and radiation + sentinel LN dissection (Both treatments either ± postop chemotherapy/tamoxifen)
What are the indications for radiation therapy after a modified radical mastectomy?	Stage IIIA Stage IIIB Pectoral muscle/fascia invasion Positive internal mammary LN Positive surgical margins ≥4 positive axillary LNs postmenopausal
What breast carcinomas are candidates for lumpectomy and radiation (breast-conserving therapy)?	Stages I and II (tumors <5 cm)
What approach may allow a patient with stage IIIA cancer to have breast-conserving surgery?	NEOadjuvant chemotherapy—if the preop chemo shrinks the tumor
What is the treatment of inflammatory carcinoma of the breast?	**Chemotherapy first!** Then often followed by radiation, mastectomy, or both
What is "lumpectomy and radiation"?	Lumpectomy (segmental mastectomy: removal of a **part** of the breast); axillary node dissection; and a course of radiation therapy **after** operation, over a period of several weeks
What are other contraindications to lumpectomy and radiation?	Previous radiation to the chest Positive margins Collagen vascular disease (e.g., scleroderma) Extensive DCIS (often seen as diffuse microcalcification) **Relative contraindications:** Lesion that cannot be seen on the mammograms (i.e., early recurrence will be missed on follow-up mammograms) Very small breast (no cosmetic advantage)

What is a modified radical mastectomy?	Breast, axillary nodes (level II, I), and nipple–areolar complex are removed Pectoralis major and minor muscles are **not** removed (Auchincloss modification) Drains are placed to drain lymph fluid
Where are the drains placed with an MRM?	1. Axilla 2. Chest wall (breast bed)
When should the drains be removed?	<30 cc/day drainage
How can the long thoracic and thoracodorsal nerves be identified during an axillary dissection?	Nerves can be stimulated with forceps, which results in contraction of the latissimus dorsi (thoracodorsal nerve) or anterior serratus (long thoracic nerve)
What is a sentinel node biopsy?	Instead of removing all the axillary LNs, the **primary** draining or "sentinel" LN is removed
How is the sentinel LN found?	Inject blue dye and/or technetium-labeled sulfur colloid (best results with both)
What follows a positive sentinel node biopsy?	Removal of the rest of the axillary LNs
What is now considered the standard of care for LN evaluation in women with T1 or T2 tumors (stages I and IIA) and clinically negative axillary LNs?	Sentinel LN dissection
What do you do with a mammotome biopsy that returns as "atypical hyperplasia"?	Open needle localization biopsy as many will have DCIS or invasive cancer
How does tamoxifen work?	Binds estrogen receptors
What is the treatment for local recurrence in breast after lumpectomy and radiation?	"Salvage" mastectomy
Can tamoxifen prevent breast cancer?	**Yes.** In the Breast Cancer Prevention Trial of 13,000 women at increased risk of developing breast cancer, tamoxifen reduced risk by ≈50% across all ages
What are common options for breast reconstruction?	TRAM flap, implant, latissimus dorsi flap

What is a TRAM flap?

Transverse Rectus Abdominis Myocutaneous flap

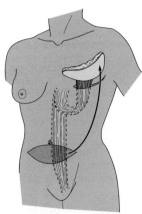

What are side effects of tamoxifen?

Endometrial cancer (2.5× relative risk), DVT, pulmonary embolus, cataracts, hot flashes, mood swings

Give the common adjuvant therapy for the following patients with breast cancer. (These are rough guidelines; check for current guidelines, as they are always changing; ER = estrogen receptor.)

Premenopausal, node +, ER −   Chemotherapy

Premenopausal, node +, ER −   Chemotherapy and tamoxifen

Premenopausal, node −, ER +   Tamoxifen and/or chemotherapy

Postmenopausal, node +, ER +   Tamoxifen, ± chemotherapy

Postmenopausal, node +, ER −   Chemotherapy, ± tamoxifen

DCIS

What does DCIS stand for?

Ductal Carcinoma In Situ

Normal duct   **Ductal carcinoma in situ**

What is DCIS also known as?	Intraductal carcinoma
Describe DCIS?	Cancer cells in the duct without invasion (in situ: cells do not penetrate the basement membrane)
What are the signs/symptoms?	Usually none; usually nonpalpable
What are the mammographic findings?	Microcalcifications
How is the diagnosis made?	Core or open biopsy
What is the most aggressive histologic type?	Comedo
What is the risk of LN metastasis with DCIS?	<2% (usually when microinvasion is seen)
What is the major risk with DCIS?	Subsequent development of infiltrating ductal carcinoma in the **same breast**
What is the treatment for DCIS in the following cases?	
Tumor <1 cm (low grade)	Remove with 1-cm margins and XRT
Tumor >1 cm	Perform lumpectomy with 1-cm margins and radiation **or** total mastectomy (**no** axillary dissection)
What is a total (simple) mastectomy?	Removal of the breast and nipple without removal of the axillary nodes (always remove nodes with invasive cancer)
When must a simple mastectomy be performed for DCIS?	Diffuse breast involvement (e.g., diffuse microcalcifications), >1 cm and contraindication to radiation
What is the role of axillary node dissection with DCIS?	No role in true DCIS (i.e., without microinvasion); some perform a sentinel LN dissection for high-grade DCIS
What is adjuvant Rx for DCIS?	1. Tamoxifen if ER+ 2. Postlumpectomy XRT
What is a memory aid for the breast in which DCIS breast cancer arises?	Cancer arises in the **same** breast as DCIS (Think: **D**CIS = **D**irectly in same breast)

LCIS

What is LCIS?

Lobular Carcinoma In Situ (carcinoma cells in the lobules of the breast without invasion)

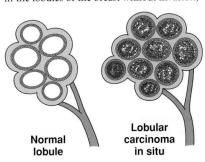

Normal lobule

Lobular carcinoma in situ

What are the signs/symptoms?

There are none

What are the mammographic findings?

There are none

How is the diagnosis made?

LCIS is found **incidentally** on biopsy

What is the major risk?

Carcinoma of **either** breast

Which breast is most at risk for developing an invasive carcinoma?

Equal risk in both breasts! (Think of LCIS as a **risk marker** for future development of cancer in either breast)

What percentage of women with LCIS develops an invasive breast carcinoma?

≈30% in the 20 years after diagnosis of LCIS!

What type of invasive breast cancer do patients with LCIS develop?

Most commonly, **infiltrating ductal carcinoma, with equal distribution** in the contralateral and ipsilateral breasts

What medication may lower the risk of developing breast cancer in LCIS?

Tamoxifen for 5 years will lower the risk up to 50%, but with an increased risk of endometrial cancer and clots; it must be an individual patient determination

What is the treatment of LCIS?

Close follow-up (or bilateral simple mastectomy in high-risk patients)

What is the major difference in the subsequent development of invasive breast cancer with DCIS and LCIS?

LCIS cancer develops in *either* breast; DCIS cancer develops in the ipsilateral breast

How do you remember which breast is at risk for invasive cancers in patients with LCIS?

Think: **LCIS = L**iberally in either breast

MISCELLANEOUS

What is the most common cause of bloody nipple discharge in a young woman?	Intraductal papilloma
What is the most common breast tumor in patients <30 years?	Fibroadenoma
What is Paget's disease of the breast?	Scaling rash/dermatitis of the nipple caused by invasion of skin by cells from a ductal carcinoma

MALE BREAST CANCER

What is the incidence of breast cancer in men?	<1% of all breast cancer cases (1/150)
What is the average age at diagnosis?	65 years of age
What are the risk factors?	Increased estrogen Radiation Gynecomastia from increased estrogen Estrogen therapy Klinefelter's syndrome (XXY) *BRCA2* carriers
Is benign gynecomastia a risk factor for male breast cancer?	No
What type of breast cancer do men develop?	Nearly 100% of cases are ductal carcinoma (men do not usually have breast lobules)
What are the signs/symptoms of breast cancer in males?	Breast mass (most are painless), breast skin changes (ulcers, retraction), and nipple discharge (usually blood or a blood-tinged discharge)
What is the most common presentation?	Painless breast mass
How is breast cancer in males diagnosed?	Biopsy and mammogram
What is the treatment?	1. Mastectomy 2. Sentinel LN dissection of clinically negative axilla 3. Axillary dissection if clinically positive axillary LN

BENIGN BREAST DISEASE

What is the most common cause of green, straw-colored, or brown nipple discharge?

Fibrocystic disease

What is the most common cause of breast mass after breast trauma?

Fat necrosis

What must be ruled out with spontaneous galactorrhea (± amenorrhea)?

Prolactinoma (check pregnancy test and prolactin level)

CYSTOSARCOMA PHYLLODES

What is it?

Mesenchymal tumor arising from breast lobular tissue; most are benign (**Note:** "Sarcoma" is a misnomer, as the vast majority are benign; 1% of breast cancers)

What is the usual age of the patient with this tumor?

35 to 55 years (usually older than the patient with fibroadenoma)

What are the signs/symptoms?

Mobile, smooth breast mass that resembles a fibroadenoma on exam, mammogram/ U/S findings

How is it diagnosed?

Through core biopsy or excision

What is the treatment?

If benign, wide local excision; if malignant, simple total mastectomy

What is the role of axillary dissection with cystosarcoma phyllodes tumor?

Only if clinically palpable axillary nodes, as the malignant form rarely spreads to nodes (most common site of metastasis is the lung)

Is there a role for chemotherapy with cystosarcoma phyllodes?

Consider chemotherapy if large tumor >5 cm and "stromal overgrowth"

FIBROADENOMA

What is it?

Benign tumor of the breast consisting of stromal overgrowth, collagen arranged in "swirls"

What is the clinical presentation of a fibroadenoma?

Solid, mobile, **well-circumscribed** round breast mass, usually <40 years of age

How is fibroadenoma diagnosed?

Negative needle aspiration looking for fluid; U/S; core biopsy

What is the treatment?

Surgical resection for large or growing lesions; small fibroadenomas can be observed closely

What is this tumor's claim to fame?	Most common breast tumor in women <30 years

FIBROCYSTIC DISEASE

What is it?	Common benign breast condition consisting of fibrous (rubbery) and cystic changes in the breast
What are the signs/symptoms?	Breast pain or tenderness that varies with the menstrual cycle; cysts; and fibrous ("nodular") fullness
How is it diagnosed?	Through breast exam, history, and aspirated cysts (usually straw-colored or green fluid)
What is the treatment for symptomatic fibrocystic disease?	Stop caffeine Pain medications (NSAIDs) Vitamin E, evening primrose oil (danazol and OCP as last resort)
What is done if the patient has a breast cyst?	Needle drainage: If aspirate is bloody or a palpable mass remains after aspiration, an open biopsy is performed If the aspirate is straw-colored or green, the patient is followed closely; then, if there is recurrence, a second aspiration is performed Re-recurrence usually requires open biopsy

MASTITIS

What is it?	Superficial infection of the breast (cellulitis)
In what circumstance does it most often occur?	Breastfeeding
What bacteria are most commonly the cause?	*Staphylococcus aureus*
How is mastitis treated?	Stop breastfeeding and use a breast pump instead; apply heat; administer antibiotics
Why must the patient with mastitis have close follow-up?	To make sure that she does not have inflammatory breast cancer!

BREAST ABSCESS

What are the causes?	Mammary ductal ectasia (stenosis of breast duct) and mastitis
What is the most common bacteria?	Nursing = *S. aureus* Nonlactating = mixed infection

What is the treatment of breast abscess?	Antibiotics (e.g., dicloxacillin) Needle or open drainage with cultures taken Resection of involved ducts if recurrent Breast pump if breastfeeding
What is lactational mastitis?	Infection of the breast during breastfeeding—most commonly caused by *S. aureus;* treat with antibiotics and follow for abscess formation
What must be ruled out with a breast abscess in a nonlactating woman?	Breast cancer!

MALE GYNECOMASTIA

What is it?	Enlargement of the male breast
What are the causes?	**Medications** Drugs (marijuana) Liver failure Increased estrogen Decreased testosterone
What is the major differential diagnosis in the older patient?	Male breast cancer
What is the treatment?	Stop or change medications; correct underlying cause if there is a hormonal imbalance; and perform biopsy or subcutaneous mastectomy (i.e., leave nipple) if refractory to conservative measures and time

RAPID-FIRE REVIEW

Name the most likely diagnosis:

45-year-old female with itching of the right nipple for 6 months and a right breast mass	Paget's disease (infiltrating ductal carcinoma with spread to the nipple)
60-year-old male with nipple discharge	Male breast cancer
36-year-old female with a right breast mass after hitting her right breast on a door handle	Fat necrosis
39-year-old female with bilateral milky breast discharge, decreased lateral vision fields, and pituitary mass	Prolactinoma

28-year-old female with unilateral green-brown nipple discharge increasing immediately before menses	Fibrocystic disease
25-year-old female with bloody nipple discharge	Ductal papilloma
56-year-old female with a red breast, no fever, no leukocytosis; on exam, the skin looks swollen like an orange	Inflammatory breast cancer with peau d'orange (orange peel skin) on exam
40-year-old female without a palpable breast mass has "microcalcifications" on mammogram	Ductal Carcinoma In Situ (DCIS)
2 weeks' s/p modified radical mastectomy a 45-year-old female with infiltrating ductal cancer of the right breast returns to the clinic and complains of her right scapula "sticking out"	Winged scapula due to injury to the long thoracic nerve

Name the diagnostic modality:

28-year-old female with history of bloody nipple discharge mammogram is negative	Galactography to look for ductal papilloma

Chapter 56 | Endocrine

ADRENAL GLAND

Anatomy

Where is the drainage of the LEFT adrenal vein?	Left renal vein
Where is the drainage of the RIGHT adrenal vein?	Inferior vena cava (IVC)

Normal Adrenal Physiology

What is CRH?	Corticotropin-Releasing Hormone: released from anterior hypothalamus and causes release of ACTH from anterior pituitary

What is ACTH?	AdrenoCorticoTropic Hormone: released normally by anterior pituitary, which in turn causes adrenal gland to release cortisol
What feeds back to inhibit ACTH secretion?	Cortisol

Cushing's Syndrome

What is Cushing's syndrome?	Excessive **cortisol** production (Think: Cushing's = **C**ortisol)
What is the most common cause?	Iatrogenic (i.e., prescribed prednisone)
What is the second most common cause?	Cushing's disease (most common noniatrogenic cause)
What is Cushing's disease?	Cushing's syndrome caused by excess production of ACTH by anterior **pituitary**

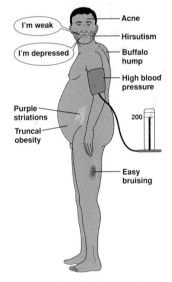

What is an ectopic ACTH source?	Tumor not found in the pituitary that secretes ACTH, which in turn causes adrenal gland to release cortisol without the normal negative feedback loop
What are the signs/symptoms of Cushing's syndrome?	Truncal obesity, hirsutism, "moon" facies, acne, "buffalo hump," purple striae, hypertension, diabetes, weakness, depression, easy bruising, myopathy
How can cortisol levels be indirectly measured over a short duration?	By measuring urine cortisol or the breakdown product of cortisol, 17-hydroxycorticosteroid (**17-OHCS**), in the urine

What is a direct test of serum cortisol?	Serum cortisol level (highest in the morning and lowest at night in healthy patients)
What initial tests should be performed in Cushing's syndrome?	Electrolytes Serum cortisol Urine-free cortisol, urine 17-OHCS Low-dose dexamethasone suppression test
What is the low-dose dexamethasone suppression test?	Dexamethasone is a synthetic cortisol that results in negative feedback on ACTH secretion and subsequent cortisol secretion in healthy patients; patients with **Cushing's syndrome** do **not** suppress their cortisol secretion
After the dexamethasone test, what is next?	Check ACTH levels

In ACTH-dependent Cushing's syndrome, how do you differentiate between a pituitary versus an ectopic ACTH source?	High-dose dexamethasone test:
	  Pituitary source—cortisol is suppressed
	  Ectopic ACTH source—no cortisol suppression

What is the most common site of ectopic ACTH-producing tumor?	>66% are oat cell tumors of the lung (#2 is carcinoid)
How are the following tumors treated?	
Adrenal adenoma	Adrenalectomy (almost always **unilateral**)
Adrenal carcinoma	Surgical excision (only 33% of cases are operable)
Ectopic ACTH-producing tumor	Surgical excision, if feasible
Cushing's DISEASE	Transsphenoidal adenomectomy
What is a complication of BILATERAL adrenalectomy?	Nelson's syndrome—occurs in 10% of patients after bilateral adrenalectomy
What is Nelson's syndrome?	Functional pituitary adenoma producing excessive ACTH and mass effect producing visual disturbances, hyperpigmentation, amenorrhea, with elevated ACTH levels (Think: **N**elson = **N**uclear reaction in the pituitary)

Adrenal Incidentaloma

What is an incidentaloma?	Tumor found in the adrenal gland **incidentally** on a CT scan performed for an unrelated reason
What is the incidence of incidentalomas?	4% of all CT scans (9% of autopsies)
What is the most common cause of incidentaloma?	Nonfunctioning adenoma (>75% of cases)

What is the risk factor for carcinoma?	Solid tumor >6 cm in diameter
What is the treatment?	Controversial for smaller/medium-sized tumors, but almost all surgeons would agree that resection is indicated for solid incidentalomas >6 cm in diameter because of risk of cancer
What tumor must be ruled out prior to biopsy or surgery for any adrenal mass?	Pheochromocytoma (24-hour urine for catecholamine, VMA, metanephrines)

Pheochromocytoma

What is it?	Tumor of the adrenal **MEDULLA** and sympathetic ganglion (from chromaffin cell lines) that produces **catecholamines** (norepinephrine > epinephrine)
What is the incidence?	Cause of hypertension in ≈**1**/500 hypertensive patients (≈10% of US population has hypertension)
Which age group is most likely to be affected?	Any age (children and adults); average age is 40 to 60 years
What are the associated risk factors?	MEN-II, family history, von Recklinghausen disease, von Hippel–Lindau disease
What are the signs/symptoms?	"Classic" triad: 1. Palpitations 2. Headache 3. Episodic diaphoresis Also, hypertension (50%), pallor → flushing, anxiety, weight loss, tachycardia, hyperglycemia

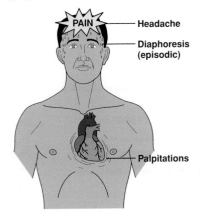

PAIN — Headache

Diaphoresis (episodic)

Palpitations

How can the pheochromocytoma SYMPTOMS triad be remembered?	Think of the first three letters in the word **PHE**ochromocytoma: **P**alpitations **H**eadache **E**pisodic diaphoresis
What is the most common sign of pheochromocytoma?	Hypertension
What diagnostic tests should be performed?	Urine screen: Vanillyl**M**andelic **A**cid (**VMA**), **metanephrine**, and normetanephrine (all breakdown products of the catechols) Urine/serum epinephrine/norepinephrine levels
What are the other common lab findings?	Hyperglycemia (epinephrine increases glucose, norepinephrine decreases insulin) Polycythemia (resulting from intravascular volume depletion)
What is the most common site of a pheochromocytoma?	Adrenal >90%
What are the other sites for pheochromocytoma?	Organ of Zuckerkandl, thorax (mediastinum), bladder, scrotum

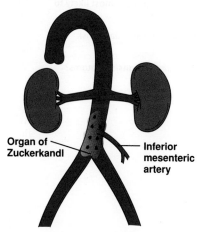

Organ of Zuckerkandl   **Inferior mesenteric artery**

What are the tumor localization tests?	CT scan, MRI, ^{131}I-**MIBG**, PET scan, OctreoScan (^{111}In-pentetreotide scan)
What does ^{131}I-MIBG stand for?	Iodine^{131} **M**eta**I**odo**B**enzyl**G**uanidine
How to remember MIBG and pheochromocytoma?	Think: **MIBG** = **My Big** = and thus "My Big Pheo" = **MIBG Pheo**
How does the ^{131}I-MIBG scan work?	^{131}I-MIBG is a norepinephrine analog that collects in adrenergic vesicles and, thus, in pheochromocytomas

What is the role of PET scan?	Positron Emission Tomography is helpful in localizing pheochromocytomas that do not accumulate MIBG
What is the scan for imaging adrenal cortical pheochromocytoma?	NP-59 (cholesterol analog)
What is the localizing option if a tumor is not seen on CT scan, MRI, or I-MIBG?	IVC venous sampling for catecholamines (gradient will help localize the tumor)
What is the tumor site if epinephrine is elevated?	Must be adrenal or near the adrenal gland (e.g., organ of Zuckerkandl), because nonadrenal tumors lack the capability to methylate norepinephrine to epinephrine
Can histology be used to determine malignancy?	No; only distant metastasis or invasion can determine malignancy
What is the classic pheochromocytoma "rule of 10's"?	**10% malignant** **10% bilateral** **10% in children** **10% multiple tumors** **10% extra-adrenal**
What is the preoperative/medical treatment?	**Increase intravascular volume** with α-blockade (e.g., phenoxybenzamine or prazosin) to allow reduction in catecholamine-induced vasoconstriction and resulting volume depletion; treatment should start as soon as diagnosis is made ± β-blockers
How can you remember phenoxybenzamine as a medical treatment of pheochromocytoma?	**PHE**ochromocytoma = **PHE**noxybenzamine
What is the surgical treatment?	Tumor resection with early ligation of venous drainage (lower possibility of catecholamine release/crisis by tying off drainage) and minimal manipulation
What are the possible perioperative complications?	Anesthetic challenge: hypertensive crisis with manipulation (treat with nitroprusside), hypotension with total removal of the tumor, cardiac dysrhythmias
In the patient with pheochromocytoma, what must be ruled out?	MEN type II (almost all cases are bilateral)

What is the organ of Zuckerkandl?	Body of embryonic chromaffin cells around the abdominal aorta (near the inferior mesenteric artery); normally atrophies during childhood, but is the most common site of extra-adrenal pheochromocytoma

Conn's Syndrome

What is it?	Primary hyper**aldosteronism** due to high aldosterone production
How do you remember what Conn's syndrome is?	**CON**n's disease = **HYPERAL**dosterone = "**CON HYPER AL**"

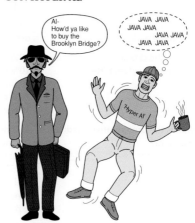

What are the common sources?	**Adrenal adenoma** or **adrenal hyperplasia;** aldosterone is abnormally secreted by an adrenal adenoma (66%) > hyperplasia > carcinoma
What is the normal physiology for aldosterone secretion?	BP in the renal afferent arteriole is low Low sodium and hyperkalemia cause **renin** secretion from juxtaglomerular cells Renin then converts angiotensinogen to angiotensin I Angiotensin-converting enzyme in the lung then converts angiotensin I to angiotensin II Angiotensin II then causes the adrenal glomerulosa cells to secrete **aldosterone**

What is the normal physiologic effect of aldosterone?	Aldosterone causes sodium retention for exchange of potassium in the kidney, resulting in fluid retention and increased BP
What are the signs/symptoms?	**Hypertension**, headache, polyuria, weakness
What are the two classic clues of Conn's syndrome?	1. Hypertension 2. Hypokalemia
What diagnostic tests should be ordered?	1. Plasma aldosterone concentration 2. Plasma renin activity
What ratio of these diagnostic tests is associated with primary hyperaldosteronism?	Aldosterone-to-renin ratio of >30
What diagnostic tests should be performed?	CT scan, adrenal venous sampling for aldosterone levels, saline infusion
What is the saline infusion test?	Saline infusion will decrease aldosterone levels in normal patients but not in Conn's syndrome
What is the preoperative treatment?	Spironolactone, K^+ supplementation
What is spironolactone?	Antialdosterone medication (works at the kidney tubule)
What are the causes of Conn's syndrome?	Adrenal adenoma (66%) Bilateral idiopathic adrenal hyperplasia (30%) Adrenal cancer (<1%)
What is the treatment of the following conditions?	
Adenoma	Unilateral adrenalectomy (laparoscopic)
Unilateral hyperplasia	Unilateral adrenalectomy (laparoscopic)
Bilateral hyperplasia	Spironolactone (usually no surgery)
What are the renin levels in patients with PRIMARY hyperaldosteronism?	Normal or low (key point!)

ADDISON'S DISEASE

What is it?	Acute adrenal insufficiency
What are the electrolyte findings?	HYPERkalemia, hyponatremia
How do you remember what ADDISON's disease is?	Think: **ADD**ison's disease = **AD**renal **D**own

INSULINOMA

What is it?	Insulin-producing tumor arising from β cells
What is the incidence?	#1 islet cell neoplasm; half of β-cell tumors of the pancreas produce insulin
What are the associated risks?	Associated with MEN-I syndrome (**PPP** = **P**ituitary, **P**ancreas, **P**arathyroid tumors)
What are the signs/symptoms?	**Sympathetic nervous system symptoms resulting from hypoglycemia:** palpitations, diaphoresis, tremulousness, irritability, weakness
What are the neurologic symptoms?	Personality changes, confusion, obtundation, seizures, coma
What is Whipple's triad?	1. Hypoglycemic symptoms produced by fasting 2. Blood glucose <50 mg/dL during symptomatic attack 3. Relief of symptoms by administration of glucose
What lab tests should be performed?	Glucose and insulin levels during fast; C-peptide and proinsulin levels (if self-injection of insulin is a concern, as insulin injections have **no** proinsulin or C-peptides)
What diagnostic tests should be performed?	Fasting hypoglycemia with inappropriately high levels of insulin 72-**hour fast**, then check glucose and insulin levels every 6 hours (monitor very closely because patient can develop hypoglycemic crisis)
What is the diagnostic fasting insulin-to-glucose ratio?	>0.4
What localizing tests should be performed?	CT scan, A-gram, endoscopic U/S, venous catheterization (to sample blood along portal and splenic veins to measure insulin and localize tumor), intraoperative U/S
What is the medical treatment?	Diazoxide, to suppress insulin release
What is the surgical treatment?	Surgical resection
What is the prognosis?	≈80% of patients have a benign solitary adenoma that is cured by surgical resection

GLUCAGONOMA

What is it?	Glucagon-producing tumor
Where is it located?	Pancreas (usually in the tail)
What are the symptoms?	**Necrotizing migratory erythema** (usually below the waist), glossitis, stomatitis, diabetes, weight loss
What are the skin findings?	Necrotizing migratory erythema is a red, often psoriatic-appearing rash with serpiginous borders over the trunk and limbs
What test is used for localization?	CT scan
What is the most likely anatomic location?	Tail of the pancreas
What is the medical treatment of necrotizing migratory erythema?	Zinc, somatostatin, IV amino acids, fatty acids
What is the treatment?	Surgical resection

SOMATOSTATINOMA

What is it?	Pancreatic tumor that secretes somatostatin
What is the diagnostic triad?	1. **D**iabetes 2. **D**iarrhea (steatorrhea) 3. Gallstones
What is used to make the diagnosis?	CT scan and somatostatin level
What is the treatment?	Resection (do not enucleate)

ZOLLINGER–ELLISON SYNDROME (Z-E SYNDROME)

What is it?	**Gastrinoma:** non–β-islet cell tumor of the pancreas (or other locale) that produces gastrin, causing gastric hypersecretion of HCl acid, resulting in GI **ulcers**
What is the incidence?	1/1,000 in patients with peptic ulcer disease, but nearly 2% in patients with **recurrent ulcers**

What is the associated syndrome?	MEN-I syndrome
What percentage of patients with Z-E syndrome has MEN-I syndrome?	≈25% (75% of cases of Z-E syndrome are "sporadic")
What percentage of patients with MEN-I will have Z-E syndrome?	≈50%
With gastrinoma, what lab tests should be ordered to screen for MEN-I?	1. Calcium level 2. Parathyroid hormone level
What are the signs/symptoms?	Peptic ulcers, diarrhea, weight loss, abdominal pain
What causes the diarrhea?	Massive acid hypersecretion and destruction of digestive enzymes
What are the signs?	**PUD** (epigastric pain, hematemesis, melena, hematochezia), GERD, diarrhea, **recurrent ulcers**, ulcers in unusual locations (e.g., proximal jejunum)
What are the possible complications?	GI hemorrhage/perforation, gastric outlet obstruction/stricture, metastatic disease
Which patients should have a gastrin level checked?	Those with recurrent ulcer; ulcer in unusual position (e.g., jejunum) or refractory to medical management; before any operation for ulcer
What lab tests should be performed?	Fasting gastrin level Postsecretin challenge gastrin level Calcium (screen for MEN-I) Chem-7
What are the associated gastrin levels?	NL fasting = 100 pg/mL Z-E syndrome fasting = 200 to 1000 pg/mL
What is the secretin-stimulation test?	IV secretin is administered and the gastrin level is determined; patients with Z-E syndrome have a paradoxical increase in gastrin

What are the classic secretin stimulation results?	**Lab results with secretin challenge:**
	    NL—Decreased gastrin
	    Z-E syndrome—Increased gastrin
	        (increased by >200 pg/mL)

How can you remember the diagnostic stimulation test for Z-E syndrome?

Think: **"Secret Z-E GAS": SECRETin = Z-E GAS**trin

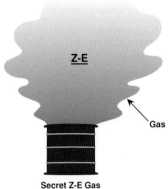

Secret Z-E Gas

What tests are used to evaluate ulcers?

EGD, UGI, or both

What tests are used to localize the tumor?

Octreotide scan (somatostatin receptor scan), abdominal CT scan, MRI, endoscopic ultrasonography (EUS)

What is the most common site?

Pancreas

What is the most common NONpancreatic site?

Duodenum

What are some other sites?

Stomach, lymph nodes, liver, kidney, ovary

Define "Passaro's triangle":

A.k.a. "gastrinoma triangle," a triangle drawn from the following points:
1. Cystic duct/CBD junction
2. Junction of the second and third portions of the duodenum
3. Neck of the pancreas

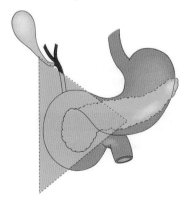

What percentage of gastrinomas is in Passaro's triangle?	≈80%
What is the medical treatment?	H$_2$ blockers, omeprazole, somatostatin
What is the surgical treatment needed for each of the following?	
Tumor in head of pancreas	1. Enucleation of tumor 2. Whipple procedure if main pancreatic duct is involved
Tumor in body or tail of pancreas	Distal pancreatectomy
Tumor in duodenum	Local resection
Unresectable tumor	Highly selective vagotomy
What percentage has malignant tumors?	66%
What is the most common site of metastasis?	Liver
What is the treatment of patients with liver metastasis?	Excision, if technically feasible
What is the prognosis with the following procedures?	
Complete excision	90% 10-year survival
Incomplete excision	25% 10-year survival

MULTIPLE ENDOCRINE NEOPLASIA

What is it also known as?	MEN syndrome
What is it?	Inherited condition of propensity to develop multiple endocrine tumors
How is it inherited?	Autosomal dominant (but with a significant degree of variation in penetrance)
Which patients should be screened for MEN?	All family members of patients diagnosed with MEN

MEN TYPE I

What is the gene defect in MEN type I?	Chromosome 11 (Think: 11 = 1)

What are the most common tumors and their incidences?

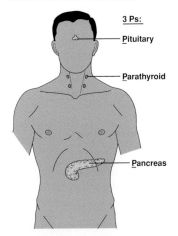

3 Ps:
Pituitary
Parathyroid
Pancreas

"PPP":
    Parathyroid hyperplasia (≈90%)
    Pancreatic islet cell tumors (≈66%)
        Gastrinoma: Z-E syndrome (50%)
        Insulinoma (20%)
    Pituitary tumors (≈50%)

How can tumors for MEN-I be remembered?

Think: type **I** = **P**rimary, **P**rimary, **P**rimary = **PPP** = **P**arathyroid, **P**ancreas, **P**ituitary

How can the P's associated with MEN-I be remembered?

All the P's are followed by a vowel: PA, PA, PI

What are the highest-yield screening lab tests for MEN-I?

1. Calcium
2. PTH
3. Gastrin
4. Prolactin (in females)

What percentage of patients with MEN-I has parathyroid hyperplasia?

≈90%

What percentage of patients with MEN-I has a gastrinoma?

≈50%

What other tumors (in addition to PPP) are associated with MEN-I?

Adrenal (30%) and thyroid (15%) adenomas

Men Type IIA

What is the gene defect in MEN type IIa?

RET (Think: re**T** = **T**wo)

What are the most common tumors and their incidences?

"MPH":
    Medullary thyroid carcinoma (100%);
        Calcitonin secreted
    Pheochromocytoma (>33%);
        Catecholamine excess
    Hyperparathyroidism (≈50%);
        Hypercalcemia

How can the tumors involved with MEN-IIa be remembered?	Think: type **2** = **2 MPH** or **2 M**iles **P**er **H**our = **MPH** = **M**edullary, **P**heochromocytoma, **H**yperparathyroid
How can the P of MPH be remembered?	Followed by the consonant "H"—**PH**EOCHROMOCYTOMA (Remember, the P's of MEN-I are followed by vowels)
What percentage of patients with MEN-IIa has medullary carcinoma of the thyroid?	100%
What are the best screening lab tests for MEN-II?	1. Calcitonin level (± stimulation) 2. Calcium levels 3. PTH 4. Catecholamines and metabolites (metanephrine and normetanephrine) 5. RET gene testing

Men Type IIB

What are the most common abnormalities, their incidences, and symptoms?	"MMMP": **M**ucosal neuromas (100%)—in the nasopharynx, oropharynx, larynx, and conjunctiva **M**edullary thyroid carcinoma (≈85%)— more aggressive than in MEN-IIa **M**arfanoid body habitus (long/lanky) **P**heochromocytoma (≈50%) and found bilaterally
How can the features of MEN-IIb be remembered?	**MMMP** (Think: **3M P**lastics)
How can you remember that MEN-IIb is marfanoid habitus?	Think: "**TO BE** marfanoid" = **II B** marfanoid
What is the anatomic distribution of medullary thyroid carcinoma in MEN-II?	**Almost always bilateral** (non–MEN-II cases are almost always **unilateral!**)
What are the physical findings/signs of MEN-IIb?	Mucosal neuromas (e.g., mouth, eyes) Marfanoid body habitus Pes cavus/planum (large arch of foot/ flat-footed) Constipation
What is the major difference between MEN-IIa and MEN-IIb?	MEN-IIa = parathyroid hyperplasia MEN-IIb = **no** parathyroid hyperplasia (and neuromas, marfanoid habitus, pes cavus [extensive arch of foot], etc.)

What type of parathyroid disease is associated with MEN-I and MEN-IIa?

Hyperplasia (treat with removal of all parathyroid tissue with autotransplant of some of the parathyroid tissue to the forearm)

RAPID-FIRE REVIEW

Name the diagnostic stimulation test for the following:

Conn's disease	Captopril (plasma aldosterone >15 µg/dL) or high-sodium diet (no suppression of plasma renin activity)
Insulinoma	Fasting glucose
Z-E syndrome	Secretin
Adrenal insufficiency	ACTH stimulation test (corticotropin 250 µg)
Pituitary versus ectopic/ adrenal source of hypercortisolism	High-dose dexamethasone suppression test: most pituitary causes will suppress
	Metyrapone test: most pituitary causes will result in an increase in ACTH

Name the diagnostic modality:

37-year-old with history of palpitations, episodic diaphoresis, and his blood pressure is 210/110	MIBG (metaiodobenzylguanidine) scan, CT scan (and/or MRI), and urine VMA/ metanephrines/catecholes for workup for pheochromocytoma

What is the treatment?

39-year-old female with Cushing's disease	Transsphenoidal adenomectomy
44-year-old female develops headaches and cannot see right or left peripherally	Pituitary prolactinoma

Name the radiographic test for localizing the following:

Conn's disease	CT scan, adrenal vein sampling for aldosterone and cortisol
Pheochromocytoma	MIBG
Glucagonoma	CT scan
Carcinoid	^{111}In-octreotide scintigraphy, MIBG
Gastrinoma (Zollinger–Ellison syndrome)	^{111}In-octreotide scintigraphy, CT scan, endoscopic U/S, MRI

Chapter 57 | Thyroid Gland

THYROID DISEASE

Anatomy

Identify the following structures:

1. Pyramidal lobe
2. Right lobe
3. Isthmus
4. Left lobe

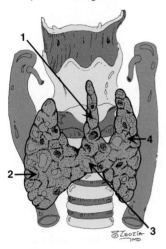

What is the arterial blood supply to the thyroid?

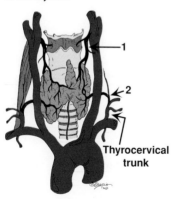

Two arteries:

1. Superior thyroid artery (first branch of the external carotid artery)
2. Inferior thyroid artery (branch of the thyrocervical trunk) (IMA artery rare)

What is the venous drainage of the thyroid?

Three veins:
1. Superior thyroid vein
2. **Middle** thyroid vein
3. Inferior thyroid vein

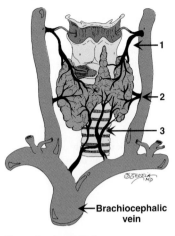

Brachiocephalic vein

Name the thyroid lobe appendage coursing toward the hyoid bone from around the thyroid isthmus

Pyramidal lobe

What percentage of patients has a pyramidal lobe?

≈50%

Name the lymph node (LN) group around the pyramidal thyroid lobe.

Delphian LN group

What is the thyroid isthmus?

Midline tissue border between the left and right thyroid lobes

Which ligament connects the thyroid to the trachea?

Ligament of Berry

Which paired nerves must be carefully identified during a thyroidectomy?

Recurrent laryngeal nerves, which are found in the tracheoesophageal grooves and dive behind the cricothyroid muscle; damage to these nerves paralyzes laryngeal abductors and causes hoarseness if unilateral, and airway obstruction if bilateral

What other nerve is at risk during a thyroidectomy and what are the symptoms?

Superior laryngeal nerve; if damaged, patient will have a deeper and quieter voice (unable to hit high pitches)

What is the name of the famous opera singer whose superior laryngeal nerve was injured during thyroidectomy?

Urban legend has it that it was Amelita Galli-Curci, but no objective data support such a claim (*Ann Surg* 2001;233:588)

Physiology

What is TRH?	**T**hyrotropin-**R**eleasing **H**ormone released from the hypothalamus; causes release of TSH
What is TSH?	**T**hyroid-**S**timulating **H**ormone released by the anterior pituitary; causes release of thyroid hormone from the thyroid
What are the thyroid hormones?	T3 and T4
What is the most active form of thyroid hormone?	T3
What is a negative feedback loop?	T3 and T4 feedback negatively on the anterior pituitary (causing decreased release of TSH in response to TRH)
What is Synthroid® (levothyroxine): T3 or T4?	T4
What is the half-life of Synthroid® (levothyroxine)?	7 days
What do parafollicular cells secrete?	Calcitonin

Thyroid Nodule

What percentage of people has a thyroid nodule?	≈5%
What is the differential diagnosis of a thyroid nodule?	Multinodular goiter Adenoma Hyperfunctioning adenoma Cyst Thyroiditis Carcinoma/lymphoma Parathyroid carcinoma
Name three types of nonthyroidal neck masses:	1. Inflammatory lesions (e.g., abscess, lymphadenitis) 2. Congenital lesions (i.e., thyroglossal duct [midline], branchial cleft cyst [lateral]) 3. Malignant lesions: lymphoma, metastases, squamous cell carcinoma
What studies can be used to evaluate a thyroid nodule?	U/S—solid or cystic nodule **F**ine-**N**eedle **A**spirate (**FNA**) → cytology ^{123}I scintiscan—hot or cold nodule
What is the DIAGNOSTIC test of choice for thyroid nodule?	FNA

What is the percentage of false-negative results on FNA for thyroid nodule?	≈5%
What is meant by a "hot" versus a "cold" nodule?	Nodule uptake of IV ^{131}I or ^{99}mT **Hot**—Increased ^{123}I uptake = functioning/hyperfunctioning nodule **Cold**—Decreased ^{123}I uptake = nonfunctioning nodule
What are the indications for a ^{123}I scintiscan?	1. Nodule with multiple "nondiagnostic" FNAs with low TSH 2. Nodule with thyrotoxicosis and low TSH
What is the role of thyroid suppression of a thyroid nodule?	Diagnostic and therapeutic; administration of thyroid hormone suppresses TSH secretion, and up to half of the benign thyroid nodules will disappear!
In evaluating a thyroid nodule, which of the following suggest thyroid carcinoma?	
History	1. Neck radiation 2. Family history (thyroid cancer, MEN-II) 3. Young age (especially children) 4. Male > female
Signs	1. Single nodule 2. Cold nodule 3. Increased calcitonin levels 4. Lymphadenopathy 5. Hard, immobile nodule
Symptoms	1. Voice change (vocal cord paralysis) 2. Dysphagia 3. Discomfort (in neck) 4. Rapid enlargement
What is the most common cause of thyroid enlargement?	Multinodular goiter
What are indications for surgery with multinodular goiter?	Cosmetic deformity, compressive symptoms, cannot rule out cancer
What is Plummer's disease?	Toxic multinodular goiter

Malignant Thyroid Nodules

What percentage of cold thyroid nodules is malignant?	≈25% in adults
What percentage of multinodular masses is malignant?	≈1%

What is the treatment of a patient with a history of radiation exposure, thyroid nodule, and negative FNA?

Most experts would remove the nodule surgically (because of the high risk of radiation) with thyroid lobectomy

What should be done with thyroid cyst aspirate?

Send to cytopathology

Thyroid Carcinoma

What are the FIVE main types of thyroid carcinoma and their relative percentages?

1. Papillary carcinoma: 80% (**P**opular = **P**apillary)
2. Follicular carcinoma: 10%
3. Medullary carcinoma: 5%
4. Hürthle cell carcinoma: 4%
5. Anaplastic/undifferentiated carcinoma: 1% to 2%

What are the signs/symptoms?

Mass/nodule, lymphadenopathy; most are **euthyroid**

What comprises the workup?

FNA, thyroid U/S, TSH, calcium level, CXR, ± ^{123}I scintiscan

What oncogenes are associated with thyroid cancers?

Ras gene family and RET protooncogene

Papillary Adenocarcinoma

What is papillary carcinoma's claim to fame?

Most common thyroid cancer (Think: **P**apillary = **P**opular) = 80% of all thyroid cancers

What is the environmental risk?

Radiation exposure

What is the average age?

30 to 40 years

What is the sex distribution?

Female > male; 2:1

What are the associated histologic findings?

Psammoma bodies (Remember, **P** = **P**sammoma = **P**apillary)

Describe the route and rate of spread:

Most spread via lymphatics (cervical adenopathy); spread occurs slowly

^{131}I uptake?

Good uptake

What is the 10-year survival rate?

≈95%

What is the treatment for?

<1.5 cm and no history of neck radiation exposure

Options:
1. Thyroid lobectomy and isthmectomy
2. Near-total thyroidectomy
3. Total thyroidectomy

>1.5 cm, bilateral, + cervical node metastasis O.R. a history of radiation exposure	Total thyroidectomy

What is the treatment for the following?

Lateral palpable cervical LNs	Selective neck dissection (ipsilateral)
Central	Central neck dissection
Do positive cervical nodes affect the prognosis?	NO!

What is a "lateral aberrant thyroid" in papillary cancer?	Misnomer—it is metastatic papillary carcinoma to a LN
What postoperative medication should be administered?	Thyroid hormone replacement, to suppress TSH
What is a postoperative treatment option for papillary carcinoma?	Postoperative ^{131}I scan can locate residual tumor and distant metastasis that can be treated with ablative doses of ^{131}I
What is the most common site of distant metastases?	Pulmonary (lungs)

What are the "Ps" of papillary thyroid cancer (7)?

Papillary cancer:
1. **P**opular (most common)
2. **P**sammoma bodies
3. **P**alpable LNs (spreads most commonly by lymphatics, seen in ≈33% of patients)
4. **P**ositive ^{131}I uptake
5. **P**ositive prognosis
6. **P**ostoperative ^{131}I scan to diagnose/treat metastases
7. **P**ulmonary metastases

Follicular Adenocarcinoma

What percentage of thyroid cancers does it comprise?	≈10%
Describe the nodule consistency:	Rubbery, encapsulated
What is the route of spread?	Hematogenous, more aggressive than papillary adenocarcinoma
What is the male-to-female ratio?	1:3
^{131}I uptake?	Good uptake
What is the overall 10-year survival rate?	≈85%
Can the diagnosis be made by FNA?	No; tissue structure is needed for a diagnosis of cancer

What histologic findings define malignancy in follicular cancer?	Capsular or blood vessel invasion
What is the most common site of distant metastasis?	Bone
What is the treatment for follicular cancer?	Total thyroidectomy
What is the postoperative treatment option if malignant?	Postoperative ^{131}I scan for diagnosis/treatment
What are the "Fs" of follicular cancer (4)?	Follicular cancer: 1. **F**ar-away metastasis (spreads hematogenously) 2. **F**emale (3:1) 3. **F**NA ... NOT (FNA CANNOT diagnose cancer) 4. **F**avorable prognosis

Hürthle Cell Thyroid Cancer

What is it?	Thyroid cancer of the Hürthle cells
What percentage of thyroid cancers does it comprise?	≈5%
What is the cell of origin?	Follicular cells
^{131}I uptake?	No uptake
How is the diagnosis made?	FNA can identify cells, but malignancy can be determined only by tissue histology (like follicular cancer)
What is the route of metastasis?	Lymphatic > hematogenous
What is the treatment?	Total thyroidectomy
What is the 10-year survival rate?	80%

Medullary Carcinoma

What percentage of all thyroid cancers does it comprise?	≈5%
With what other conditions is it associated?	MEN type II; autosomal dominant genetic transmission
Histology?	Amyloid (a**M**yloid = **M**edullary)
What does it secrete?	Calcitonin (tumor marker)
What is the appropriate stimulation test?	Pentagastrin (causes an increase in calcitonin)

What is the route of spread?	Lymphatic and hematogenous distant metastasis
How is the diagnosis made?	FNA
^{131}I uptake?	Poor uptake
What is the associated genetic mutation?	RET protooncogene
What is the female-to-male ratio?	Female > male; 1.5:1
What is the 10-year survival rate?	80% without LN involvement 45% with LN spread
What should all patients with medullary thyroid cancer also be screened for?	MEN II: pheochromocytoma, hyperparathyroidism
If medullary thyroid carcinoma and pheochromocytoma are found, which one is operated on first?	Pheochromocytoma
What is the treatment?	Total thyroidectomy and median LN dissection Modified neck dissection, if lateral cervical nodes are positive
What are the "Ms" of medullary carcinoma (4)?	Medullary cancer: 1. MEN II 2. aMyloid 3. Median LN dissection 4. Modified neck dissection if lateral nodes are positive

Anaplastic Carcinoma

What is it also known as?	Undifferentiated carcinoma
What is it?	Undifferentiated cancer arising in ≈75% of previously differentiated thyroid cancers (most commonly, follicular carcinoma)
What percentage of all thyroid cancers does it comprise?	≈2%
What is the gender preference?	Women > men
What are the associated histologic findings?	Giant cells, spindle cells
^{131}I uptake?	Very poor uptake
How is the diagnosis made?	FNA (large tumor)
What is the major differential diagnosis?	Thyroid lymphoma (much better prognosis!)

What is the treatment of the following disorders?

Small tumors

Total thyroidectomy + XRT/chemotherapy

Airway compromise

Debulking surgery and tracheostomy, XRT/chemotherapy

What is the prognosis?

Dismal, because most patients are at stage IV at presentation (3% alive at 5 years)

Miscellaneous

What laboratory value must be followed postoperatively after a thyroidectomy?

Calcium decreased secondary to parathyroid damage

What is the differential diagnosis of postoperative dyspnea after a thyroidectomy?

Neck hematoma (remove sutures and clot at the **bedside**)

Bilateral recurrent laryngeal nerve damage

What is a "lateral aberrant rest" of the thyroid?

Misnomer: It is **papillary** cancer of an LN from metastasis

Benign Thyroid Disease

What is the most common cause of hyperthyroidism?

Graves' disease

What is Graves' disease?

Diffuse goiter with hyperthyroidism, exophthalmos, and pretibial myxedema

What is the etiology?

Caused by circulating **antibodies** that stimulate TSH receptors on follicular cells of the thyroid

What is the female-to-male ratio?

6:1

What specific physical finding is associated with Graves'?

Exophthalmos

How is the diagnosis made?

Increased T3, T4, and anti-TSH receptor antibodies, decreased TSH, global uptake of ^{131}I radionuclide

What are treatment option modalities for Graves' disease?

1. **Medical blockade:** iodide, propranolol, propylthiouracil (PTU), methimazole, Lugol's solution (potassium iodide)
2. **Radioiodide ablation:** most popular therapy
3. **Surgical resection** (bilateral subtotal thyroidectomy)

What are the possible indications for surgical resection?

Suspicious nodule; if patient is noncompliant or refractory to medicines, pregnant, a child, or if patient refuses radioiodide therapy

What is the major complication of radioiodide or surgery for Graves' disease?	Hypothyroidism
What does PTU stand for?	**P**ropyl**T**hio**U**racil
How does PTU work?	1. Inhibits incorporation of iodine into T4/T3 (by blocking peroxidase oxidation of iodide to iodine) 2. Inhibits peripheral conversion of T4 to T3
How does methimazole work?	Inhibits incorporation of iodine into T4/T3 **only** (by blocking peroxidase oxidation of iodide to iodine)

Toxic Multinodular Goiter

What is it also known as?	Plummer's disease
What is it?	Multiple thyroid nodules with one or more nodules producing thyroid hormone, resulting in hyperfunctioning thyroid (hyperthyroidism or a "toxic" thyroid state)
What medication may bring on hyperthyroidism with a multinodular goiter?	Amiodarone (or any iodine-containing medication/contrast)
How is the hyperfunctioning nodule(s) localized?	^{131}I radionuclide scan
What is the treatment?	Surgically remove hyperfunctioning nodule(s) with lobectomy or near total thyroidectomy

Thyroiditis

What are the features of acute thyroiditis?	Painful, swollen thyroid; fever; overlying skin erythema; dysphagia
What is the cause of ACUTE thyroiditis?	Bacteria (usually *Streptococcus* or *Staphylococcus*), usually caused by a thyroglossal fistula or anatomic variant
What is the treatment of ACUTE thyroiditis?	Antibiotics, drainage of abscess, needle aspiration for culture; most patients need definitive surgery later to remove the fistula
What are the features of SUBACUTE thyroiditis?	Glandular swelling, tenderness, often follows URI, elevated ESR
What is the cause of SUBACUTE thyroiditis?	Viral infection
What is the treatment of SUBACUTE thyroiditis?	Supportive: NSAIDS, ± steroids

What is De Quervain's thyroiditis?	Just another name for subacute thyroiditis caused by a virus (Think: De Quer**V**ain = **V**irus)
How can the differences between etiologies of ACUTE and SUBACUTE thyroiditis be remembered?	Alphabetically: **A** before **S, B** before **V** (i.e., **A**cute before **S**ubacute and **B**acterial before **V**iral; thus, **A**cute = **B**acterial and **S**ubacute = **V**iral)
What are the common causative bacteria in acute suppurative thyroiditis?	*Streptococcus* or *Staphylococcus*
What are the two types of chronic thyroiditis?	1. Hashimoto's thyroiditis 2. Riedel's thyroiditis
What is the etiology of Hashimoto's disease?	Autoimmune (Think: Hashim**OTO** = **AUTO**; thus, Hashimoto = autoimmune)
What is Riedel's thyroiditis?	Benign inflammatory thyroid enlargement **with fibrosis** of thyroid Patients present with painless, large thyroid Fibrosis may involve surrounding tissues
What is the treatment for Riedel's thyroiditis?	Surgical tracheal decompression, thyroid hormone replacement as needed—possibly steroids/tamoxifen, if refractory

RAPID-FIRE REVIEW

Name the diagnostic stimulation test for the following:	
Medullary thyroid carcinoma?	Pentagastrin (also calcium)
Name the most likely diagnosis:	
60-year-old female with a thyroid mass, + follicular cells on biopsy, + capsular invasion, + vascular invasion	Thyroid follicular carcinoma
42-year-old female with thyroid mass, + amyloid on histology, hypercalcemia	Medullary thyroid carcinoma
25-year-old male with thyroid mass, + psammoma bodies on histology	Papillary thyroid carcinoma
Hypothyroidism, "woody" hard thyroid, tracheal compression	Riedel's thyroiditis

17-year-old female with upper respiratory tract infection followed by fever, neck pain, dysphagia, tender thyroid gland, + strep cultures	Acute suppurative thyroiditis
28-year-old female with tender thyroid, hypothyroidism, elevated antimicrosomal antibodies, increased antithyroglobulin antibodies	Hashimoto's thyroiditis

Chapter 58 | Parathyroid

ANATOMY

How many parathyroids are there?	Usually **four** (two superior and two inferior)
What percentage of patients has five parathyroid glands?	≈5% (Think: 5 = 5)
What percentage of patients has three parathyroid glands?	≈10%
What is the usual position of the inferior parathyroid glands?	Posterior and lateral behind the thyroid and below the inferior thyroid artery
What is the most common site of an "extra" gland?	Thymus gland
What percentage of patients has a parathyroid gland in the mediastinum?	≈1%
If only three parathyroid glands are found at surgery, where can the fourth be hiding?	Thyroid gland Thymus/mediastinum Carotid sheath Tracheoesophageal groove Behind the esophagus
What is the embryologic origin of the following structures?	
Superior parathyroid glands	Fourth pharyngeal pouch
Inferior parathyroid glands	Third pharyngeal pouch (counterintuitive)
What supplies blood to all four parathyroid glands?	Inferior thyroid artery

What is the most common cause of hypercalcemia in outpatients?	Hyperparathyroidism

PHYSIOLOGY

What cell type produces PTH?	Chief cells produce ParaThyroid Hormone (**PTH**)
What are the major actions of PTH?	**Increases** blood **calcium** levels (takes from bone breakdown, GI absorption, increased resorption from kidney, excretion of phosphate by kidney), **decreases** serum phosphate
How does vitamin D work?	Increases intestinal absorption of calcium and phosphate
Where is calcium absorbed?	Duodenum and proximal jejunum

HYPERPARATHYROIDISM (HPTH)

What is primary HPTH?	Increased secretion of PTH by parathyroid gland(s); marked by elevated calcium, low phosphorus
What is secondary HPTH?	Increased serum PTH resulting from calcium wasting caused by **renal failure or decreased GI calcium absorption,** rickets or osteomalacia; calcium levels are usually **low**
What is tertiary HPTH?	Persistent HPTH after correction of secondary hyperparathyroidism; results from autonomous PTH secretion not responsive to the normal negative feedback due to elevated Ca^{2+} levels
What are the methods of imaging the parathyroids?	Surgical operation U/S **Sestamibi scan** ^{201}TI (technetium)–thallium subtraction scan CT scan/MRI A-gram (rare) Venous sampling for PTH (rare)
What are the indications for a localizing preoperative study?	**Reoperation** for recurrent hyperparathyroidism
What is the most common cause of primary HPTH?	Adenoma (>85%)

What are the etiologies of primary HPTH and percentages?	**Adenoma** ($\approx$85%) Hyperplasia ($\approx$10%) Carcinoma ($\approx$1%)
What is the incidence of primary HPTH in the United States?	$\approx$1/1,000 to 4,000
What are the risk factors for primary HPTH?	Family history, MEN-I and MEN-IIa, irradiation

What are the signs/symptoms of primary HPTH hypercalcemia?	**"Stones, bones, groans, and psychiatric overtones":**
	    Stones: Kidney stones
	    Bones: Bone pain, pathologic fractures, subperiosteal resorption
	    Groans: Muscle pain and weakness, pancreatitis, gout, constipation
	    Psychiatric overtones: Depression, anorexia, anxiety
	    Other symptoms: Polydipsia, weight loss, HTN (10%), polyuria, lethargy

What is the "33-to-1" rule?	Most patients with primary HPTH have a ratio of serum (Cl^-) to phosphate $\geq$33
What plain x-ray findings are classic for HPTH?	Subperiosteal bone resorption (usually in hand digits; said to be "pathognomonic" for HPTH!)
How is primary HPTH diagnosed?	Labs—elevated PTH (hypercalcemia, $\downarrow$ phosphorus, $\uparrow$ chloride); urine calcium should be checked for familial hypocalciuric hypercalcemia
What is familial hypocalciuric hypercalcemia?	Familial (autosomal dominant) inheritance of a condition of **asymptomatic** hypercalcemia and low urine calcium, with or without elevated PTH; in contrast, hypercalcemia from HPTH results in high levels of urine calcium *Note:* Surgery to remove parathyroid glands is not indicated for this diagnosis
How many of the glands are USUALLY affected by the following conditions?	
Hyperplasia	4
Adenoma	1
Carcinoma	1

What is the differential diagnosis of hypercalcemia?

"CHIMPANZEES":
Calcium overdose
Hyperparathyroidism (1°/2°/3°),
Hyperthyroidism, Hypocalciuric
    Hypercalcemia (familial)
Immobility/Iatrogenic (thiazide diuretics)
Metastasis/Milk-alkali syndrome (rare)
Paget's disease (bone)
Addison's disease/acromegaly
Neoplasm (colon, lung, breast, prostate,
    multiple myeloma)
Zollinger–Ellison syndrome
Excessive vitamin D
Excessive vitamin A
Sarcoid

What is the initial medical treatment of hypercalcemia (1° HPTH)?

Medical—IV fluids, furosemide—**NOT** thiazide diuretics

Although most recommend surgery for asymptomatic 1° HHPTH, when is it considered mandatory?

"ROACH":
Renal insufficiency (CR ↓ by 30%)
Osteoporosis (T score < −2.5)
Age <50
Calcium >1 mg/dL above upper limit of
    normal
Hypercalciuria (>400 mg/day Ca^{2+}
    excretion)

What is the definitive treatment of HPTH in the following cases?

    Primary HPTH resulting from HYPERPLASIA

Neck exploration removing all parathyroid glands and leaving at least 30 mg of parathyroid tissue placed in the forearm muscles (nondominant arm, of course!)

    Primary HPTH resulting from parathyroid ADENOMA

Surgically remove adenoma (send for frozen section) and biopsy all abnormally enlarged parathyroid glands (some experts biopsy all glands)

    Primary HPTH resulting from parathyroid CARCINOMA

Remove carcinoma, ipsilateral thyroid lobe, and all enlarged lymph nodes (modified radical neck dissection for LN metastases)

    Secondary HPTH

Correct calcium and phosphate; perform renal transplantation (no role for parathyroid surgery)

    Tertiary HPTH

Correct calcium and phosphate; perform surgical operation to remove all parathyroid glands and reimplant 30 to 40 mg in the forearm if **REFRACTORY** to medical management

Why place 30 to 40 mg of sliced parathyroid gland in the forearm?	To retain parathyroid function; if HPTH recurs, remove some of the parathyroid gland from the easily accessible forearm
What must be ruled out in the patient with HPTH from hyperplasia?	MEN type I and MEN type IIa
What carcinomas are commonly associated with hypercalcemia?	**Breast cancer metastases,** prostate cancer, kidney cancer, lung cancer, pancreatic cancer, multiple myeloma
What is the most likely diagnosis if a patient has a PALPABLE neck mass, hypercalcemia, and elevated PTH?	Parathyroid carcinoma (vast majority of other causes of primary HPTH have nonpalpable parathyroids)

PARATHYROID CARCINOMA

What is it?	Primary carcinoma of the parathyroid gland
What is the number of glands usually affected?	1
What are the signs/symptoms?	Hypercalcemia, elevated PTH, **PALPABLE** parathyroid gland (50%), pain in neck, recurrent laryngeal nerve paralysis (change in voice), hypercalcemic crisis (usually associated with calcium levels >14)
What is the common tumor marker?	Human Chorionic Gonadotropin (**HCG**)
What is the treatment?	Surgical resection of parathyroid mass with ipsilateral thyroid lobectomy, ipsilateral lymph node resection
What percentage of all cases of primary HPTH is caused by parathyroid carcinoma?	1%

Postoperative Complications of Parathyroidectomy

What are the possible postoperative complications after a parathyroidectomy?	Recurrent nerve injury (unilateral: voice change; bilateral: airway obstruction), neck hematoma (open at bedside if breathing is compromised), hypocalcemia, superior laryngeal nerve injury
What is "hungry bone syndrome"?	Severe hypocalcemia seen after surgical correction of HPTH as chronically calcium-deprived bone aggressively absorbs calcium
What are the signs/symptoms of postoperative hypocalcemia?	Perioral tingling, paresthesia, + Chvostek's sign, + Trousseau's sign, + tetany

What is the treatment of hypoparathyroidism?	Acute: IV calcium Chronic: PO calcium, and vitamin D
What is parathyromatosis?	Multiple small hyperfunctioning parathyroid tissue masses found over the neck and mediastinum—thought to be from congenital rests or spillage during surgery—remove surgically (RARE)

RAPID-FIRE REVIEW

What is the correct diagnosis:

Palpable parathyroid gland and hypercalcemia	Parathyroid carcinoma
50-year-old female with parathyroid hyperplasia, jejunal ulcers, loss of peripheral vision	MEN-I (parathyroid hyperplasia, gastrinoma, pituitary tumor)
45-year-old female with palpable neck mass and hypercalcemia with elevated parathyroid hormone	Parathyroid carcinoma
34-year-old female with a symptomatic hypercalcemia with low calcium level in her urine	Familial hypocalciuric hypercalcemia

Name the radiographic test for localizing the following:

Hyperfunctioning parathyroid	^{99m}Tc-sestamibi scintigraphy

Chapter 59 | Spleen and Splenectomy

Which arteries supply the spleen?	Splenic artery (a branch of the celiac trunk) and the short gastric arteries that arise from the gastroepiploic arteries

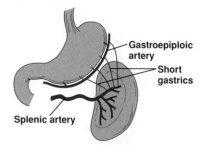

Gastroepiploic artery

Short gastrics

Splenic artery

What is the venous drainage of the spleen?	**Portal** vein, via the splenic vein and the left gastroepiploic vein
What is said to "tickle" the spleen?	Tail of the pancreas
What percentage of people has an accessory spleen?	≈20%
What is "delayed splenic rupture"?	Subcapsular hematoma or pseudoaneurysm may rupture sometime after blunt trauma, causing "delayed splenic rupture"; rupture classically occurs ≈2 weeks post injury and presents with shock/abdominal pain
What are the signs/symptoms of ruptured/injured spleen?	Hemoperitoneum and Kehr's sign, LUQ abdominal pain, Ballance's sign
What is Kehr's sign?	Left shoulder pain seen with splenic rupture
How is a spleen injury diagnosed?	Abdominal CT scan, **if the patient is stable;** DPL or FAST exam if the patient is unstable
What is the treatment?	1. Nonoperative in a stable patient with an isolated splenic injury without hilar involvement/complete rupture 2. If patient is unstable, DPL/FAST laparotomy with splenorrhaphy or splenectomy 3. Embolization is an option in selected patients
What is a splenorrhaphy?	Splenic salvage operation: wrapping Vicryl® mesh, aid of topical hemostatic agents or partial splenectomy, sutures (buttressed)
What are the other indications for splenectomy?	
Malignant diseases	Hodgkin's staging not conclusive by CT scan (rare) Splenic tumors (primary/metastatic/locally invasive) Hypersplenism caused by other leukemias/non-Hodgkin's lymphomas
Anemias	Medullary fibrosis with myeloid metaplasia Hereditary elliptocytosis Sickle cell anemia (rare, most autosplenectomize) Pyruvate kinase deficiency Autoimmune hemolytic anemia Hereditary spherocytosis Thalassemias (e.g., β-thalassemia major, a.k.a. "Cooley's")

Thrombocytopenia	**ITP** (**I**diopathic **T**hrombocytopenic **P**urpura) **TTP** (**T**hrombotic **T**hrombocytopenic **P**urpura)
Is G6PD deficiency an indication for splenectomy?	NO
What are the possible postsplenectomy complications?	Thrombocytosis, subphrenic abscess, atelectasis, pancreatitis, gastric dilation, and **O**verwhelming **P**ost**S**plenectomy **S**epsis (**OPSS**), pancreatic injury (tail)
What causes OPSS?	Increased susceptibility to fulminant bacteremia, meningitis, or pneumonia because of loss of splenic function
What is the incidence of OPSS in adults?	<1%
What is the incidence and overall mortality of OPSS in children?	1% to 2% with 50% mortality rate
What is the typical presentation of OPSS?	Fever, lethargy, common cold, sore throat, URI followed by confusion, shock, and coma with death ensuing within 24 hours in up to 50% of patients
What are the common organisms associated with OPSS?	**Encapsulated:** *Streptococcus pneumoniae, Neisseria meningitidis, Haemophilus influenzae*
What is the most common bacteria in OPSS?	*S. pneumoniae*
What is the preventive treatment of OPSS?	Vaccinations for pneumococcus, *H. influenzae,* and meningococcus Prophylactic penicillin for all minor infections/illnesses and immediate medical care if febrile illness develops
What is the best time to give immunizations to splenectomy patients?	**Preoperatively,** if at all possible If emergent, then *2 weeks* postoperatively
What lab tests are abnormal after splenectomy?	WBC count increases by 50% over the baseline; marked **thrombocytosis** occurs; RBC smear is abnormal
What are the findings on postsplenectomy RBC smear?	Peripheral smear will show Pappenheimer bodies, Howell–Jolly bodies, and Heinz bodies
What is the most common cause of splenic vein thrombosis?	Pancreatitis

What opsonins does the spleen produce?	**PRO**perdin, **TUF**tsin (Think: "**PRO**fessionally **TUF** spleen")
What is the most common cause of ISOLATED GASTRIC varices?	Splenic vein thrombosis (usually from pancreatitis)
What is the treatment of gastric varices caused by splenic vein thrombosis?	Splenectomy
Which patients develop hyposplenism?	Patients with ulcerative colitis
What vaccinations should every patient with a splenectomy receive?	Pneumococcus Meningococcus *H. influenzae* type B
What is hypersplenism?	Hyperfunctioning spleen Documented loss of blood elements (WBC, Hct, platelets) Large spleen (splenomegaly) Hyperactive bone marrow (trying to keep up with loss of blood elements)
What is splenomegaly?	Enlarged spleen
What is idiopathic thrombocytopenic purpura (ITP)?	Autoimmune (antiplatelet antibodies IgG in >90% of patients) platelet destruction leading to troublesome bleeding and purpura
What is the most common cause of failure to correct thrombocytopenia after splenectomy for ITP?	Missed accessory spleen
What are the "Is" of ITP (4)?	1. Immune etiology (IgG antiplatelets ABs) 2. Immunosuppressive treatment (initially treated with steroids) 3. Immune globulin 4. Improvement with splenectomy (75% of patients have improved platelet counts after splenectomy)
What is TTP?	Thrombotic Thrombocytopenic Purpura
What is the treatment of choice for TTP?	Plasmapheresis (splenectomy reserved as a last resort—very rare)
What is the most common physical finding of portal hypertension?	Splenomegaly

Chapter 60 | Surgically Correctable HTN

What is it?

Hypertension caused by conditions that are amenable to surgical correction

What percentage of patients with HTN has a surgically correctable cause?

≈7%

What diseases that cause HTN are surgically correctable?

Think **"CAN I CHURP?"**:

Cushing's syndrome
Aortic coarctation
Neuroblastoma/neoplasia

Increased intracranial pressure

Conn's syndrome (primary hyperaldosteronism)
Hyperparathyroidism/hyperthyroidism
Unilateral renal parenchymal disease
Renal artery stenosis
Pheochromocytoma

Chapter 61 | Soft Tissue Sarcomas and Lymphomas

SOFT TISSUE SARCOMAS

Name the following types of malignant sarcoma:

Fat

Liposarcoma

Gastrointestinal

GIST (**G**astro**I**ntestinal **S**tromal **T**umor)

Myofibroblast

Malignant fibrous histiocytoma

Striated muscle

Rhabdomyosarcoma

Vascular endothelium

Angiosarcoma

Fibroblast

Fibrosarcoma

Lymph vessel

Lymphangiosarcoma

Peripheral nerve

Malignant neurilemmoma or schwannoma

AIDS

Kaposi's sarcoma

Lymphedema

Lymphangiosarcoma

What are the signs/symptoms?	Soft tissue mass; pain from compression of adjacent structures, often noticed after minor trauma to area of mass
How do most sarcomas metastasize?	Hematogenously (i.e., via blood)
What is the most common location and route of metastasis?	**Lungs** via hematogenous route
What are the three most common malignant sarcomas in adults?	Fibrous histiocytoma (25%) Liposarcoma (20%) Leiomyosarcoma (15%)
What are the two most common sarcomas in children?	Rhabdomyosarcoma (≈50%), fibrosarcoma (20%)
What is the most common sarcoma of the retroperitoneum?	Liposarcoma
How is the diagnosis made?	Imaging workup—MRI is superior to CT scan at distinguishing the tumor from adjacent structures Mass <3 cm: excisional biopsy **Mass >3 cm:** incisional biopsy or **core biopsy**
What is excisional biopsy?	Biopsy by removing the **entire** mass
What is incisional biopsy?	Biopsy by removing a **piece** of the mass
What is the orientation of incision for incisional biopsy of a suspected extremity sarcoma?	**Longitudinal,** not transverse, so that the incision can be incorporated in a future resection if biopsy for sarcoma is positive
What determines histologic grade of sarcomas?	1. Differentiation 2. Mitotic count 3. Tumor necrosis Grade 1 = well differentiated Grade 2 = moderately differentiated Grade 3 = poorly differentiated
What is a pseudocapsule and what is its importance?	Outer layer of a sarcoma that represents compressed malignant cells
What is the most important factor in the prognosis?	**Histologic grade** of the primary lesion
What is the treatment?	Surgical resection and radiation (with or without chemotherapy)
What surgical margins are obtained?	2 cm (1 cm minimum)
What is the "limb-sparing" surgery for extremity sarcoma?	Avoidance of amputation with local resection and chemoradiation
What is the treatment of pulmonary metastasis?	Surgical resection for isolated lesions

GI Lymphoma

What is it?	Non-Hodgkin's lymphoma arising in the GI tract
What is the risk factor for gastric lymphoma?	*Helicobacter pylori*
What are the signs/symptoms?	Abdominal pain, obstruction, GI hemorrhage, GI tract perforation, fatigue
What is the treatment of intestinal lymphoma?	Surgical resection with removal of draining lymph nodes and chemotherapy
What is the most common site of primary GI tract lymphoma?	Stomach (66%)

Chapter 62 | Skin Lesions

What are the most common skin cancers?	1. Basal cell carcinoma (75%) 2. Squamous cell carcinoma (20%) 3. Melanoma (4%)
What is the most common fatal skin cancer?	Melanoma
What is malignant melanoma?	A redundancy! All melanomas are considered malignant!

SQUAMOUS CELL CARCINOMA

What is it?	Carcinoma arising from epidermal cells
What are the most common sites?	Head, neck, and hands
What are the risk factors?	Sun exposure, pale skin, chronic inflammatory process, immunosuppression, xeroderma pigmentosum, arsenic
What is a precursor skin lesion?	Actinic keratosis
What are the signs/symptoms?	Raised, slightly pigmented skin lesion; ulceration/exudate; chronic scab; itching
How is the diagnosis made?	Small lesion—excisional biopsy Large lesions—incisional biopsy
What is the treatment?	Small lesion (<1 cm): Excise with 0.5-cm margin Large lesion (>1 cm): Resect with 1- to 2-cm margins of normal tissue (large lesions may require skin graft/flap)

What is the dreaded sign of metastasis?	Palpable lymph nodes (remove involved lymph node basin)
What is Marjolin's ulcer?	Squamous cell carcinoma that arises in an area of chronic inflammation (e.g., chronic fistula, burn wound, osteomyelitis)
What is the prognosis?	Excellent if totally excised (95% cure rate); most patients with positive lymph node metastasis eventually die from metastatic disease
What is the treatment for solitary metastasis?	Surgical resection

BASAL CELL CARCINOMA

What is it?	Carcinoma arising in the germinating basal cell layer of epithelial cells
What are the risk factors?	Sun exposure, fair skin, radiation, chronic dermatitis, xeroderma pigmentosum
What are the most common sites?	Head, neck, and hands
What are the signs/symptoms?	Slow-growing skin mass (chronic, scaly); scab; ulceration, with or without pigmentation, often described as "pearl-like"
How is the diagnosis made?	Excisional or incisional biopsy
What is the treatment?	Resection with 5-mm margins (2-mm margin in cosmetically sensitive areas)
What is the risk of metastasis?	Very low (recur locally)

MISCELLANEOUS SKIN LESIONS

What is an epidermal inclusion cyst?	**EIC** = Benign subcutaneous cyst filled with epidermal cells (should be removed surgically) filled with waxy material; no clinical difference from a sebaceous cyst
What is a sebaceous cyst?	Benign subcutaneous cyst filled with sebum (waxy, paste-like substance) from a blocked sweat gland (should be removed with a small area of skin that includes the blocked gland); may become infected; much less common than EIC
What is actinic keratosis?	Premalignant skin lesion from sun exposure; seen as a scaly skin lesion (surgical removal eliminates the 20% risk of cancer transformation)

What is seborrheic keratosis?	Benign pigmented lesion in the elderly; observe or treat by excision (especially if there is any question of melanoma), curettage, or topical agents
How to remember actinic keratosis versus seborrheic keratosis malignant potential?	Actinic **K**eratosis = **AK** = **A**sset **K**icker = premalignant (20% convert to carcinoma) Seborrheic **K**eratosis = **SK** = **S**oft **K**icker = benign
What is Bowen's disease of the skin?	Squamous carcinoma in situ (should be removed or destroyed, thereby removing the problem)
What is "Mohs" surgery?	Mohs technique or surgery: repeats thin excision until margins are clear by microscopic review (named after Dr. Mohs)—used to minimize collateral skin excision (e.g., on the face)

Chapter 63 | Melanoma

What is it?	Neoplastic disorder produced by malignant transformation of the melanocyte; melanocytes are derived from neural crest cells
Which patients are at greatest risk?	White patients with blonde/red hair, fair skin, freckling, a history of blistering sunburns, blue/green eyes, actinic keratosis Male > female
What are the three most common sites?	1. Skin 2. Eyes 3. Anus (Think: **SEA** = **S**kin, **E**yes, **A**nus)
What is the most common site in African Americans?	Palms of the hands, soles of the feet (acral lentiginous melanoma)
What characteristics are suggestive of melanoma?	Usually a pigmented lesion with an irregular border, irregular surface, or irregular coloration Other clues: darkening of a pigmented lesion, development of pigmented satellite lesions, irregular margins or surface elevations, notching, recent or rapid enlargement, erosion or ulceration of surface, pruritus

What are the "ABCDEs" of melanoma?	**A**symmetry **B**order irregularity **C**olor variation **D**iameter >6 mm and **D**ark lesion **E**volution (changes over time)
What are the associated risk factors?	Severe sunburn before age 18, giant congenital nevi, family history, race (White), ultraviolet radiation (sun), multiple dysplastic nevi
How does location differ in men and women?	Men get more lesions on the trunk; women on the extremities
Which locations are unusual?	Noncutaneous regions, such as mucous membranes of the vulva/vagina, anorectum, esophagus, and choroidal layer of the eye
What is the most common site of melanoma in men?	Back (33%)
What is the most common site of melanoma in women?	Legs (33%)
What are the four major histologic types?	1. Superficial spreading 2. Lentigo maligna 3. Acral lentiginous 4. Nodular

Define the following terms:

Superficial spreading melanoma	Occurs in both sun-exposed and nonexposed areas; **most common** of all melanomas (75%)
Lentigo maligna melanoma	Malignant cells that are superficial, found usually in elderly patients on the head or neck Called "Hutchinson's freckle" if noninvasive Least aggressive type; very good prognosis Accounts for <10% of all melanomas
Acral lentiginous melanoma	Occurs on the palms, soles, subungual areas, and mucous membranes Accounts for ≈5% of all melanomas (most common melanoma in African American patients; ≈50%)
Nodular melanoma	Vertical growth predominates Lesions are usually dark Most aggressive type/worst prognosis Accounts for ≈15% of all melanomas
Amelanotic melanoma	Melanoma from melanocytes but with obvious lack of pigment
What is the most common type of melanoma?	Superficial spreading (≈75%) (Think: **SUPER**ficial = **SUPER**ior)

What type of melanoma arises in Hutchinson's freckle?	Lentigo maligna melanoma
What is Hutchinson's freckle?	Lentigo maligna melanoma in the radial growth phase without vertical extension (noninvasive); usually occurs on the faces of elderly women
What are the common sites of metastasis?	Nodes (local) Distant: lung, liver, bone, heart, and brain Melanoma has a specific attraction for small bowel mucosa Brain metastases are a common cause of death
What are the metastatic routes?	Both lymphatic and hematogenous
How is the diagnosis made?	Excisional biopsy (complete removal leaving only normal tissue) or incisional biopsy for very large lesions (*Note:* Early diagnosis is crucial!)
What is the role of shave biopsy?	No role
What is the "sentinel node" biopsy?	Inject Lymphazurin® blue dye, colloid with a radiolabel, or both around the melanoma; the first lymph node (LN) in the draining chain is identified as the "sentinel lymph node" and reflects the metastatic status of the group of LNs
When is elective LN dissection recommended?	Controversial—possible advantage in melanomas 1 to 2 mm in depth but jury still out; sentinel node biopsy if >1 mm is becoming very common
Melanoma "tumor marker"?	S-100
What is the recommended size of the surgical margin for depth of invasion of the following?	
Melanoma in situ	0.5-cm margin
≤1 mm thick	1-cm margin
1 to 4 mm thick	2-cm margin
>4 mm thick	3-cm margin
What is the treatment for digital melanoma?	Amputation
What is the treatment of palpable LN metastasis?	Lymphadenectomy
What factors determine the prognosis?	Depth of invasion and metastasis are the most important factors

What is the workup to survey for metastasis in the patient with melanoma?	Physical exam, LFTs, CXR (bone scan/CT scan/MRI reserved for symptoms)
What is the treatment of intestinal metastasis?	Surgical resection to prevent bleeding/obstruction
What is FDA-approved adjuvant therapy?	Interferon α-2b (for stages IIB/III)
What is the treatment of unresectable brain metastasis?	Radiation
What is the treatment of isolated adrenal metastasis?	Surgical resection
What is the treatment of isolated lung metastasis?	Surgical resection
What is the most common symptom of anal melanoma?	Bleeding
What is the treatment of anal melanoma?	APR or wide excision (no survival benefit from APR, but better local control)
What is the median survival with distant metastasis?	$\approx$6 months

Chapter 64 | Surgical Intensive Care

INTENSIVE CARE UNIT (ICU) BASICS

How is an ICU note written?	By **systems:** Neurologic (e.g., GCS, MAE, pain control) Pulmonary (e.g., vent settings) CVS (e.g., pressors) GI (gastrointestinal) Heme (CBC) FEN (e.g., Chem-10, nutrition) Renal (e.g., urine output, BUN, Cr) ID (e.g., T_{max}, WBC, antibiotics) Assessment Plan (***Note:*** Physical exam included in each section)
What is the best way to report urine output in the ICU?	24 hours/last shift/last 3 hourly rate = "urine output has been 2 L over the last 24 hours, 350 last shift, and 45, 35, 40 cc over the last 3 hours"

What are the possible causes of fever in the ICU?	Central line infection Pneumonia/atelectasis UTI, urosepsis Intra-abdominal abscess Sinusitis DVT Thrombophlebitis Drug fever Fungal infection, meningitis, wound infection Endocarditis
What is the most common bacteria in ICU pneumonia?	Gram-negative rods
What is the acronym for the basic ICU care checklist (Dr. Vincent)?	"FAST HUG": Feeding Analgesia Sedation Thromboembolic prophylaxis Head-of-bed elevation (pneumonia prevention) Ulcer prevention Glucose control

INTENSIVE CARE UNIT FORMULAS AND TERMS YOU SHOULD KNOW

What is CO?	Cardiac Output: HR (heart rate) × SV (stroke volume)
What is the normal CO?	4 to 8 L/min
What factors increase CO?	Increased contractility, heart rate, and preload; decreased afterload
What is CI?	Cardiac Index: CO/BSA (body surface area)
What is the normal CI?	2.5 to 3.5 L/min/m^2
What is SV?	Stroke Volume: the amount of blood pumped out of the ventricle each beat; simply, end-diastolic volume minus the end-systolic volume **or** CO/HR
What is the normal SV?	60 to 100 cc
What is CVP?	Central Venous Pressure: indirect measurement of intravascular volume status
What is the normal CVP?	4 to 11

What is PCWP?	**P**ulmonary **C**apillary **W**edge **P**ressure: indirectly measures left atrial pressure, which is an estimate of intravascular volume (LV filling pressure)
What is the normal PCWP?	5 to 15
What is anion gap?	$Na^+ - (Cl^- + HCO_3^-)$
What are the normal values for anion gap?	10 to 14
Why do you get an increased anion gap?	Unmeasured acids are unmeasured anions in the equation that are part of the "counterbalance" to the sodium cation
What are the causes of increased anion gap acidosis in surgical patients?	Think **"SALUD"**: **S**tarvation **A**lcohol (ethanol/methanol) **L**actic acidosis **U**remia (renal failure) **D**KA
Define MODS:	**M**ultiple **O**rgan **D**ysfunction **S**yndrome
What is SVR?	**S**ystemic **V**ascular **R**esistance: (MAP − CVP)/CO × 80 (Remember, P = F × R, **P**ower **FoR**ward; and calculating resistance: **R = P/F**)
What is SVRI?	**S**ystemic **V**ascular **R**esistance **I**ndex: SVR/BSA
What is the normal SVRI?	1,500 to 2,400
What is MAP?	**M**ean **A**rterial **P**ressure: diastolic blood pressure + **1/3 (systolic pressure − diastolic pressure)** (*Note:* Not the mean between diastolic and systolic blood pressure because diastole lasts longer than systole)
What is PVR?	**P**ulmonary **V**ascular **R**esistance: PA (MEAN) − PCWP/CO × 80 (PA is pulmonary artery pressure and LA is left atrial or PCWP pressure)
What is the normal PVR value?	100 ± 50
What is the formula for arterial oxygen content?	Hemoglobin × O_2 saturation (SaO_2) × 1.34
What is the basic formula for oxygen delivery?	CO × (oxygen content)
What is the full formula for oxygen delivery?	CO × (1.34 × Hgb × SaO_2) × 10
What factors can increase oxygen delivery?	Increased CO by increasing SV, HR, or both; increased O_2 content by increasing the hemoglobin content, SaO_2, or both

What is mixed venous oxygen saturation?	Svo_2; simply, the O_2 saturation of the blood in the right ventricle or pulmonary artery; an indirect measure of peripheral oxygen supply and demand
Which lab values help assess adequate oxygen delivery?	Svo_2 (low with inadequate delivery), lactic acid (elevated with inadequate delivery), pH (acidosis with inadequate delivery), base deficit
What is FENa?	Fractional Excretion of Sodium (**Na$^+$**): $(U_{Na^+} \times P_{cr}/P_{Na^+} \times U_{cr}) \times 100$
What is the memory aid for calculating FENa?	Think: **YOU NEED PEE = U (U**rine) **N (Na$^+$) P (P**lasma); $U_{Na^+} \times P_{cr}$; for the denominator, switch everything, $P_{Na^+} \times U_{cr}$ (cr = creatinine)
What is the prerenal FENa value?	<1.0; renal failure from decreased renal blood flow (e.g., cardiogenic, hypovolemia, arterial obstruction, etc.)

LAB VALUES ACUTE RENAL FAILURE

BUN-to-Cr ratio?	
Prerenal	>20:1
Renal ATN	<20:1
FENa?	
Prerenal	<1
Renal ATN	>1
Urine osmolality?	
Prerenal	>500
Renal ATN	<350
Urine Na$^+$?	
Prerenal	<20
Renal ATN	>40
Urine SG (Specific Gravity)?	
Prerenal	>1.020
How long do Lasix® effects last?	6 hours = **LASIX** = **LA**sts **SIX** hours
What is the formula for flow/pressure/resistance?	Remember **P**ower Fo**R**ward: **P**ressure = **F**low × **R**esistance
What is the "10-for-0.08 rule" of acid–base?	For every increase of $Paco_2$ by **10** mm Hg, the pH falls by **0.08**

What is the "40, 50, 60 for 70, 80, 90 rule" for O_2 sats?	PaO_2 of **40, 50, 60** corresponds roughly to an O_2 sat of **70, 80, 90**, respectively
One liter of O_2 via nasal cannula raises Fio_2 by how much?	$\approx 3\%$
What is pure respiratory acidosis?	Low pH (acidosis), increased $Paco_2$, normal bicarbonate
What is pure respiratory alkalosis?	High pH (alkalosis), decreased $Paco_2$, normal bicarbonate
What is pure metabolic acidosis?	Low pH, low bicarbonate, normal $Paco_2$
What is pure metabolic alkalosis?	High pH, high bicarbonate, normal $Paco_2$

How does the body compensate for each of the following?

Respiratory acidosis	Increased bicarbonate
Respiratory alkalosis	Decreased bicarbonate
Metabolic acidosis	Decreased $Paco_2$
Metabolic alkalosis	Increased $Paco_2$
What does MOF stand for?	**M**ultiple **O**rgan **F**ailure
What does SIRS stand for?	**S**ystemic **I**nflammatory **R**esponse **S**yndrome

SICU DRUGS

Dopamine

What is the site of action and effect at the following levels?

Low dose (1–3 µg/kg/min)	+ + dopa agonist; **renal vasodilation** (a.k.a. "renal dose dopamine")
Intermediate dose (4–10 µg/kg/min)	$+ \alpha_1$, $+ + \beta_1$; positive inotropy and some vasoconstriction
High dose (>10 µg/kg/min)	$+ + + \alpha_1$ agonist; marked afterload increase from arteriolar vasoconstriction
Has "renal dose" dopamine been shown to decrease renal failure?	NO

Dobutamine

What is the site of action?	$+ + + \beta_1$ agonist, $+ + \beta_2$
What is the effect?	$\uparrow$ Inotropy; $\uparrow$ chronotropy, decrease in systemic vascular resistance

Isoproterenol

What is the site of action?	$+++\beta_1$ and β_2 agonist
What is the effect?	↑ Inotropy; ↑ chronotropy; (+ vasodilation of skeletal and mesenteric vascular beds)

Epinephrine (EPI)

What is the site of action?	$++\alpha_1, \alpha_2, ++++\beta_1$, and β_2 agonist
What is the effect?	↑ Inotropy; ↑ chronotropy
What is the effect at high doses?	Vasoconstriction

Norepinephrine (NE)

What is the site of action?	$+++\alpha_1, \alpha_2, +++\beta_1$, and β_1 agonist
What is the effect?	↑ Inotropy; ↑ chronotropy; ++ increase in blood pressure
What is the effect at high doses?	Severe vasoconstriction

Vasopressin

What is the action?	Vasoconstriction (increases MAP, SVR)
What are the indications?	Hypotension, especially refractory to other vasopressors (low-dose infusion—0.01–0.04 units per minute) or as a bolus during ACLS (40 u)

Sodium Nitroprusside (SNP)

What is the site of action?	$+++$ venodilation; $+++$ arteriolar dilation
What is the effect?	Decreased preload and afterload (allowing blood pressure titration)
What is the major toxicity of SNP?	**Cyanide** toxicity

INTENSIVE CARE PHYSIOLOGY

Define the following terms:

Preload	Load on the heart muscle that stretches it to end-diastolic volume (end-diastolic pressure) = intravascular volume
Afterload	Load or resistance the heart must pump against = vascular tone = SVR
Contractility	Force of heart muscle contraction
Compliance	Distensibility of heart by the preload

What is the Frank–Starling curve?	Cardiac output increases with increasing preload up to a point
What factors influence mixed venous oxygen saturation?	Oxygen **delivery** (hemoglobin concentration, arterial oxygen saturation, cardiac output) and oxygen **extraction** by the peripheral tissues
What lab test for tissue ischemia is based on the shift from aerobic to anaerobic metabolism?	Serum lactic acid levels

Define the following terms:

Dead space	That part of the inspired air that does not participate in gas exchange (e.g., the gas in the large airways/ET tube not in contact with capillaries) (Think: space = air)
Shunt fraction	That fraction of pulmonary venous blood that does not participate in gas exchange (Think: shunt = blood)
What causes increased dead space?	Overventilation (emphysema, excessive PEEP) or underperfusion (pulmonary embolus, low cardiac output, pulmonary artery vasoconstriction)
At high shunt fractions, what is the effect of increasing Fio_2 on arterial PO_2?	At high shunt fractions (>50%), changes in Fio_2 have almost no effect on arterial PO_2 because the blood that does "see" the O_2 is already at maximal O_2 absorption; thus, increasing the Fio_2 has no effect (Fio_2 can be minimized to prevent oxygen toxicity)
Define ARDS:	**A**cute **R**espiratory **D**istress **S**yndrome: lung inflammation causing respiratory failure
What is the ARDS diagnostic triad?	A "CXR": **C: C**apillary wedge pressure <18 **X: X**-ray of chest with bilateral infiltrates **R: R**atio of Pao_2 to Fio_2 <300 (a.k.a. "P/F ratio")

Define ARDS?

Mild	P/F ratio 200 to 300
Moderate	P/F ratio 100 to 200
Severe	P/F ratio ≤100
What does the classic chest x-ray look like with ARDS?	Bilateral fluffy infiltrates
How can you remember the Pao_2-to-Fio_2, or PF, ratio?	Think: "**PUFF**" ratio: **PF** ratio = $Pao_2:Fio_2$ ratio

At what concentration does O_2 toxicity occur?	Fio_2 of >60% × 48 hours; thus, try to keep Fio_2 <60% at all times
What are the ONLY ventilatory parameters that have been shown to decrease mortality in ARDS patients?	Low tidal volumes (≤6 cc/kg) and low plateau pressures <30
What else has been shown to decrease mortality in severe ARDS?	Prone positioning
What are the main causes of carbon dioxide retention?	Hypoventilation, increased dead space ventilation, and increased carbon dioxide production (as in hypermetabolic states)
Why are carbohydrates minimized in the diet/TPN of patients having difficulty with hypercapnia?	**R**espiratory **Q**uotient (**RQ**) is the ratio of CO_2 production to O_2 consumption and is highest for carbohydrates (1.0) and lowest for fats (0.7)

HEMODYNAMIC MONITORING

Why are indwelling arterial lines used for blood pressure monitoring in critically ill patients?	Because of the need for frequent measurements, the inaccuracy of frequently repeated cuff measurements, the inaccuracy of cuff measurements in hypotension, and the need for frequent arterial blood sampling/labs
What happens with a line tracing with hypovolemia?	Variation with arterial line tracing with inspiration

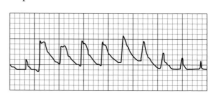

What is a Swan–Ganz (PA) catheter?	Pulmonary capillary pressure after balloon occlusion of the pulmonary artery, which is equal to left atrial pressure because there are no valves in the pulmonary system
	Left atrial pressure is essentially equal to left ventricular end-diastolic pressure (LVEDP): left heart preload, and, thus, intravascular volume status

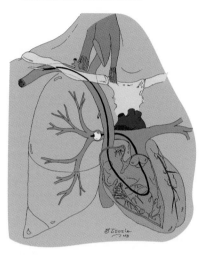

What is the primary use of the PCWP?	As an indirect measure of preload = intravascular volume

MECHANICAL VENTILATION

What is ventilation?	Air through the lungs; monitored by PCO_2
What is oxygenation?	Oxygen delivery to the alveoli; monitored by O_2 sats and PO_2
What can increase ventilation to decrease PCO_2?	Increased respiratory rate (RR), increased tidal volume (minute ventilation)
What is minute ventilation?	Volume of gas ventilated through the lungs (RR × tidal volume)
What is tidal volume?	Volume delivered with each breath; should be 6 to 8 cc/kg on the ventilator
Are ventilation and oxygenation related?	Basically no; you can have an O_2 sat of 100% and a PCO_2 of 150; O_2 sats do not tell you anything about the PCO_2 (key point!)

What can increase PO$_2$ (oxygenation) in the ventilated patient?	Increased Fio$_2$ Increased PEEP
What can decrease PCO$_2$ in the ventilated patient?	Increased RR Increased tidal volume (i.e., increase minute ventilation)

Define the following modes:

IMV	**I**ntermittent **M**andatory **V**entilation: mode with intermittent mandatory ventilations at a predetermined rate; patients can also breathe on their own above the mandatory rate **without** help from the ventilator
SIMV	**S**ynchronous **IMV:** mode of IMV that delivers the mandatory breath synchronously with patient's initiated effort; if no breath is initiated, the ventilator delivers the predetermined mandatory breath
A-C	**A**ssist-**C**ontrol ventilation: mode in which the ventilator delivers a breath when the patient initiates a breath, or the ventilator "assists" the patient to breathe; if the patient does not initiate a breath, the ventilator takes "control" and delivers a breath at a predetermined rate
CPAP	**C**ontinuous **P**ositive **A**irway **P**ressure: positive pressure delivered **continuously** (during expiration and inspiration) by ventilator, but no volume breaths (patient breathes on own)
Pressure support	Pressure is delivered only **with an initiated breath;** pressure support decreases the work of breathing by overcoming the resistance in the ventilator circuit
APRV	**A**irway **P**ressure **R**elease **V**entilation: high airway pressure intermittently released to a low airway pressure (shorter period of time)
HFV	**H**igh-**F**requency **V**entilation: rapid rates of ventilation with small tidal volumes
PEEP	**P**ositive **E**nd-**E**xpiratory **P**ressure: positive pressure maintained at the end of a breath; keeps alveoli open

What is "physiologic PEEP"?	PEEP of 5 cm H$_2$O; thought to approximate normal pressure in normal nonintubated people caused by the closed glottis

What are the typical initial ventilator settings?	
Mode	Synchronous intermittent mandatory ventilation
Tidal volume	6 to 8 mL/kg
Ventilator rate	10 breaths/min
Fio_2	100% and wean down
PEEP	5 cm H_2O From these parameters, change according to blood gas analysis
What is a normal I:E (inspiratory-to-expiratory time)?	1:2
When would you use an inverse I:E ratio (e.g., 2:1, 3:1, etc.)?	To allow for longer inspiration in patients with poor compliance, to allow for "alveolar recruitment"
When would you use a prolonged I:E ratio (e.g., 1:4)?	COPD, to allow time for complete exhalation (prevents "breath stacking")
What clinical situations cause increased airway resistance?	Airway or endotracheal tube obstruction, bronchospasm, ARDS, mucous plug, CHF (pulmonary edema)
What are the presumed advantages of PEEP?	Prevention of alveolar collapse and atelectasis, improved gas exchange, increased pulmonary compliance, decreased shunt fraction
What parameters must be evaluated in deciding if a patient is ready to be extubated?	Patient alert and able to protect airway, gas exchange (Pao_2 >70, $Paco_2$ <50), tidal volume (>5 cc/kg), minute ventilation (<10 L/min), negative inspiratory pressure (<−20 cm H_2O, or more negative), Fio_2 ≤40%, PEEP 5, PH >7.25, RR <35, Tobin index <105
What is the Rapid-Shallow Breathing (a.k.a. "Tobin") index?	**R**ate: **T**idal volume ratio; Tobin index <105 is associated with successful extubation (Think: **R**espiratory **T**herapist = **RT** = **R**ate: **T**idal volume)
What is a possible source of fever in a patient with an NG or nasal endotracheal tube?	Sinusitis (diagnosed by sinus films/CT scan)
What is the 35–45 rule of blood gas values?	Normal values: pH = 7.35–7.45 PCO_2 = 35–45
Which medications can be delivered via an endotracheal tube?	Think **"NAVEL":** **N**arcan **A**tropine **V**asopressin **E**pinephrine **L**idocaine

What conditions should you think of with ↑ peak airway pressure and ↓ urine output?

1. Tension pneumothorax
2. Abdominal compartment syndrome

RAPID-FIRE REVIEW

What is the diagnosis?

48-year-old male with pancreatitis now with acute onset of respiratory failure, PaO_2-to-FiO_2 ratio of 89, nl heart echo, bilateral pulmonary edema on CXR	Severe ARDS
67-year-old female with severe diverticulitis now with acute onset of respiratory failure, PaO_2-to-FiO_2 ratio of 234, nl heart echo, bilateral pulmonary edema on CXR	Mild ARDS
22-year-old male s/p MCC 48-year-old now with bleeding through liver and pelvic packs; TEG reveals a progressive narrowing of the TEG tracing over time (small tail)	Hyperfibrinolysis
22-year-old female s/p fall with severe TBI, urine output 30 to 50 cc/hr, CVP 15, sodium of 128	SIADH
45-year-old with severe pancreatitis, now with increasing peak airway pressures, decreased urine output, and hypotension	Abdominal compartment syndrome
70-year-old male with severe sepsis on three pressors (vasopressors), antibiotics, refractory to fluid bolus and progressively increasing doses of pressors	Adrenal insufficiency
44-year-old male with pulmonary contusions s/p several infusions of KCl for hypokalemia but with no increase in postinfusion potassium level	Hypomagnesemia

44-year-old female with severe pancreatitis on ventilator ABG reveals pH of 7.2, PO₂ of 100, PCO₂ of 65, bicarbonate 26	Respiratory acidosis (uncompensated)
65-year-old male s/p pulmonary contusion on a ventilator, ABG reveals pH 7.35, PO₂ 80, PCO₂ of 60, bicarbonate of 35	Compensated respiratory acidosis
34-year-old female s/p liver injury from an MVC on the ventilator, ABG reveals pH 7.23, PO₂ 105, PCO₂ 40, bicarbonate 17	Metabolic acidosis
76-year-old male with severe diverticulitis on ventilator, pH 7.35, PO₂ 76, PCO₂ 25, bicarbonate 16	Metabolic acidosis with respiratory compensation
45-year-old "found down" with pH of 7.17, PCO₂ 39, PO₂ 90, sodium 140, chloride 108, bicarbonate 26	Normal anion gap metabolic acidosis $(140 - 108 - 26 = 6)$
56-year-old female "found down" with pH of 7.19, sodium 140, bicarbonate 18, chloride 100	Increased anion gap acidosis $(140 - 18 - 100 = 22)$

What is the treatment?

34-year-old female s/p MVC with carotid dissection on CTA	Antiplatelet (aspirin and/or Plavix®) or anticoagulation (enoxaparin or IV heparin or PO anticoagulation medication, classically Coumadin®) therapy
25-year-old male s/p crush injury with CK of 45,000, dark urine	Myoglobinuria: IV fluid hydration, ± bicarbonate IV
DVT prophylaxis for 34-year-old trauma patient with acute renal failure	Unfractionated heparin
78-year-old male in ICU develops SVT and hypotensive 75/palp	Synchronized cardioversion
80-year-old male s/p Hartmann's procedure for severe fecal diverticulitis, now with urine output of 10 ccs per hour, FENA <1%, creatinine 1.7, BUN-to-Cr ratio of >20, urine sodium of 8	Prerenal acute renal failure, treat with IV volume

Chapter 65 | Vascular Surgery

What must be present for a successful arterial bypass operation?	1. Inflow (e.g., patent aorta) 2. Outflow (e.g., open distal popliteal artery) 3. Run off (e.g., patent trifurcation vessels down to the foot)
What is the major principle of safe vascular surgery?	Get **proximal** and **distal** control of the vessel to be worked on!
What does it mean to "POTTS" a vessel?	Place a vessel loop twice around a vessel so that if you put tension on the vessel loop, it will occlude the vessel
What is the suture needle orientation through graft versus diseased artery in a graft to artery anastomosis?	Needle "in-to-out" of the lumen in diseased artery to help **tack down the plaque** and the needle "out-to-in" on the graft
What are the three layers of an artery?	1. Intima 2. Media 3. Adventitia
Which arteries supply the blood vessel itself?	Vasa vasorum
What is a true aneurysm?	Dilation (>2× nL diameter) of all three layers of a vessel
What is a false aneurysm (a.k.a. "pseudoaneurysm")?	Dilation of artery not involving all three layers
What is "ENDOVASCULAR" repair?	Placement of a catheter in artery and then deployment of a graft intraluminally

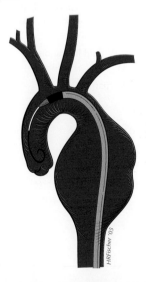

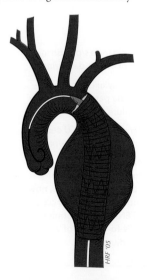

PERIPHERAL VASCULAR DISEASE

What is peripheral vascular disease (PVD)?	Occlusive atherosclerotic disease in the lower extremities
What is the most common site of arterial atherosclerotic occlusion in the lower extremities?	Occlusion of the SFA in Hunter's canal
What are the symptoms of PVD?	Intermittent claudication, rest pain, erectile dysfunction, sensorimotor impairment, tissue loss
What is intermittent claudication?	Pain, cramping, or both of the lower extremity, usually the calf muscle, after walking a specific distance; then the pain/cramping resolves after stopping for a specific amount of time while standing; this pattern is reproducible
What is rest pain?	Pain in the foot, usually over the distal metatarsals; this pain arises at rest (classically at night, awakening the patient)
What classically resolves rest pain?	Hanging the foot over the side of the bed or standing; gravity affords some extra flow to the ischemic areas
What are the signs of PVD?	Absent pulses, bruits, muscular atrophy, decreased hair growth, thick toenails, tissue necrosis/ulcers/infection
What is the site of a PVD ulcer versus a venous stasis ulcer?	PVD arterial insufficiency ulcer—usually on the toes/foot Venous stasis ulcer—medial malleolus (ankle)
What is the ABI?	**A**nkle to **B**rachial **I**ndex (**ABI**); simply, the ratio of the systolic blood pressure at the ankle to the systolic blood pressure at the arm (brachial artery) A:B; ankle pressure taken with Doppler; the ABI is noninvasive
What ABIs are associated with normals, claudicators, and rest pain?	Normal ABI: ≥ 1.0 Claudicator ABI: <0.6 Rest pain ABI: <0.4
Who gets false ABI readings?	Patients with calcified arteries, especially those with diabetes
What are PVRs?	**P**ulse **V**olume **R**ecordings; pulse wave forms are recorded from lower extremities representing volume of blood per heartbeat at sequential sites down leg Large wave form means good collateral blood flow (Noninvasive using pressure cuffs)

Prior to surgery for chronic PVD, what diagnostic test will every patient receive?

A-gram (arteriogram: dye in vessel and x-rays) maps disease and allows for best treatment option (i.e., angioplasty vs. surgical bypass vs. endarterectomy)

Gold standard for diagnosing PVD

What is the bedside management of a patient with PVD?

1. Sheep skin (easy on the heels)
2. Foot cradle (keeps sheets/blankets off the feet)
3. Skin lotion to avoid further cracks in the skin that can go on to form a fissure and then an ulcer

What are the indications for surgical treatment in PVD?

Use the acronym **"STIR"**:

    Severe claudication refractory to conservative treatment that affects quality of life/livelihood (e.g., can't work because of the claudication)

    Tissue necrosis

    Infection

    Rest pain

What is the treatment of claudication?

For the vast majority, conservative treatment, including exercise, smoking cessation, treatment of HTN, diet, aspirin, with or without Trental® (pentoxifylline)

How can the medical conservative treatment for claudication be remembered?

Use the acronym **"PACE"**:

    Pentoxifylline

    Aspirin

    Cessation of smoking

    Exercise

How does aspirin work?

Inhibits platelets (inhibits cyclooxygenase and platelet aggregation)

How does Trental® (pentoxifylline) work?

Results in increased RBC deformity and flexibility (Think: pento**X**ifylline = RBC fle**X**ibility)

What is the risk of limb loss with claudication?

5% limb loss at 5 years (Think: 5 in 5), 10% at 10 years (Think: 10 in 10)

What is the risk of limb loss with rest pain?

>50% of patients will have amputation of the limb at some point

In the patient with PVD, what is the main postoperative concern?

Cardiac status, because most patients with PVD have coronary artery disease; ≈20% have an AAA

MI is the most common cause of postoperative death after a PVD operation

What are the treatment options for severe PVD?

1. Surgical graft bypass
2. Angioplasty—balloon dilation
3. Endarterectomy—remove diseased intima and media
4. Surgical patch angioplasty (place patch over stenosis)

What is a FEM-POP bypass?

Bypass SFA occlusion with a graft from the **FEM**oral artery to the **POP**liteal artery

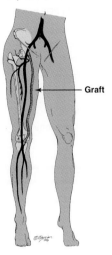

Graft

What is a FEM-DISTAL bypass?

Bypass from the **FEM**oral artery to a **DISTAL** artery (peroneal artery, anterior tibial artery, or posterior tibial artery)

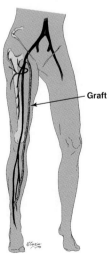

Graft

What graft material has the longest patency rate?	Autologous vein graft
What is an "in situ" vein graft?	Saphenous vein is more or less left in place, all branches are ligated, and the vein valves are broken with a small hook or cut out; a vein can also be used if reversed so that the valves do not cause a problem
What type of graft is used for above-the-knee FEM-POP bypass?	Either vein or Gore-Tex® graft; vein still has better patency
What type of graft is used for below-the-knee FEM-POP or FEM-DISTAL bypass?	Must use vein graft; prosthetic grafts have a prohibitive thrombosis rate
What is DRY gangrene?	Dry necrosis of tissue without signs of infection ("mummified tissue")
What is WET gangrene?	Moist necrotic tissue with signs of infection
What is blue toe syndrome?	Intermittent painful blue toes (or fingers) due to microemboli from a proximal arterial plaque

LOWER EXTREMITY AMPUTATIONS

What are the indications?	Irreversible tissue ischemia (no hope for revascularization bypass) and necrotic tissue, severe infection, severe pain with no bypassable vessels, or if patient is not interested in a bypass procedure
Identify the level of the following amputations:	1. **A**bove-the-**K**nee **A**mputation (**AKA**) 2. **B**elow-the-**K**nee **A**mputation (**BKA**) 3. Symes amputation 4. Transmetatarsal amputation 5. Toe amputation

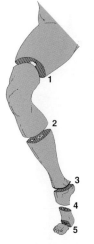

What is a Ray amputation?	Removal of toe and head of metatarsal

ACUTE ARTERIAL OCCLUSION

What is it?	Acute occlusion of an artery, usually by embolization; other causes include acute thrombosis of an atheromatous lesion, vascular trauma
What are the classic signs/ symptoms of acute arterial occlusion?	"Six Ps": 1. **P**ain 2. **P**aralysis 3. **P**allor 4. **P**aresthesia 5. **P**olar (some say **P**oikilothermia—you pick) 6. **P**ulselessness (You **must** know these!)
What is the classic timing of pain with acute arterial occlusion from an embolus?	Acute onset; the patient can classically tell you exactly when and where it happened
What is the immediate preoperative management?	1. Anticoagulate with IV heparin (bolus followed by constant infusion) 2. A-gram
What are the sources of emboli?	1. Heart—85% (e.g., clot from AFib, clot forming on dead muscle after MI, endocarditis, myxoma) 2. Aneurysms 3. Atheromatous plaque (atheroembolism)
What is the most common cause of embolus from the heart?	**AFib**
What is the most common site of arterial occlusion by an embolus?	Common femoral artery (SFA is the most common site of arterial occlusion from atherosclerosis)
What diagnostic studies are in order?	1. A-gram 2. ECG (looking for MI, AFib) 3. Echocardiogram (±) looking for clot, MI, valve vegetation
What is the treatment?	Surgical embolectomy via cutdown and Fogarty balloon (bypass is reserved for embolectomy failure)
What is a Fogarty?	Fogarty balloon catheter—catheter with a balloon tip that can be inflated with saline; used for embolectomy
How is a Fogarty catheter used?	Insinuate the catheter with the balloon deflated past the embolus and then inflate the balloon and pull the catheter out; the balloon brings the embolus with it

How many mm in diameter is a 12-French Fogarty catheter?	Simple: To get mm from French measurements, divide the French number by π, or 3.14; thus, a 12-French catheter is 12/3 = 4 mm in diameter
What must be looked for postoperatively after reperfusion of a limb?	**Compartment syndrome,** hyperkalemia, renal failure from myoglobinuria, MI
What is compartment syndrome?	Leg (calf) is separated into compartments by very unyielding fascia; **tissue swelling** from reperfusion can increase the intracompartmental pressure
What are the signs/symptoms of compartment syndrome?	Classic signs include pain, especially after passive flexing/extension of the foot, paralysis, paresthesias, and pallor; **pulses are present** in most cases because systolic pressure is much higher than the minimal 30 mm Hg needed for the syndrome!
Can a patient have a pulse and compartment syndrome?	**YES!**
How is the diagnosis made?	History/suspicion, compartment pressure measurement
What is the treatment of compartment syndrome?	Treatment includes opening compartments via bilateral calf-incision fasciotomies of all four compartments in the calf

ABDOMINAL AORTIC ANEURYSMS

What is it also known as?	AAA, or "triple A"
What is it?	Abnormal dilation of the abdominal aorta (>1.5–2× normal), forming a true aneurysm

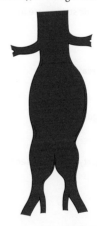

What is the male-to-female ratio?	≈6:1
What is the common etiology?	Believed to be **atherosclerotic** in 95% of cases; 5% inflammatory
What is the most common site?	Infrarenal (95%)
What is the incidence?	5% of all adults >60 years of age
What percentage of patients with AAA has a peripheral arterial aneurysm?	20%
What are the risk factors?	**Atherosclerosis**, hypertension, smoking, male gender, advanced age, connective tissue disease
What are the symptoms?	Most AAAs are **asymptomatic** and discovered during routine abdominal exam by primary care physicians; in the remainder, symptoms range from vague epigastric discomfort to back and abdominal pain
What are the risk factors for rupture?	Increasing aneurysm diameter, COPD, HTN, recent rapid expansion, large diameter, hypertension, symptomatic
What are the signs of rupture?	Classic triad of ruptured AAA: 1. Abdominal pain 2. Pulsatile abdominal mass 3. Hypotension
What is the risk of rupture per year based on AAA diameter size?	<5 cm = 4% 5 to 7 cm = 7% >7 cm = 20%
Where does the aorta bifurcate?	At the level of the **umbilicus;** therefore, when palpating for an AAA, palpate above the umbilicus and below the xiphoid process
What are the diagnostic tests?	Use U/S to follow AAA clinically; other tests involve contrast CT scan and A-gram; A-gram will assess lumen patency and iliac/renal involvement
What are the indications for surgical repair of AAA?	**AAA >5.5 cm** in diameter, if the patient is not an overwhelming high risk for surgery; also, rupture of the AAA, any size AAA with rapid growth, symptoms/embolization of plaque
What is the treatment?	Endovascular repair for most
What is endovascular repair?	Repair of the AAA by femoral catheter-placed stents

MESENTERIC ISCHEMIA

Chronic Mesenteric Ischemia

What is it?	Chronic intestinal ischemia from long-term occlusion of the intestinal arteries; most commonly results from atherosclerosis; usually in two or more arteries because of the extensive collaterals
What are the symptoms?	Weight loss, postprandial abdominal pain, anxiety/fear of food because of postprandial pain, ± heme occult, ± diarrhea/vomiting
What is "intestinal angina"?	Postprandial pain from gut ischemia
What are the signs?	Abdominal bruit is commonly heard
How is the diagnosis made?	A-gram, duplex, MRA
What is the classic finding on A-gram?	Two of the three mesenteric arteries are occluded, and the third patent artery has atherosclerotic narrowing
What are the treatment options?	Bypass, endarterectomy, angioplasty, stenting

Acute Mesenteric Ischemia

What is it?	Acute onset of intestinal ischemia
What are the causes?	1. **Emboli** to a mesenteric vessel from the heart 2. **Acute thrombosis** of long-standing atherosclerosis of mesenteric artery
What are the causes of emboli from the heart?	**AFib,** MI, cardiomyopathy, valve disease/endocarditis, mechanical heart valve
What drug has been associated with acute intestinal ischemia?	Digitalis
To which intestinal artery do emboli preferentially go?	Superior Mesenteric Artery (**SMA**)
What are the signs/symptoms of acute mesenteric ischemia?	Severe pain—classically **"pain out of proportion to physical exam,"** no peritoneal signs until necrosis, vomiting/diarrhea/hyperdefecation, ± heme stools

MEDIAN ARCUATE LIGAMENT SYNDROME

What is it?	Mesenteric ischemia resulting from narrowing of the celiac axis vessels by extrinsic compression by the median arcuate ligament

What is the median arcuate ligament composed of?	Diaphragm hiatus fibers
What are the symptoms?	Postprandial pain, weight loss
What are the signs?	Abdominal bruit in almost all patients
How is the diagnosis made?	A-gram
What is the treatment?	Release arcuate ligament surgically

CAROTID VASCULAR DISEASE

Anatomy

Identify the following structures:

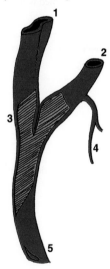

1. Internal carotid artery
2. External carotid artery
3. Carotid "bulb"
4. Superior thyroid artery
5. Common carotid artery
(Shaded area: common site of plaque formation)

What are the signs/symptoms?	Amaurosis fugax, TIA, RIND, CVA
Define the following terms:	
Amaurosis fugax	Temporary monocular blindness ("curtain coming down"): seen with microemboli to retina; example of TIA
TIA	**T**ransient **I**schemic **A**ttack: focal neurologic deficit with resolution of all symptoms within 24 hours
RIND	**R**eversible **I**schemic **N**eurologic **D**eficit: transient neurologic impairment (without any lasting sequelae) lasting 24 to 72 hours

CVA	CerebroVascular Accident (stroke): neurologic deficit with permanent brain damage
What is the risk of a CVA in patients with TIA?	≈10% a year
What is the noninvasive method of evaluating carotid disease?	**Carotid ultrasound/Doppler:** gives general location and degree of stenosis
What is the gold standard invasive method of evaluating carotid disease?	A-gram
What is the surgical treatment of carotid stenosis?	Carotid EndArterectomy (**CEA**): the removal of the diseased intima and media of the carotid artery, often performed with a shunt in place
What are the indications for CEA in the ASYMPTOMATIC patient?	Carotid artery stenosis >60% (greatest benefit is probably in patients with >80% stenosis)
What are the indications for CEA in the SYMPTOMATIC (CVA, TIA, RIND) patient?	Carotid stenosis >50%
Before performing a CEA in the symptomatic patient, what study other than the A-gram should be performed?	Head CT
In bilateral high-grade carotid stenosis, on which side should the CEA be performed in the asymptomatic, right-handed patient?	Left CEA first, to protect the dominant hemisphere and speech center
What is the dreaded complication after a CEA?	Stroke (CVA)
What are the possible postoperative complications after a CEA?	CVA, MI, hematoma, wound infection, hemorrhage, hypotension/hypertension, thrombosis, vagus nerve injury (change in voice), hypoglossal nerve injury (tongue deviation toward side of injury—"wheelbarrow" effect), intracranial hemorrhage
What is the mortality rate after CEA?	≈1%
What is the perioperative stroke rate after CEA?	Between 1% (asymptomatic patient) and 5% (symptomatic patient)
What is the postoperative medication?	Aspirin (inhibits platelets by inhibiting cyclooxygenase)

What is the most common cause of death during the early postoperative period after a CEA?	MI
Define "Hollenhorst plaque":	Microemboli to retinal arterioles seen as bright defects

CLASSIC CEA INTRAOPERATIVE QUESTIONS

What thin muscle is cut right under the skin in the neck?	Platysma muscle
What are the extracranial branches of the internal carotid artery?	None
Which vein crosses the carotid bifurcation?	Facial vein
What is the first branch of the external carotid?	Superior thyroidal artery
Which muscle crosses the common carotid proximally?	Omohyoid muscle
Which muscle crosses the carotid artery distally?	Digastric muscle (Think: **D**igastric = **D**istal)
Which nerve crosses ≈1 cm distal to the carotid bifurcation?	Hypoglossal nerve; cut it and the tongue will deviate toward the side of the injury (the "wheelbarrow effect")

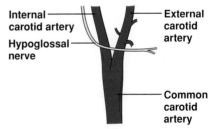

Which nerve crosses the internal carotid near the ear?	Facial nerve (marginal branch)
What is in the carotid sheath?	1. Carotid artery 2. Internal jugular vein 3. **Vagus** nerve (lies posteriorly in 98% of patients and anteriorly in 2%) 4. Deep cervical lymph nodes

SUBCLAVIAN STEAL SYNDROME

What is it?

Arm fatigue and vertebrobasilar insufficiency from obstruction of the left subclavian artery or innominate proximal to the vertebral artery branch point; ipsilateral arm movement causes increased blood flow demand, which is met by retrograde flow from the vertebral artery, thereby "stealing" from the vertebrobasilar arteries

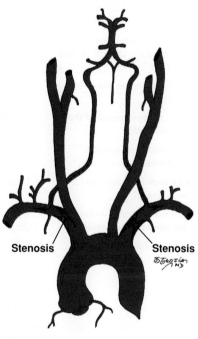

Stenosis   **Stenosis**

Which artery is most commonly occluded?

Left subclavian

What are the symptoms?

Upper extremity claudication, syncopal attacks, vertigo, confusion, dysarthria, blindness, ataxia

What are the signs?

Upper extremity blood pressure discrepancy, bruit (above the clavicle), vertebrobasilar insufficiency

What is the treatment?

Surgical bypass or endovascular stent

RENAL ARTERY STENOSIS

What is it?

Stenosis of renal artery, resulting in decreased perfusion of the juxtaglomerular apparatus and subsequent activation of the renin-angiotensin–aldosterone system (i.e., hypertension from renal artery stenosis)

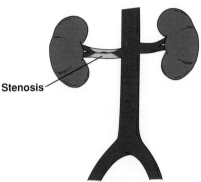

Stenosis

What antihypertensive medication is CONTRAINDICATED in patients with hypertension from renovascular stenosis?

ACE inhibitors (result in renal insufficiency)

SPLENIC ARTERY ANEURYSM

What are the causes?

Females—medial dysplasia
Males—atherosclerosis

How is the diagnosis made?

Usually by abdominal pain → U/S or CT scan, in the O.R. after rupture, or incidentally **by eggshell calcifications seen on AXR**

What is the risk factor for rupture?

Pregnancy

What are the indications for splenic artery aneurysm removal?

Pregnancy, >2 cm in diameter, symptoms, and in women of childbearing age

POPLITEAL ARTERY ANEURYSM

What is it?

Aneurysm of the popliteal artery caused by atherosclerosis and, rarely, bacterial infection

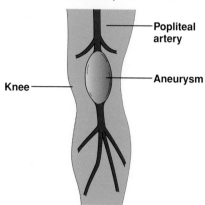

How is the diagnosis made?

Usually by physical exam → A-gram, U/S

Why examine the contralateral popliteal artery?

50% of all patients with a popliteal artery aneurysm have a popliteal artery aneurysm in the contralateral popliteal artery

Why examine the rest of the arterial tree (especially the abdominal aorta)?

75% of all patients with popliteal aneurysms have additional aneurysms elsewhere; >50% of these are located in the abdominal aorta/iliacs

What size of the following aneurysms is usually considered indications for surgical repair?

Thoracic aorta	>6.5 cm
Abdominal aorta	>5.5 cm
Iliac artery	>4 cm
Femoral artery	>2.5 cm
Popliteal artery	>2 cm

RAPID-FIRE REVIEW

What is the correct diagnosis?

65-year-old male presents with atrial fibrillation and acute onset of severe abdominal pain without peritonitis	Mesenteric ischemia from an embolus to the SMA
Tender pulsatile abdominal mass	Abdominal aortic aneurysm
Syncope with the use of the left arm	Subclavian steal syndrome

Name the most likely diagnosis:

24-year-old heavy cigarette smoker with initial onset of foot pain followed by digit necrosis	Buerger's disease
55-year-old female with calf claudication, "hourglass" stenosis on angiogram of popliteal artery, and cyst on ultrasound of posterior knee	Cystic degeneration of the popliteal artery
65-year-old female started on Coumadin® alone for atrial fibrillation develops acute DVT	Coumadin®-induced hypercoagulable state due to decreased protein C and S
72-year-old male with history of hypertension and tobacco abuse presents with 20 minutes of left eye blindness; left carotid bruit is detected on exam	TIA—amaurosis fugax
Pain on passive flexion/ extension, arm or leg pain "out of proportion to injury"	Extremity compartment syndrome
29-year-old male smoker with necrotic fingers	Buerger's disease
Skier with fingers that go from white to blue to red	Raynaud's phenomenon
19-year-old male in motorcycle crash with knee dislocation and loss of pedal pulses	Thrombosed popliteal artery
Pregnant 22-year-old with LUQ pain and hypotension	Ruptured splenic artery aneurysm
Claudication, impotence, atrophy of thigh	Leriche's syndrome

Name the diagnostic modality:

28-year-old s/p head on MVC presents with chest pain and a widened mediastinum on chest x-ray

CTA of chest to rule out aortic injury

22-year-old male s/p gunshot wound to the left leg, distal pulse intact, no pulsatile bleeding nor hematoma, ABI is 0.5 (ABI is 1.1 in right leg)

CTA or angiogram to rule out arterial injury to the extremity

What is the treatment?

45-year-old with recent fascial closure after an open abdomen develops hypotension, decreased urine output, and elevated peak airway pressures

Open fascia to treat for abdominal compartment syndrome

Chapter 66 | Pediatric Surgery

What is the motto of pediatric surgery?	"Children are NOT little adults!"

PEDIATRIC IV FLUIDS AND NUTRITION

What is the maintenance IV fluid for children?	<D5 1/4 NS + 20 mEq KCl
Why 1/4 NS?	Children (especially those <4 years of age) cannot concentrate their urine and cannot clear excess sodium
How are maintenance fluid rates calculated in children?	**4, 2, 1 per hour:** **4 cc/kg for the first 10 kg of body weight** **2 cc/kg for the second 10 kg of body weight** **1 cc/kg for every kilogram over the first 20** (e.g., the rate for a child weighing 25 kg is $4 \times 10 = 40$ plus $2 \times 10 = 20$ plus $1 \times 5 = 5$, for an IVF rate of 65 cc/hr)
What is the minimal urine output for children?	From 1 to 2 mL/kg/hr
What are the caloric requirements by age for the following patients?	
Premature infants	80 Kcal/kg/day and then go up
Children <1 year	≈100 Kcal/kg/day (90–120)
Children ages 1 to 7	≈85 Kcal/kg/day (75–90)
Children ages 7 to 12	≈70 Kcal/kg/day (60–75)
Youths ages 12 to 18	≈40 Kcal/kg/day (30–60)
What are the protein requirements by age for the following patients?	
Children <1 year	3 g/kg/day (2–3.5)
Children ages 1 to 7	2 g/kg/day (2–2.5)
Children ages 7 to 12	2 g/kg/day
Youths ages 12 to 18	1.5 g/kg/day

| How many calories are in breast milk? | 20 Kcal/30 cc (same as most formulas) |

PEDIATRIC BLOOD VOLUMES

What is the blood volume per kilogram?

Newborn infant	85 cc
Infants age 1 to 3 months	75 cc
Child	70 cc

FETAL CIRCULATION

Oxygenated blood travels through the liver to the IVC through which structure?	Ductus venosus
Oxygenated blood passes from the right atrium to the left atrium through which structure?	Foramen ovale
Unsaturated blood goes from the right ventricle to the descending aorta through which structure?	Ductus arteriosus

Define the overall fetal circulation:

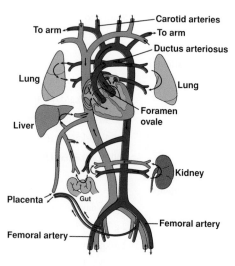

ECMO

What is ECMO?	**E**xtra**C**orporeal **M**embrane **O**xygenation: chronic cardiopulmonary bypass—for complete respiratory support
What are the indications?	Severe hypoxia, usually from congenital diaphragmatic hernia, meconium aspiration, persistent pulmonary hypertension, sepsis
What are the contraindications?	Weight <2 kg, **IVH** (**I**ntra**V**entricular **H**emorrhage in brain contraindicated because of heparin in line)

NECK

Thyroglossal Duct Cyst

What is it?	Remnant of the diverticulum formed by migration of thyroid tissue

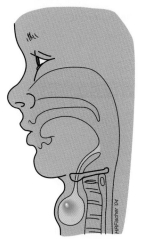

What is the average age at diagnosis?	Usually presents ≈5 years of age
How is the diagnosis made?	Ultrasound
What is the anatomic location?	Almost always in the **midline**

How to remember the position of the thyroglossal duct cyst?

Think: thyro**GLOSSAL** = **TONGUE** midline sticking out

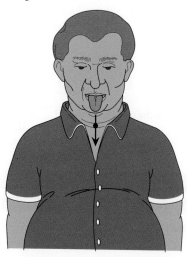

What is the treatment?

Antibiotics if infection is present, then excision, which must include the midportion of the hyoid bone and entire tract to foramen cecum (**Sistrunk** procedure)

Branchial Cleft Anomalies

What is it?

Remnant of the primitive branchial clefts in which epithelium forms a sinus tract between the pharynx (second cleft), or the external auditory canal (first cleft), and the skin of the anterior neck; if the sinus ends blindly, a cyst may form

What is the common presentation?

Infection because of communication between pharynx and external ear canal

What is the anatomic position?

Second cleft anomaly—**lateral to the midline** along anterior border of the sternocleidomastoid, anywhere from angle of jaw to clavicle

First cleft anomaly—less common than second cleft anomalies; tend to be located higher under the mandible

What is the treatment?	Antibiotics if infection is present, then surgical excision of cyst and tract once inflammation is resolved
What is the major anatomic difference between thyroglossal cyst and branchial cleft cyst?	Thyroglossal cyst = **midline** Branchial cleft cyst = **lateral** (Think: brAnchial = lAteral)

Stridor

What is stridor?	Harsh, high-pitched sound heard on breathing caused by obstruction of the trachea or larynx
What are the signs/symptoms?	Dyspnea, cyanosis, difficulty with feedings
What is the differential diagnosis?	Laryngomalacia Tracheobronchomalacia

Cystic Hygroma

What is it?	Congenital abnormality of lymph sac resulting in lymphangioma
What is the anatomic location?	Occurs in sites of primitive lymphatic lakes and can occur virtually anywhere in the body, most commonly in the floor of mouth; under the jaw; or in the neck, axilla, or thorax
What is the treatment?	Early total surgical removal because they tend to enlarge; sclerosis may be needed if the lesion is unresectable

ASPIRATED FOREIGN BODY (FB)

Which bronchus do FBs go into more commonly (left or right)?	<Age 4—50/50 Age ≥4—most go into right bronchus because it develops into a straight shot (less of an angle)
What is the most commonly aspirated object?	Peanut
What is the associated risk with peanut aspiration?	Lipoid pneumonia
How can you tell on AP CXR if a coin is in the esophagus or the trachea?	Coin in **esophagus** results in the coin lying "en face" with face of the coin viewed as a **round object** because of compression by anterior and posterior structures If coin is in the **trachea,** it is viewed as a **side projection** due to the U-shaped cartilage with membrane posteriorly

What is the treatment of tracheal or esophageal FB?	Remove FB with bronchoscope or esophagoscope

CHEST

Pectus Deformity

What heart abnormality is associated with pectus abnormality?	Mitral valve prolapse (many patients receive preoperative echocardiogram)

Pectus Excavatum

What is it?	Chest wall deformity with sternum caving inward (Think: exCAVatum = CAVE)

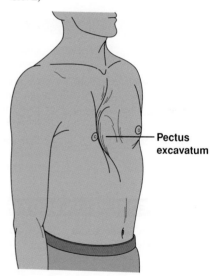

— Pectus excavatum

What is the treatment?	Open perichondrium, remove abnormal cartilage, place substernal strut; new cartilage grows back in the perichondrium in normal position; remove strut 6 months later
What is the NUSS procedure?	Placement of metal strut to elevate sternum **without** removing cartilage

Pectus Carinatum

What is it?

Chest wall deformity with sternum outward (pectus = chest, carinatum = pigeon); much less common than pectus excavatum

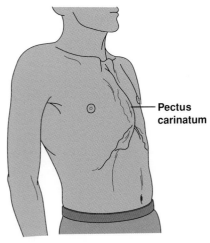

Pectus carinatum

What is the treatment?

Open perichondrium and remove abnormal cartilage
Place substernal strut
New cartilage grows into normal position
Remove strut 6 months later

Esophageal Atresia without Tracheoesophageal (TE) Fistula

What is it?

Blind-ending esophagus from atresia

What are the signs?

Excessive oral secretions and inability to keep food down

How is the diagnosis made?

Inability to pass NG tube; plain x-ray shows tube coiled in upper esophagus and no gas in abdomen

What is the definitive treatment?

Surgical with 1° anastomosis, often with preoperative stretching of blind pouch (other options include colonic or jejunal interposition graft or gastric tube formation if esophageal gap is long)

Esophageal Atresia with Tracheoesophageal (TE) Fistula

What is it?	Esophageal atresia occurring with a fistula to the trachea; occurs in >90% of cases of esophageal atresia
What is the incidence?	1 in 1,500 to 3,000 births

Define the following types of fistulas/atresias:

Type A

Esophageal atresia without TE fistula (8%)

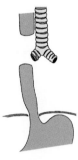

Type B

Proximal esophageal atresia with proximal TE fistula (1%)

Type C

Proximal esophageal atresia with distal TE fistula (85%); most common type

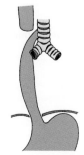

Type D   Proximal esophageal atresia with both
                                 proximal and distal TE fistulas (2%) (Think:
                                 D = **D**ouble connection to trachea)

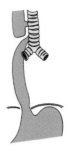

Type E   "H-type" TE fistula without esophageal
                                 atresia (4%)

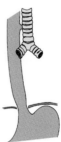

How do you remember which   Simple: Most **C**ommon type is type **C**
type is most common?

What is the initial treatment? Directed toward minimizing complications
                                 from aspiration:
                                 1. Suction blind pouch (NPO/TPN)
                                 2. Upright position of child
                                 3. Prophylactic antibiotics (Amp/gent)

What is the definitive treatment? Surgical correction via a thoracotomy,
                                 usually through the right chest with division
                                 of fistula and end-to-end esophageal
                                 anastomosis, if possible

What are the associated   **VACTERL** cluster (present in about 10% of
anomalies?   cases):
                                 Vertebral or vascular, **A**norectal, **C**ardiac,
                                 TE fistula, **E**sophageal atresia
                                 Radial limb and renal abnormalities,
                                 Lumbar and limb
                                 Previously known as **VATER**: **V**ertebral,
                                 Anus, **TE** fistula, **R**adial

What is the significance of a No air to the stomach and, thus, no
"gasless" abdomen on AXR?   tracheoesophageal fistula

Congenital Diaphragmatic Hernia

What is it?	Failure of complete formation of the diaphragm, leading to a defect through which abdominal organs are herniated
What are the types of hernias?	Bochdalek and Morgagni
What are the associated positions?	Bochdalek—posterolateral with L > R Morgagni—anterior parasternal hernia, relatively uncommon
How to remember the position of the Bochdalek hernia?	Think: BOCH DA LEK = "BACK TO THE LEFT"

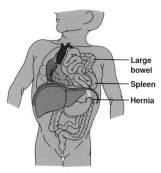

- Large bowel
- Spleen
- Hernia

What is the treatment?	NG tube, ET tube, stabilization, and if patient is stable, surgical repair; if patient is unstable: nitric oxide ± ECMO then to the O.R. when feasible

PULMONARY SEQUESTRATION

What is it?	Abnormal benign lung tissue with separate blood supply that **DOES NOT** communicate with the normal tracheobronchial airway

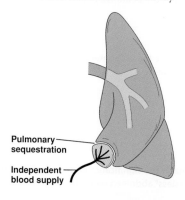

Pulmonary sequestration

Independent blood supply

What is the treatment of each type?	
Extralobar	Surgical resection
Intralobar	Lobectomy
What is the major risk during operation for sequestration?	Anomalous blood supply from below the diaphragm (can be cut and retracted into the abdomen and result in exsanguination!); always document blood supply by A-gram or U/S with Doppler flow

INGUINAL HERNIA

What is the most commonly performed procedure by US pediatric surgeons?	Indirect inguinal hernia repair
What is the most common inguinal hernia in children?	Indirect
What is an indirect inguinal hernia?	Hernia lateral to Hesselbach's triangle into the internal inguinal ring and down the inguinal canal (Think: through the abdominal wall indirectly into the internal ring and out through the external inguinal ring)
What is Hesselbach's triangle?	Triangle formed by: 1. Epigastric vessels 2. Inguinal ligament 3. Lateral border of the rectus sheath
What type of hernia goes through Hesselbach's triangle?	Direct hernia from a weak abdominal floor; rare in children (0.5% of all inguinal hernias)
What is the incidence of indirect inguinal hernia in all children?	≈3%
What is the incidence in premature infants?	Up to 30%
What is the male-to-female ratio?	6:1
What are the risk factors for an indirect inguinal hernia?	Male gender, ascites, V-P shunt, prematurity, family history, meconium ileus, abdominal wall defect elsewhere, hypo/epispadias, connective tissue disease, bladder exstrophy, undescended testicle, CF
Which side is affected more commonly?	**Right** (≈60%)
What percentage is bilateral?	≈15%

What percentage has a family history of indirect hernias?	≈10%
What are the signs/symptoms?	Groin bulge, scrotal mass, thickened cord, silk glove sign
What is the "silk glove" sign?	Hernia sac rolls under the finger like the finger of a silk glove
Why should it be repaired?	Risk of incarcerated/strangulated bowel or ovary; will not go away on its own
How is a pediatric inguinal hernia repaired?	High ligation of hernia sac (no repair of the abdominal wall floor, which is a big difference between the procedures in children vs. adults; high refers to high position on the sac neck next to the peritoneal cavity)
Which infants need overnight apnea monitoring/observation?	Premature infants; infants <3 months of age
What is the risk of recurrence after high ligation of an indirect pediatric hernia?	≈1%
Define the following terms:	
Cryptorchidism	Failure of the testicle to descend into the scrotum
Hydrocele	Fluid-filled sac (i.e., fluid in a patent processus vaginalis or in the tunica vaginalis around the testicle)
Communicating hydrocele	Hydrocele that communicates with the peritoneal cavity and thus fills and drains peritoneal fluid or gets bigger, then smaller
Noncommunicating hydrocele	Hydrocele that does not communicate with the peritoneal cavity; stays about the same size

Classic Intraoperative Questions During Repair of an Indirect Inguinal Hernia

From what abdominal muscle layer is the cremaster muscle derived?	Internal oblique muscle
From what abdominal muscle layer is the inguinal ligament (a.k.a. "Poupart's ligament") derived?	External oblique
What nerve travels with the spermatic cord?	Ilioinguinal nerve

What are the five structures in the spermatic cord?	1. Cremasteric muscle fibers 2. Vas deferens 3. Testicular artery 4. Testicular pampiniform venous plexus 5. With or without hernia sac
What is the hernia sac made of?	Basically peritoneum or a patent processus vaginalis
What attaches the testicle to the scrotum?	Gubernaculum
How can the opposite side be assessed for a hernia intraoperatively?	Many surgeons operatively explore the opposite side when they repair the affected side Laparoscope is placed into the abdomen via the hernia sac and the opposite side internal inguinal ring is examined
Name the remnant of the processus vaginalis around the testicle:	Tunica vaginalis
What is a Littre's inguinal hernia?	Hernia with a Meckel's diverticulum in the hernia sac
What may a yellow/orange tissue that is not fat be on the spermatic cord/testicle?	Adrenal rest
What is the most common organ in an inguinal hernia sac in boys?	Small intestine
What is the most common organ in an inguinal hernia sac in girls?	Ovary/fallopian tube
What lies in the inguinal canal in girls instead of the vas?	Round ligament
Where in the inguinal canal does the hernia sac lie in relation to the other structures?	Anteromedially
What is a "cord lipoma"?	Preperitoneal fat on the cord structures (pushed in by the hernia sac); not a real lipoma Should be removed surgically, if feasible
Within the spermatic cord, do the vessels or the vas lie medially?	Vas is medial to the testicular vessels
What is a small outpouching of testicular tissue off the testicle?	Testicular appendage (a.k.a. "the appendix testes"); should be removed with electrocautery
What is a "blue dot" sign?	Blue dot on the scrotal skin from a twisted testicular appendage

How is a transected vas treated?	Repair with primary anastomosis
How do you treat a transected ilioinguinal nerve?	Should not be repaired; many surgeons ligate it to inhibit neuroma formation
What happens if you cut the ilioinguinal nerve?	Loss of sensation to the medial aspect of the inner thigh and scrotum/labia; loss of cremasteric reflex

UMBILICAL HERNIA

What is it?	Fascial defect at the umbilical ring
What are the risk factors?	1. African American infant 2. Premature infant
What are the indications for surgical repair?	1. >1.5 cm defect 2. Bowel incarceration 3. >4 years of age

GERD

What is it?	**G**astro**E**sophageal **R**eflux **D**isease
What cytologic aspirate finding on bronchoscopy can diagnose aspiration of gastric contents?	Lipid-laden macrophages (from phagocytosis of fat)

What are the indications for surgery?	"**SAFE**":
	     Stricture
	     Aspiration, pneumonia/asthma
	     Failure to thrive
	     Esophagitis

What is the surgical treatment?	**Nissen** 360° fundoplication, with or without G-tube

CONGENITAL PYLORIC STENOSIS

What is it?	Hypertrophy of smooth muscle of pylorus, resulting in obstruction of outflow

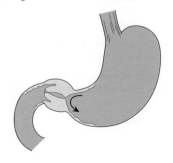

What are the associated risks?	Family history, firstborn males are affected most commonly, decreased incidence in African American population
What is the incidence?	1 in 750 births, male-to-female ratio = 4:1
What is the average age at onset?	Usually from 3 weeks after birth to about 3 months (**"3–3"**)
What are the symptoms?	Increasing frequency of regurgitation, leading to eventual nonbilious projectile vomiting
Why is the vomiting nonbilious?	Obstruction is proximal to the ampulla of Vater
What are the signs?	Abdominal mass or "olive" in epigastric region (85%), hypokalemic hypochloremic metabolic alkalosis, icterus (10%), visible gastric peristalsis, paradoxical aciduria, hematemesis (<10%)
What is the differential diagnosis?	Pylorospasm, milk allergy, increased ICP, hiatal hernia, GERD, adrenal insufficiency, uremia, malrotation, duodenal atresia, annular pancreas, duodenal web
How is the diagnosis made?	Usually by history and physical exam alone U/S—demonstrates elongated (>15 mm) pyloric channel and thickened muscle wall (>3.5 mm) If U/S is nondiagnostic, then barium swallow—shows "string sign" or "double railroad track sign"
What is the initial treatment?	Hydration and correction of alkalosis with D10 NS plus 20 mEq of KCl (**Note:** The infant's liver glycogen stores are very small; therefore, use D10; Cl⁻ and hydration will correct the alkalosis)
What is the definitive treatment?	Surgical, via Fredet–Ramstedt pyloromyotomy (division of circular muscle fibers without entering the lumen/mucosa)
What are the postoperative complications?	Unrecognized incision through the duodenal mucosa, bleeding, wound infection, aspiration pneumonia
What is the appropriate postoperative feeding?	Start feeding with Pedialyte® at 6 to 12 hours postoperatively; advance to full-strength formula over 24 hours
Which vein crosses the pylorus?	Vein of Mayo

DUODENAL ATRESIA

What is it?	Complete obstruction or stenosis of duodenum caused by an ischemic insult during development or failure of recanalization
What are the signs?	Bilious vomiting (if distal to the ampulla), epigastric distention
What is the differential diagnosis?	Malrotation with Ladd's bands, annular pancreas
How is the diagnosis made?	Plain abdominal film revealing "double bubble," with one air bubble in the stomach and the other in the duodenum
What is the treatment?	Duodenoduodenostomy or duodenojejunostomy
What are the associated abnormalities?	50% to 70% have cardiac, renal, or other GI defects; 30% have trisomy 21

MECONIUM ILEUS

What is it?	Intestinal obstruction from solid meconium concretions
What is the incidence?	Occurs in ≈15% of infants with CF
What percentage of patients with meconium ileus has cystic fibrosis (CF)?	>95%
What are the signs/symptoms of meconium ileus?	Bilious vomiting, abdominal distention, failure to pass meconium, Neuhauser's sign, peritoneal calcifications
What is the treatment?	70% nonoperative clearance of meconium using Gastrografin® enema, ± acetylcysteine, which is hypertonic and therefore draws fluid into lumen, separating meconium pellets from bowel wall (60% success rate)
What is the surgical treatment?	If enema is unsuccessful, then enterotomy with intraoperative catheter irrigation using acetylcysteine (Mucomyst®)
What should you remove during all operative cases?	Appendix
What is the long-term medical treatment?	Pancreatic enzyme replacement

MECONIUM PERITONITIS

What is it?	Sign of **intrauterine** bowel perforation; sterile meconium leads to an intense local inflammatory reaction with eventual formation of calcifications
What are the signs?	Calcifications on plain films

MECONIUM PLUG SYNDROME

What is it?	Colonic obstruction from meconium, forming a "plug"
What are the signs/symptoms?	Abdominal distention and **failure to pass meconium within the first 24 hours of life;** plain films demonstrate many loops of distended bowel and air–fluid levels
What is the nonoperative treatment?	Contrast enema is both diagnostic and therapeutic
What is the major differential diagnosis?	Hirschsprung's disease
Is meconium plug highly associated with CF?	No; <5% of patients have CF, in contrast to meconium ileus, in which nearly all have CF (95%)

ANORECTAL MALFORMATIONS

Imperforate Anus

What is it?	Congenital absence of normal anus (complete absence or fistula)
What is a "high" imperforate anus?	Rectum patent to level above puborectalis sling
What is a "low" imperforate anus?	Rectum patent to below puborectalis sling
Which type is much more common in females?	Low
What are the associated anomalies?	**V**ertebral abnormalities, **A**nal abnormalities, **C**ardiac, **TE** fistulas, **E**sophageal Atresia, **R**adial/**R**enal abnormalities, **L**umbar abnormalities (**VACTERL;** most commonly TE fistula)
What are the signs/symptoms?	No anus, fistula to anal skin or bladder, UTI, fistula to vagina or urethra, bowel obstruction, distended abdomen, hyperchloremic acidosis

How is the diagnosis made?	Physical exam, perineal ultrasound

What is the treatment of the following conditions?

Low imperforate anus with anal fistula	Dilatation of anal fistula and subsequent anoplasty
High imperforate anus	Diverting colostomy and mucous fistula; neoanus is usually made at 1 year of age

HIRSCHSPRUNG'S DISEASE

What is it also known as?	Aganglionic megacolon
What is it?	Neurogenic form of intestinal obstruction in which obstruction results from inadequate relaxation and peristalsis; absence of normal ganglion cells of the rectum and colon
What is the male-to-female ratio?	4:1
What is the anatomic location?	Aganglionosis begins at the anorectal line and involves rectosigmoid in 80% of cases (10% have involvement to splenic flexure, and 10% have involvement of entire colon)
What are the signs/symptoms?	Abdominal distention and bilious vomiting; >95% present with failure to pass meconium in the first 24 hours; may also present later with constipation, diarrhea, and decreased growth
What is the classic history?	Failure to pass meconium in the first 24 hours of life
What imaging studies should be ordered?	**AXR:** reveals dilated colon **Unprepared barium enema:** reveals constricted aganglionic segment with dilated proximal segment, but this picture may not develop for 3 to 6 weeks; BE will also demonstrate retention of barium for 24 to 48 hours (normal evacuation = 10–18 hours)
What is needed for definitive diagnosis?	Rectal biopsy
What is the "colonic transition zone"?	Transition (taper) from aganglionic small colon into the large dilated normal colon seen on BE
What is the initial treatment?	In neonates, a colostomy proximal to the transition zone prior to correction, to allow for pelvic growth and dilated bowel to return to normal size

What is a "leveling" colostomy?

Colostomy performed for Hirschsprung's disease at the level of normally innervated ganglion cells as ascertained on frozen section intraoperatively

Describe the following procedures:

Swenson

Primary anastomosis between the anal canal and healthy bowel (rectum removed)

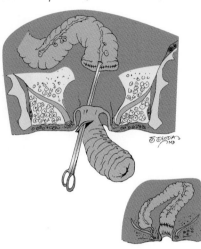

Duhamel

Anterior, aganglionic region of the rectum is preserved and anastomosed to a posterior portion of healthy bowel; a functional rectal pouch is thereby created (Think: **duha = dual** barrels side by side)

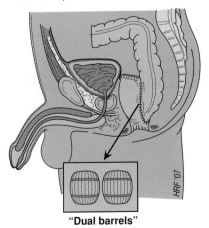

"Dual barrels"

Soave

A.k.a. "endorectal pull-through"; this procedure involves bringing proximal normal colon through the aganglionic rectum, which has been stripped of its mucosa but otherwise present (Think: **SOAVE = SAVE** the rectum, lose the mucosa)

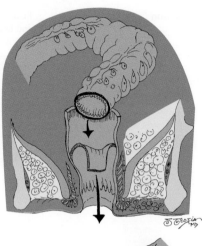

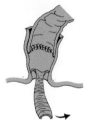

What is the prognosis?

Overall survival rate >90%; >96% of patients continent; postoperative symptoms improve with age

MALROTATION AND MIDGUT VOLVULUS

What is it?

Failure of the normal 270° counterclockwise bowel rotation, with resultant abnormal intestinal attachments and anatomic position

Where is the cecum?

With malrotation, the cecum usually ends up in the RUQ

What are Ladd's bands?

Fibrous bands that extend from the abnormally placed cecum in the RUQ, often crossing over the duodenum and causing obstruction

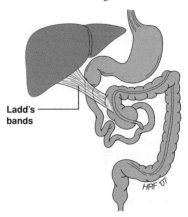

Ladd's bands

HRF '01

What is the usual age at onset?

33% are present by 1 week of age, 75% by 1 month, and 90% by 1 year

What is the usual presentation?

Sudden onset of bilious vomiting (bilious vomiting in an infant is malrotation until proven otherwise!)

Why is the vomiting bilious?

"Twist" is distal to the ampulla of Vater

How is the diagnosis made?

Upper GI contrast study showing cutoff in duodenum; BE showing abnormal position of cecum in the upper abdomen

What are the possible complications?

Volvulus with midgut infarction, leading to death or necessitating massive enterectomy **(Rapid diagnosis is essential!)**

What is the treatment?

IV antibiotics and fluid resuscitation with LR, followed by emergent laparotomy with Ladd's procedure; second-look laparotomy if bowel is severely ischemic in 24 hours to determine if remaining bowel is viable

What is the Ladd's procedure?

1. **Counterclockwise** reduction of midgut volvulus
2. Splitting of Ladd's bands
3. Division of peritoneal attachments to the cecum, ascending colon
4. Appendectomy

In what direction is the volvulus reduced—clockwise or counterclockwise?

Rotation of the bowel in a counterclockwise direction

Where is the cecum after reduction?

LLQ

What is the cause of bilious vomiting in an infant until proven otherwise?	Malrotation with midgut volvulus

OMPHALOCELE

What is it?	Defect of abdominal wall at umbilical ring; sac **covers** extruded viscera
How is it diagnosed prenatally?	May be seen on **fetal** U/S after 13 weeks' gestation, with elevated maternal AFP
What comprises the "sac"?	Peritoneum and amnion
What organ is often found protruding from an omphalocele, but is almost never found with a gastroschisis?	Liver
What is the incidence?	≈1 in 5,000 births
How is the diagnosis made?	Prenatal U/S
What are the possible complications?	Malrotation of the gut, anomalies
What is the treatment?	1. NG tube for decompression 2. IV fluids 3. Prophylactic antibiotics 4. Surgical repair of the defect
What is the treatment of a small defect (<2 cm)?	Closure of abdominal wall
What is the treatment of a medium defect (2–10 cm)?	Removal of outer membrane and placement of a silicone patch to form a "silo," temporarily housing abdominal contents; the silo is then slowly decreased in size over 4 to 7 days, as the abdomen accommodates the viscera; then the defect is closed

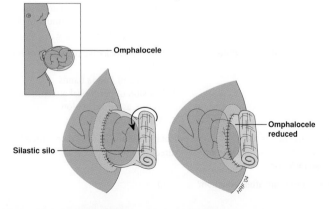

Omphalocele

Silastic silo

Omphalocele reduced

What is the treatment of "giant" defects (>10 cm)?	Skin flaps or treatment with Betadine® spray, mercurochrome, or silver sulfadiazine (Silvadene®) over defect; this allows an eschar to form, which epithelializes over time, allowing opportunity for future repair months to years later
What are the associated abnormalities?	50% of cases occur with abnormalities of the GI tract, cardiovascular system, GU tract, musculoskeletal system, CNS, and chromosomes
Of what "pentalogy" is omphalocele a part?	Pentalogy of Cantrell
What is the pentalogy of Cantrell?	"D COPS": **D**iaphragmatic defect (hernia) **C**ardiac abnormality **O**mphalocele **P**ericardium malformation/absence **S**ternal cleft

GASTROSCHISIS

What is it?	Defect of abdominal wall; sac does not cover extruded viscera
How is it diagnosed prenatally?	Possible at fetal ultrasound after 13 weeks' gestation, elevated maternal AFP
Where is the defect?	Lateral to the umbilicus (Think: g**A**strochisis = l**A**teral)
On what side of the umbilicus is the defect most commonly found?	Right
What is the usual size of the defect?	2 to 4 cm
What are the possible complications?	Thick edematous peritoneum from exposure to amniotic fluid; malrotation of the gut Other complications include hypothermia; hypovolemia from third spacing; sepsis; and metabolic acidosis from hypovolemia and poor perfusion, NEC, prolonged ileus
How is the diagnosis made?	Prenatal U/S
What is the treatment?	Primary—NG tube decompression, IV fluids (D10 LR), and IV antibiotics Definitive—surgical reduction of viscera and abdominal closure; may require staged closure with silo

What is a "silo"?	Silastic silo is a temporary housing for external abdominal contents; silo is slowly tightened over time
What is the prognosis?	>90% survival rate
What are the associated anomalies?	Unlike omphalocele, relatively uncommon except for intestinal atresia, which occurs in 10% to 15% of cases
What are the major differences compared with omphalocele?	No membrane coverings Uncommon associated abnormalities Lateral to umbilicus—not on umbilicus
How can you remember the position of omphalocele versus gastroschisis?	Think: **OM**phalocele = **ON** the umbilicus
How do you remember that omphalocele is associated with abnormalities in 50% of cases?	Think: **O**mphalocele = "**Oh** no, lots of abnormalities"

APPENDICITIS

What is it?	Obstruction of the appendiceal lumen (fecalith, lymphoid hyperplasia), producing a closed loop with resultant inflammation that can lead to necrosis and perforation
What is its claim to fame?	Most common surgical disease requiring emergency surgery in children
What is the affected age?	Very rare before 3 years of age
What is the usual presentation?	Onset of referred or **periumbilical pain** followed by **anorexia,** nausea, and vomiting (***Note:*** Unlike gastroenteritis, **pain precedes vomiting,** then migrates to the **RLQ,** where it intensifies from local peritoneal irritation) If the patient is hungry and can eat, seriously question the diagnosis of appendicitis
How is the diagnosis made?	History and physical exam
What are the signs/symptoms?	Signs of peritoneal irritation may be present—guarding, muscle spasm, rebound tenderness, obturator and psoas signs; low-grade fever rising to high grade if perforation occurs
What is the differential diagnosis?	Intussusception, volvulus, Meckel's diverticulum, Crohn's disease, ovarian torsion, cyst, tumor, perforated ulcer, pancreatitis, PID, ruptured ectopic pregnancy, mesenteric lymphadenitis

What is the common bacterial cause of mesenteric lymphadenitis?	*Yersinia enterocolitica*
What are the associated lab findings with appendicitis?	Increased WBC (>10,000 per mm^3 in >90% of cases, with a left shift in most)
What is the role of urinalysis?	To evaluate for possible pyelonephritis or renal calculus, but mild hematuria and pyuria are common in appendicitis because of ureteral inflammation
What radiographic studies may be performed?	Often none; CXR to rule out RML or RLL pneumonia; abdominal films are usually nonspecific, but calcified fecalith is present in 5% of cases; U/S, CT scan
What is the treatment?	**Nonperforated**—prompt appendectomy and cefoxitin to avoid perforation **Perforated**—triple antibiotics, fluid resuscitation, and prompt appendectomy; all pus is drained and cultures obtained, with postoperative antibiotics continued for 5 to 7 days, ±drain
How long should antibiotics be administered if nonperforated?	24 hours
How long if perforated?	Usually 5 to 7 days or until WBCs are normal and patient is afebrile
If a normal appendix is found upon exploration, what must be examined/ruled out?	Meckel's diverticulum, Crohn's disease, intussusception, gynecologic disease
What is the approximate risk of perforation?	≈25% after 24 hours from onset of symptoms ≈50% by 36 hours ≈75% by 48 hours

INTUSSUSCEPTION

What is it?	Obstruction caused by bowel telescoping into the lumen of adjacent distal bowel; may result when peristalsis carries a "leadpoint" downstream
What is its claim to fame?	Most common cause of small bowel obstruction in toddlers (<2 years old)
What is the usual age at presentation?	Disease of infancy; 60% present from 4 to 12 months of age, 80% by 2 years of age
What is the most common site?	Terminal ileum involving ileocecal valve and extending into ascending colon

What is the most common cause?	Hypertrophic Peyer's patches, which act as a lead point; many patients have prior viral illness
What are the signs/symptoms?	Alternating lethargy and irritability (colic), bilious vomiting, "currant jelly" stools, RLQ mass on plain abdominal film, empty RLQ on palpation (Dance's sign)
What is the intussuscipiens?	Recipient segment of bowel (Think: **recipients** = intussus**cipiens**)
What is the intussusceptum?	Leading point or bowel that enters the intussuscipiens
Identify locations 1 and 2:	1. Intussuscipiens 2. Intussusceptum

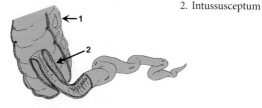

How can the spelling of intussusception be remembered?	Imagine a navy ship named "The **U.S.S. U.S.**"—INT**USSUS**CEPTION
What is the treatment?	**Air** or barium enema; 85% reduce with hydrostatic pressure (i.e., barium = meter elevation air = maximum of 120 mm Hg); if unsuccessful, then laparotomy and reduction by "milking" the ileum from the colon should be performed
What are the causes of intussusception in older patients?	Meckel's diverticulum, polyps, and tumors, all of which act as a lead point

MECKEL'S DIVERTICULUM

What is it?	Remnant of the omphalomesenteric duct/vitelline duct, which connects the yolk sac with the primitive midgut in the embryo
What is the usual location?	Between 45 and 90 cm proximal to the ileocecal valve on the antimesenteric border of the bowel
What is the major differential diagnosis?	Appendicitis
Is it a true diverticulum?	Yes; all layers of the intestine are found in the wall

What is the incidence?	2% of the population at autopsy, but >90% of these are asymptomatic
What is the gender ratio?	2 to 3 × more common in males
What is the usual age at onset of symptoms?	Most frequently in the first 2 years of life, but can occur at any age

What are the possible complications?	**Intestinal hemorrhage** (painless)—50%
	    Accounts for 50% of all lower GI bleeding in patients <2 years; bleeding results from ectopic gastric mucosa secreting acid → ulcer → bleeding
	Intestinal obstruction—25%
	    Most common complication in adults; includes volvulus and intussusception
	Inflammation (± perforation)—20%

What percentage of cases has heterotopic tissue?	>50%; usually gastric mucosa (85%), but duodenal, pancreatic, and colonic mucosa have been described
What is the most common ectopic tissue in a Meckel's diverticulum?	Gastric mucosa
What other pediatric disease entity can also present with GI bleeding secondary to ectopic gastric mucosa?	Enteric duplications
What is the most common cause of lower GI bleeding in children?	Meckel's diverticulum with ectopic gastric mucosa
What is the "rule of 2s"?	**2% are symptomatic** Found ≈**2** feet from ileocecal valve Found in **2**% of the population Most symptoms occur before age **2** One of **2** will have ectopic tissue Most diverticula are about **2** inches long Male-to-female ratio = **2**:1
What is a Meckel's scan?	Scan for ectopic gastric mucosa in Meckel's diverticulum; uses **technetium** Tc 99m **pertechnetate** IV, which is preferentially taken up by gastric mucosa

NECROTIZING ENTEROCOLITIS

What is it also known as?	NEC
What is it?	Necrosis of intestinal mucosa, often with bleeding; may progress to transmural intestinal necrosis, shock/sepsis, and death

What are the predisposing conditions?	**PREMATURITY** Stress: shock, hypoxia, RDS, apneic episodes, sepsis, exchange transfusions, PDA and cyanotic heart disease, hyperosmolar feedings, polycythemia, indomethacin
What is the pathophysiologic mechanism?	Probable splanchnic vasoconstriction with decreased perfusion, mucosal injury, and probable bacterial invasion
What is its claim to fame?	Most common cause of emergent laparotomy in the neonate
What are the signs/symptoms?	Abdominal distention, vomiting, heme+ or gross rectal bleeding, fever or hypothermia, jaundice, abdominal wall erythema (consistent with perforation and abscess formation)
What are the radiographic findings?	Fixed, dilated intestinal loops; pneumatosis intestinalis (air in the bowel wall); free air; and portal vein air (sign of advanced disease)
What are the lab findings?	Low Hct, glucose, and platelets
What is the treatment?	Most are managed medically: 1. Cessation of feedings 2. OG tube 3. IV fluids 4. IV antibiotics 5. Ventilator support, as needed
What are the surgical indications?	Free air in abdomen revealing perforation, and positive peritoneal tap revealing transmural bowel necrosis
Operation?	1. Resect 2. Stoma
What is an option for bowel perforation in <1,000-gram NEC patients?	Placement of percutaneous drain (without laparotomy!)
Is portal vein gas or pneumatosis intestinalis alone an indication for operation with NEC?	No
What are the indications for peritoneal tap?	Severe thrombocytopenia, distended abdomen, abdominal wall erythema, unexplained clinical downturn
What are the possible complications?	Bowel necrosis, gram-negative sepsis, DIC, wound infection, cholestasis, short bowel syndrome, strictures, SBO
What is the prognosis?	>80% overall survival rate

BILIARY TRACT

What is "physiologic jaundice"?	Hyperbilirubinemia in the first 2 weeks of life from inadequate conjugation of bilirubin
What enzyme is responsible for conjugation of bilirubin?	Glucuronyl transferase
How is hyperbilirubinemia from "physiologic jaundice" treated?	UV light
What is Gilbert's syndrome?	Partial deficiency of glucuronyl transferase, leading to intermittent asymptomatic jaundice in the second or third decade of life
What is Crigler–Najjar syndrome?	Rare genetic absence of glucuronyl transferase activity, causing unconjugated hyperbilirubinemia, jaundice, and death from kernicterus (usually within the first year)

Biliary Atresia

What is it?	Obliteration of extrahepatic biliary tree
What are the signs/symptoms?	Persistent jaundice (normal physiologic jaundice resolves in <2 weeks), hepatomegaly, splenomegaly, ascites and other signs of portal hypertension, acholic stools, biliuria
What are the lab findings?	Mixed jaundice is always present (i.e., both direct and indirect bilirubin increased), with an elevated serum alkaline phosphatase level
What is the differential diagnosis?	Neonatal hepatitis (TORCH); biliary hypoplasia
How is the diagnosis made?	1. U/S to rule out choledochal cyst and to examine extrahepatic bile ducts and gallbladder 2. HIDA scan—shows no excretion into the GI tract (with phenobarbital preparation) 3. Operative cholangiogram and liver biopsy
What is the treatment?	Early laparotomy by 2 months of age with a modified form of the Kasai hepatoportoenterostomy
How does a Kasai work?	Anastomosis of the porta hepatis and the small bowel allows drainage of bile via many microscopic bile ducts in the fibrous structure of the porta hepatis
What if the Kasai fails?	Revise or liver transplantation

Choledochal Cyst

What is it?

Cystic enlargement of bile ducts; most commonly arises in extrahepatic ducts, but can also arise in intrahepatic ducts

What is the usual presentation?

50% present with intermittent jaundice, RUQ mass, and abdominal pain; may also present with pancreatitis

What is the most common anatomic variant?

Common cyst

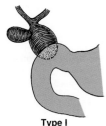

Type I

How is the diagnosis made?

U/S

What is the treatment?

Operative cholangiogram to clarify pathologic process and delineate the pancreatic duct, followed by complete resection of the cyst and a Roux-en-Y hepaticojejunostomy

What conditions are these patients at increased risk of developing?

Cholangiocarcinoma often arises in the cyst; therefore, treat by complete prophylactic resection of the cyst

Cholelithiasis

What is it?

Formation of gallstones

What are the common causes in children?

Etiology differs somewhat from that of adults; the most common cause is cholesterol stones, but the percentage of pigmented stones from hemolytic disorders is increasing

What is the treatment?

Cholecystectomy is recommended for all children with gallstones

Annular Pancreas

What is an annular pancreas?

Congenital pancreatic abnormality with complete encirclement of the duodenum by the pancreas

What are the symptoms?	Duodenal obstruction
What is the treatment?	Duodenoduodenostomy bypass of obstruction (do not resect the pancreas!)

TUMORS

What is the differential diagnosis of pediatric abdominal mass?	Wilms' tumor, neuroblastoma, hernia, intussusception, malrotation with volvulus, mesenteric cyst, duplication cyst, liver tumor (hepatoblastoma/hemangioma), rhabdomyosarcoma, teratoma

Wilms' Tumor

What is it?	Embryonal tumor of **renal** origin

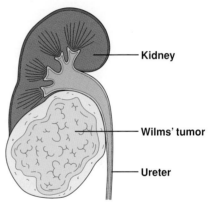

What is the incidence?	Very rare: 500 new cases in the United States per year
What is the average age at diagnosis?	Usually 1 to 5 years of age
What are the symptoms?	Usually asymptomatic except for abdominal mass; 20% of patients present with minimal blunt trauma to mass
What is the classic history?	Found during dressing or bathing
What are the signs?	Abdominal mass (most do not cross the midline); hematuria (10%–15%); HTN in 20% of cases, related to compression of juxtaglomerular apparatus; signs of Beckwith–Wiedemann syndrome
What are the diagnostic radiologic tests?	Abdominal and chest CT scan

What are the best indicators of survival?	Stage and histologic subtype of tumor; 85% of patients have favorable histology (FH); 15% have unfavorable histology (UH); overall survival for FH is 85% for all stages
What is the treatment?	Radical resection of affected kidney with evaluation for staging, followed by chemotherapy (low stages) and radiation (higher stages)
What are the associated abnormalities?	**Aniridia,** hemihypertrophy, Beckwith–Wiedemann syndrome, neurofibromatosis, horseshoe kidney
What is the Beckwith–Wiedemann syndrome?	Syndrome of: 1. Umbilical defect 2. Macroglossia (big tongue) 3. Gigantism 4. Visceromegaly (big organs) (Think: **W**ilms' = Beckwith–**W**iedemann)

Neuroblastoma

What is it?	Embryonal tumor of neural crest origin

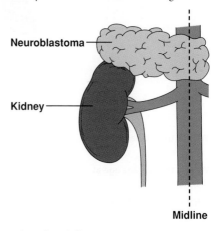

What are the anatomic locations?	**Adrenal medulla**—50% Para-aortic abdominal paraspinal ganglia—25% Posterior mediastinum—20% Neck—3% Pelvis—3%
With which types of tumor does a patient with Horner's syndrome present?	Neck, superior mediastinal tumors

What is the average age at diagnosis?	≈50% are diagnosed by 2 years of age ≈90% are diagnosed by 8 years of age
What are the signs?	Asymptomatic abdominal mass (palpable in 50% of cases), respiratory distress (mediastinal tumors), Horner's syndrome (upper chest or neck tumors), proptosis (with orbital metastases), subcutaneous tumor nodules, HTN (20%–35%)
Labs?	24-hour urine to measure VMA, HVA, and metanephrines (elevated in >85%); neuron-specific enolase, N-*myc* oncogene, DNA ploidy
What are the diagnostic radiologic tests?	CT scan, MRI, I-MIBG, somatostatin receptor scan
What is the classic abdominal plain x-ray finding?	Calcifications (≈50%)
How do you access bone marrow involvement?	Bone marrow aspirate
What is the difference in position of tumors in neuroblastoma versus Wilms' tumors?	Neuroblastoma may cross the midline, but Wilms' tumors do so only rarely

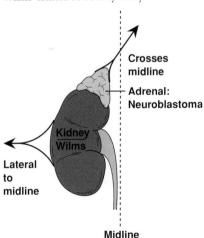

Crosses midline

Adrenal: Neuroblastoma

Kidney Wilms

Lateral to midline

Midline

What is the treatment?	Resection ± chemotherapy ± XRT
Which oncogene is associated with neuroblastoma?	N-*myc* oncogene Think: **N**-*myc* = **N**euroblastoma

Rhabdomyosarcoma

What is its claim to fame?	Most common sarcoma in children
What is the age distribution?	Bimodal: 1. 2 to 5 years 2. 15 to 19 years
What are the most common sites?	1. Head and neck (40%) 2. GU tract (20%) 3. Extremities (20%)
What are the signs/symptoms?	Mass
How is the diagnosis made?	Tissue biopsy, CT scan, MRI, bone marrow
What is the treatment?	
Resectable	Surgical excision, ± chemotherapy and radiation therapy
Unresectable	Neoadjuvant chemo/XRT, then surgical excision

Hepatoblastoma

What is it?	Malignant tumor of the liver (derived from embryonic liver cells)
What is the average age at diagnosis?	Presents in the first 3 years of life
How is the diagnosis made?	Physical exam—abdominal distention; **RUQ mass that moves with respiration** Elevated serum α-fetoprotein and ferritin (can be used as tumor markers) CT scan of abdomen, which often predicts resectability
What percentage will have an elevated α-fetoprotein level?	≈90%
What is the treatment?	Resection by lobectomy or trisegmentectomy is the treatment of choice (plus postoperative chemotherapy); large tumors may require preoperative chemotherapy and **subsequent** hepatic resection
What is the overall survival rate?	≈50%
What is the major difference in age presentation between hepatoma and hepatoblastoma?	Hepatoblastoma presents at <3 years of age; hepatoma presents at >3 years of age and in adolescents

PEDIATRIC TRAUMA

What is the leading cause of death in pediatric patients?	Trauma
How are the vast majority of splenic and liver injuries treated in children?	Observation (i.e., nonoperatively)
What is a common simulator of peritoneal signs in the blunt pediatric trauma victim?	Gastric distention (place an NG tube)
How do you estimate normal systolic blood pressure (SBP) in a child?	80 + 2 × age (e.g., a 5-year-old child should have an SBP of ≈90)
What is the 20–20–10 rule for fluid resuscitation of the unstable pediatric trauma patient?	First give a **20** cc/kg LR bolus followed by a second bolus of **20** cc/kg LR bolus if needed; if the patient is still unstable after the second LR bolus, then administer a **10** cc/kg bolus of **blood**
What is the treatment for duodenal hematoma?	Observation with NGT and TPN

RAPID-FIRE REVIEW

What are the differences between omphalocele and gastroschisis in terms of the following characteristics?	
Anomalies	Common in omphalocele (50%), uncommon in gastroschisis
Peritoneal/amnion covering (sac)	Always with omphalocele—never with gastroschisis
Position of umbilical cord	On the sac with omphalocele, from skin to the left of the gastroschisis defect
Thick bowel	Common with gastroschisis, rare with omphalocele (unless sac ruptures)
Protrusion of liver	Common with omphalocele, almost never with gastroschisis
Large defect	Omphalocele
What is the usual age at presentation of the following conditions?	
Pyloric stenosis	3 weeks to 3 months (3–3)

Intussusception	4 months to 2 years (>80%)
Wilms' tumor	1 to 5 years
Malrotation	Birth to 1 year (>85%)
Neuroblastoma	≈50% present by 2 years >80% present by 8 years
Hepatoblastoma	<3 years
Appendicitis	>3 years (but must be considered at *any* age!)

What is the correct diagnosis?

Newborn with bilious vomiting	Malrotation
Nonbilious vomiting in an infant <2 months old	Pyloric stenosis
"Currant jelly" stool in young child	Intussusception
To pass meconium within the first 24 hours of life	Hirschsprung's disease
Inability to pass an NGT in a newborn	Esophageal atresia
"Gasless" abdomen in a newborn	Esophageal atresia
Newborn with pneumatosis intestinalis	NEC (necrotizing enterocolitis)

Name the most likely diagnosis:

8-year-old male with acute scrotal pain; a small "blue dot" is seen through the scrotal skin	Testicular appendage torsion
6-year-old child with finger clubbing and history of cyanosis as an infant develops anxiety/increase in respiratory rate and cyanosis with strenuous exercise that is relieved by "squatting down"	Tetralogy of Fallot
8-year-old male with a history of claudication when running, epistaxis, decreased LE pulses, and headaches	Aortic coarctation
6-year-old female with purpuric rash, abdominal pain, hematuria, and joint pain	Schönlein–Henoch purpura

17-year-old male presents with thigh pain; x-ray reveals bony mass with a "sunburst" pattern	Osteosarcoma
16-year-old female with knee pain; x-ray reveals a periosteum "onion skinning"	Ewing's sarcoma
17-year-old female with history of breast mass, exam reveals a rubbery smooth mass	Fibroadenoma
Newborn male with excessive salivation and inability to pass an NGT	Esophageal atresia

Name the diagnostic modality:

1-day-old male with no urination	Voiding cystogram looking for posterior urethral valves

Chapter 67 | Plastic Surgery

Define the following terms:

Langer's lines

Natural skin lines of minimal tension (e.g., lines across the forehead), incisions perpendicular to Langer's lines result in larger scars than incision parallel to the lines

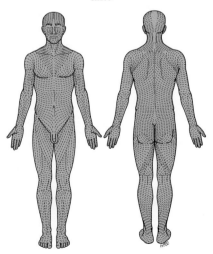

WOUND HEALING

What are the phases of wound healing?	Think: "In Every Fresh Cut" = **IEFC:** 1. Inflammation 2. Epithelialization 3. Fibroplasia 4. Contraction
What are the actions of the following phases?	
Inflammation	Vasoconstriction followed by vasodilation, capillary leak
Epithelialization	Epithelial coverage of wound
Fibroplasia	Fibroblasts and accumulation of collagen, elastin, and reticulin
Wound contraction	Myofibroblasts contract wound
In which structures does the epithelium grow from superficial burns/wounds?	Epithelial lining of sweat glands and hair follicles
In full-thickness burns?	From wound margins, grows in <1 cm from wound edge because no sweat glands or hair follicles remain; this epithelium has no underlying dermis

Wound Contraction

Which contracts more: a split-thickness (STSG) or a full-thickness skin graft (FTSG)?	STSG contracts up to 41% in surface area, whereas an FTSG contracts little, if at all
What generalized conditions inhibit wound healing?	Anemia Malnutrition Steroids Cancer Radiation Hypoxia Sepsis Diabetes
What helps wound healing in patients taking steroids?	Vitamin A is thought to counteract the deleterious effect of steroids on wound healing
When does a wound gain more than 90% of its maximal tensile strength?	After ≈6 weeks

Define the following terms:

Hypertrophic scar	Hypertrophic scar **within** original wound margins
Keloid	Proliferative scar tumor progressively enlarging scar **beyond** original wound margins
Why not clean lacerations with Betadine®?	Betadine® is harmful and inhibits normal healthy tissue

SKIN GRAFTS

What is an STSG?	Split thickness: includes the epidermis and a variable amount of the dermis
How thick is it?	10/1,000 to 18/1,000 of an inch
What is an FTSG?	Full thickness: includes the entire epidermis and dermis
What are the prerequisites for a skin graft to take?	Bed must be vascularized; a graft to a bone or tendon will not take Bacteria must be <100,000 Shearing motion and fluid beneath the graft must be minimized
What is a better bed for a skin graft: fascia or fat?	Fascia (much better blood supply)
How do you increase surface area of an STSG?	Mesh it (also allows for blood/serum to be removed from underneath the graft)
How does an STSG get nutrition for the first 24 hours?	Imbibition

FLAPS

What is a simple advancement flap?

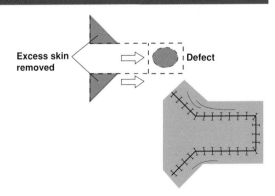

What is a rotational flap?

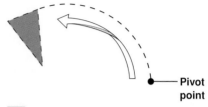

What is a "free flap"?

Flap separated from all vascular supply that requires microvascular anastomosis (microscope)

What is a TRAM flap?

Transverse Rectus Abdominis Myocutaneous flap (see page 289)

What is a "Z-plasty"?

Reorients and lengthens a scar

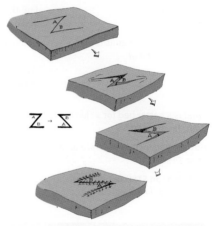

What is a "V-Y advancement flap"?

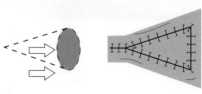

Chapter 68 | Hand Surgery

Who operates on hands?	Plastic surgeons **and** orthopedic surgeons
What are the bones of the hand?	Phalanges (fingers) Metacarpal bones Carpal bones
What is the distal finger joint?	Distal InterPhalangeal (**DIP**) joint
What is the middle finger joint?	Proximal InterPhalangeal (**PIP**) joint
What is the proximal finger joint?	Metacarpal Phalangeal (**MP**) joint
What are the "intrinsic" hand muscles?	Lumbricals, interosseous muscle
What is ADDuction and ABDuction of the fingers?	**ADD**uction is to midline and **ABD**uction is separation from midline

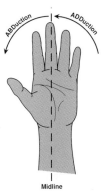

Where is "no man's land"?	Zone extending from the distal palmar crease to just beyond the PIP joint (zone 2)

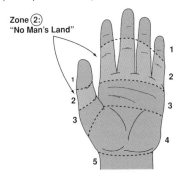

What is the significance of the "no man's land"?	Flexor tendon injuries here have a poor prognosis

SENSORY SUPPLY TO THE HAND

What is the ulnar nerve distribution?

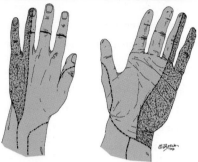

What is the radial nerve distribution?

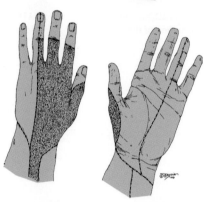

What is the median nerve distribution?

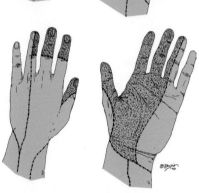

How can radial nerve motor function be tested?
1. Wrist and MCP extension
2. Abduction and extension of thumb

How can ulnar nerve motor function be tested?
1. Spread fingers apart against resistance
2. Check ability to cross index and middle fingers

How can median nerve function be tested?

1. Touch the thumb to the pinky (distal median nerve)
2. Squeeze examiner's finger (proximal median nerve)

How can the flexor digitorum PROFUNDUS (FDP) apparatus be tested?

Check isolated flexion of the finger DIP joint

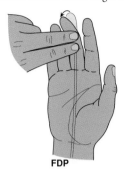

FDP

How can the flexor digitorum SUPERFICIALIS (FDS) apparatus be tested?

Check isolated flexion of the finger at the MP joint

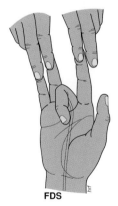

FDS

Where do the digital arteries run?

On medial and lateral sides of the digit

What hand laceration should be left unsutured?

Lacerations from human bites or animal bites

Should a clamp ever be used to stop a laceration bleeder?

No; use pressure and then tourniquet for definitive repair if bleeding does not cease because **nerves run with blood vessels!**

What is a felon?

Infection in the **tip** of the finger pad (Think: **f**elon = **f**ingerprints = in**f**ection in pad); treat by incision and drainage

What is a paronychia?

Infection on the **side** of the fingernail (nail fold); treat by incision and drainage

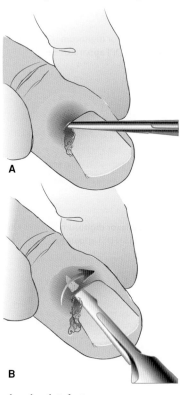

A

B

What is tenosynovitis?

Tendon sheath infection

What are Kanavel's signs?

Four signs of tenosynovitis:
1. Affected finger held in flexion
2. Pain over volar aspect of affected finger tendon sheath upon palpation
3. Swelling of affected finger (fusiform)
4. Pain on passive extension of affected finger

Most common bacteria in tenosynovitis and paronychia:

Staphylococcus aureus

How are human and animal hand bites treated?

Débridement/irrigation/administration of antibiotics; **leave wound open**

What unique bacteria are found in human bites?

Eikenella corrodens

What unique bacteria are found in dog and cat bites?

Pasteurella multocida

What is the most common hand/wrist tumor?	Ganglion cyst
What is an extremely painful type of subungual tumor?	Glomus tumor (subungual: under the nail)
What is a "boxer's fracture"?	Fracture of the fourth or fifth metacarpal
What is a "drop finger" injury?	Laceration of extensor tendon over the MP joint

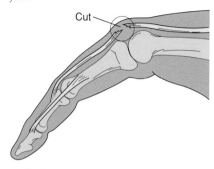

What is the classic deformity resulting from laceration of the extensor tendon over the DIP joint?	Mallet finger

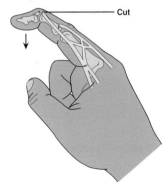

What is the classic deformity resulting from laceration of the extensor tendon over the PIP joint?	Boutonnière deformity

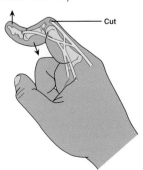

What is a "Jersey finger"?

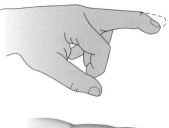

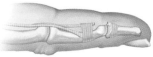

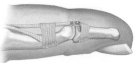

What is the "safe position" of hand splinting?

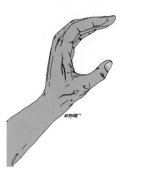

What is Dupuytren's contracture?

Fibrosis of palmar fascia, causing contracture of and inability to extend digits

What is "gamekeeper's thumb"?

Injury to the ulnar collateral ligament of the thumb

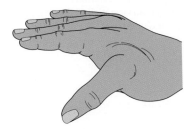

How should a subungual hematoma be treated?

Release pressure by burning a hole in the nail (use handheld disposable battery-operated coagulation probe)

CARPAL TUNNEL SYNDROME

What is it?

Compression of the median nerve in the carpal tunnel

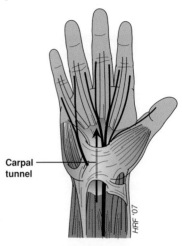

Carpal tunnel

HRF '07

What is the most common cause?

Synovitis

What are other causes?

"MEDIAN TRAPS":
> **M**edian artery (persistent)
> **E**dema of pregnancy
> **D**iabetes
> **I**diopathic
> **A**cromegaly
> **N**eoplasm (e.g., ganglioneuroma)

> **T**hyroid (myxedema)
> **R**heumatoid arthritis
> **A**myloid
> **P**neumatic drill usage
> **S**LE

What are the symptoms?

Pain and numbness in the median nerve distribution

What are the signs?

Tinel's sign (symptoms with percussion over median nerve), Phalen's test (symptoms with flexion of wrists), thenar atrophy, Wartenberg's sign

What is Wartenberg's sign?

With hand resting on a surface, the fifth digit ("pinky") rests in ABduction compared to the other four fingers

What is the workup?

EMG, nerve conduction study

What is initial treatment?	Nonoperative, rest, wrist splint, NSAIDs
What are the indications for surgery?	Refractory symptoms, thenar atrophy, thenar weakness
What surgery is performed?	Release transverse carpal ligament

RAPID-FIRE REVIEW

Name the most likely diagnosis:

| 34-year-old male carpenter develops a decrease in coordination in his hammer hand (right hand); he wakes in the middle of the night with right hand pain and "pins and needles" in the right thumb/index/middle fingers | Carpel tunnel syndrome |

Chapter 69 | Otolaryngology: Head and Neck Surgery

EAR

Otitis Externa (Swimmer's Ear)

What is it?	Generalized infection involving the external ear canal and often the tympanic membrane (TM)
What is the usual cause?	Prolonged water exposure and damaged squamous epithelium of the ear canal (e.g., swimming, hearing aid use)
What are the typical pathogens?	Most frequently *Pseudomonas,* may be *Proteus, Staphylococcus,* occasionally *Escherichia coli,* fungi (*Aspergillus, Candida*), or virus (herpes zoster or herpes simplex)
What are the signs/symptoms?	Ear pain (otalgia); swelling of external ear, ear canal, or both; erythema; pain on manipulation of the auricle; debris in canal; otorrhea

What is the treatment?	Keep the ear dry; mild infections respond to cleaning and dilute acetic acid drops; most infections require complete removal of all debris and topical antibiotics with or without hydrocortisone (anti-inflammatory)

Malignant Otitis Externa (MOE)

What is it?	Fulminant **bacterial** otitis externa
Is it malignant cancer?	NO!
Who is affected?	Most common scenario: elderly patient with poorly controlled diabetes (other forms of immunosuppression do not appear to predispose patients to MOE)
What are the causative organisms?	Usually *Pseudomonas aeruginosa*
What is the classic feature?	Nub of granulation tissue on the floor of the external ear canal at the bony–cartilaginous junction
What are the other signs/ symptoms?	Severe ear pain, excessive purulent discharge, and usually **exposed bone**
What are the diagnostic tests?	1. CT scan: shows erosion of bone, inflammation 2. Technetium-99 scan: temporal bone inflammatory process 3. Gallium-tagged white blood cell scan: to follow and document resolution
What are the complications?	Invasion of surrounding structures to produce a cellulitis, osteomyelitis of temporal bone, mastoiditis; later, a facial nerve palsy, meningitis, or brain abscess
What is the treatment?	Control of diabetes, meticulous local care with extensive débridement, hospitalization and IV antibiotics (anti-*Pseudomonas:* usually an aminoglycoside plus a penicillin)

Tumors of the External Ear

What are the most common types?	Squamous cell most common; occasionally, basal cell carcinoma or melanoma
From what location do they usually arise?	Auricle, but occasionally from the external canal
What is the associated risk factor?	Excessive sun exposure

What is the treatment of the following conditions?

Cancers of the auricle	Usually wedge excision
Extension to the canal	May require excision of the external ear canal or partial temporal bone excision
Middle ear involvement	Best treated by en bloc temporal bone resection and lymph node dissection

Tympanic Membrane Perforation

What is the etiology?

Usually the result of trauma (direct or indirect) or secondary to middle ear infection; often occurs secondary to slap to the side of the head (compression injury), explosions

What are the symptoms?

Pain, bleeding from the ear, conductive hearing loss, tinnitus

What are the signs?

Clot in the meatus, visible tear in the TM

What is the treatment?

Keep dry; use topical antibiotics if there is evidence of infection or contamination

What is the prognosis?

Most (90%) heal spontaneously, although larger perforations may require surgery (e.g., fat plug, temporalis fascia, or tragal cartilage tympanoplasty)

Cholesteatoma

What is it?

Epidermal inclusion cyst of the middle ear or mastoid, containing desquamated keratin debris; may be acquired or congenital

What are the causes?

Negative middle ear pressure from eustachian tube dysfunction (primary acquired) or direct growth of epithelium through a TM perforation (secondary acquired)

What other condition is it often associated with?

Chronic middle ear infection

What is the usual history?

Chronic ear infection with chronic, malodorous drainage

What is the appearance?

Grayish white, shiny keratinous mass behind or involving the TM; often described as a "pearly" lesion

What is the treatment?

Surgery (tympanoplasty/mastoidectomy) aimed at eradication of disease and reconstruction of the ossicular chain

Bullous Myringitis

What is it?	Vesicular infection of the TM and adjacent deep canal
What are the causative agents?	Unknown; viral should be suspected because of frequent association with viral URI (in some instances, *Mycoplasma pneumoniae* has been cultured)
What are the symptoms?	Acute, severe ear pain; low-grade fever; and bloody drainage
What are the findings on otoscopic examination?	Large, reddish blebs on the TM, wall of the meatus, or both
Is hearing affected?	Rarely; occasional reversible sensorineural loss
What is the treatment?	Oral antibiotics (erythromycin if *Mycoplasma* is suspected); topical analgesics may be used, with resolution of symptoms usually occurring in 36 hours

Acute Suppurative Otitis Media (OM)

What is it?	Bacterial infection of the middle ear, often following a viral URI; may be associated with a middle ear effusion
What is the cause?	Dysfunction of the eustachian tube that allows bacterial entry from nasopharynx; often associated with an occluded eustachian tube, although it is uncertain whether this is a cause or a result of the infection
What are the predisposing factors?	Young age, male gender, bottle feeding, crowded living conditions (e.g., day care), cleft palate, Down's syndrome, cystic fibrosis
What is the etiology?	1. *Streptococcus pneumoniae* (33% of cases) 2. *Haemophilus influenzae* 3. *Moraxella catarrhalis* 4. *Staphylococcus* 5. β-Hemolytic strep 6. *P. aeruginosa* 7. Viral/no culture
What is the etiology in infants <6 months?	1. *Staphylococcus aureus* 2. *E. coli* 3. *Klebsiella*
What are the symptoms?	Otalgia, fever, decreased hearing, infant pulls on ear, increased irritability; as many as 25% of patients are asymptomatic

What are the signs?	Early, redness of the TM; later, TM bulging with the loss of the normal landmarks; finally, impaired TM mobility on pneumatic otoscopy
If pain disappears instantly, what may have happened?	TM perforation!
What are the complications?	TM perforation, acute mastoiditis, meningitis, brain abscess, extradural abscess, labyrinthitis; if recurrent or chronic, OM may have adverse effects on speech and cognitive development as a result of decreased hearing
What is the treatment?	10-day course of antibiotics; amoxicillin is the first-line agent; if the patient is allergic to PCN, trimethoprim/sulfamethoxazole or erythromycin should be administered
What is the usual course?	Symptoms usually resolve in 24 to 36 hours
What are the indications for myringotomy and PE tube placement?	1. Persistent middle ear effusion over 3 months 2. Debilitated or immunocompromised patient 3. >3 episodes over 6 months (especially if bilateral)
What is a PE tube?	**P**neumatic **E**qualization tube (tube placed through TM)
What is a Bezold's abscess?	Abscess behind the superior attachment of the sternocleidomastoid muscle resulting from extension of a mastoid infection
What are causes of chronic OM?	Mixed, *S. aureus, P. aeruginosa*
What are the signs/symptoms of chronic OM?	Otorrhea and hearing loss

Otosclerosis

What is it?	Genetic disease characterized by abnormal spongy and sclerotic bone formation in the temporal bone around the footplate of the stapes, thus preventing its normal movement
What is the inheritance pattern?	Autosomal dominant with incomplete one-third penetrance
What are the symptoms?	Painless, progressive hearing loss (may be unilateral or bilateral), tinnitus
What is the usual age of onset?	Second through fourth decade

How is the diagnosis made?	Normal TM with conductive hearing loss and no middle-ear effusion (though may be mixed or even sensorineural if bone of cochlea is affected)
What is Schwartze's sign?	Erythema around the stapes from hypervascularity of new bone formation
What is the treatment?	Frequently surgical (stapedectomy with placement of prosthesis), hearing aids, or observation; sodium fluoride may be used if a sensorineural component is present or for preoperative stabilization

MISCELLANEOUS

Facial Nerve Paralysis

What are the causes?	Bell's palsy Trauma Cholesteatoma Tumor (carcinoma, glomus jugulare) Herpes zoster inflammation of geniculate ganglion (Ramsay-Hunt syndrome) Peripheral lesions are usually parotid gland tumors
What is the most common cause of bilateral facial nerve palsy?	Lyme disease (*Borrelia burgdorferi*)

Bell's Palsy

What is it?	Sudden onset, unilateral facial weakness or paralysis in absence of CNS, ear, or cerebellopontine angle disease (i.e., no identifiable cause)

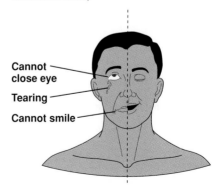

Cannot close eye

Tearing

Cannot smile

What is the clinical course?	Acute onset, with greatest muscle weakness reached within 3 weeks
What is the incidence?	Most common cause of **unilateral** facial weakness/paralysis
What is the pathogenesis?	Unknown; most widely accepted hypothesis is viral etiology (herpes virus); ischemic and immunologic factors are also implicated
What is the common preceding event?	URI
What are the signs/symptoms?	Pathology is related to swelling of the facial nerve; may present with total facial paralysis, altered lacrimation, increased tearing on affected side, change in taste if region above chorda tympani is affected, dry mouth, and hyperacusis
What is the treatment?	Usually none is required, as most cases resolve spontaneously in 1 month; protect eye with drops and tape closed as needed; most otolaryngologists advocate steroids and acyclovir Surgical decompression of CN VII is indicated if paralysis progresses or tests indicate deterioration
What is the prognosis?	Overall, 90% of patients recover completely; if paralysis is incomplete, 95% to 100% will recover without sequelae

Ménière's Disease

What is it?	Disorder of the membranous labyrinth, causing fluctuating sensorineural hearing loss, episodic vertigo, nystagmus, tinnitus, and aural fullness, N/V
What is the classic triad?	**"H, T, V":** 1. Hearing loss 2. Tinnitus 3. Vertigo
What is the medical treatment?	Salt restriction, diuretics (thiazides), antinausea agents; occasionally diazepam is added; 80% of patients respond to medical management, antihistamines
What are the indications for surgery?	Surgery is offered to those who fail medical treatment or who have incapacitating vertigo (60%–80% effective)

Glomus Tumors

What are they?	Benign, slow-growing tumors arising in glomus bodies found in the adventitial layer of blood vessels; often associated with cranial nerves IX and X in the middle ear
What is the usual location?	Middle ear, jugular bulb, course of CN IX to XII
How common are they?	Most common benign tumor of the temporal bone
What is the treatment?	Surgical resection, radiation therapy for poor operative candidates or for recurrences

NOSE AND PARANASAL SINUSES

Epistaxis

What is it?	Bleeding from the nose
What are the predisposing factors?	Trauma, anticoagulants, "nose picking," sinus infection, allergic or atrophic rhinitis, blood dyscrasias, tumor, environmental extremes (hot, dry climates; winters)
What is the usual cause?	Rupture of superficial mucosal blood vessels (Kiesselbach's plexus if anterior, sphenopalatine artery if posterior)
What is the most common type?	Anterior (90%); usually the result of trauma
Which type is more serious?	Posterior; usually occurs in the elderly or is associated with a systemic disorder (hypertension, tumor, arteriosclerosis)
What is the treatment?	Direct pressure; if this fails, proceed to nasal packing
What is the treatment of last resort?	Ligation or embolization of the sphenopalatine artery (posterior) or ethmoidal artery (anterior)

Acute Sinusitis

What is the typical history?	Previously healthy patient with unrelenting progression of a viral URI or allergic rhinitis beyond the normal 5- to 7-day course
What are the symptoms?	Periorbital pressure/pain, nasal obstruction, nasal/postnasal mucopurulent discharge, fatigue, fever, headache

What are the signs?	Tenderness over affected sinuses, pus in the nasal cavity; may also see reason for obstruction (septal deviation, spur, tight osteomeatal complex); transillumination is unreliable
What is the pathophysiology?	Thought to be secondary to decreased ciliary action of the sinus mucosa and edema causing obstruction of the sinus ostia, lowering intrasinus oxygen tension and predisposing patients to bacterial infection
What are the causative organisms?	Up to 50% of patients have negative cultures and cause is presumably (initially) viral; pneumococcus, *S. aureus*, group A streptococci, and *H. influenzae* are the most common bacteria cultured
What is the treatment?	14-day course of antibiotics (penicillin G, amoxicillin, Ceclor®, and Augmentin® are commonly used), topical and systemic decongestants, and saline nasal irrigation
What is the treatment for fungal sinusitis?	Fungal sinusitis is commonly caused by *Mucor* and seen in immunosuppressed patients; treatment is IV antifungals (e.g., amphotericin or caspofungin) and surgical débridement of all necrotic tissue

Chronic Sinusitis

What is it?	Infection of nasal sinuses lasting >4 weeks, or pattern of recurrent acute sinusitis punctuated by brief asymptomatic periods
What is the pathology?	Permanent mucosal changes secondary to inadequately treated acute sinusitis, consisting of mucosal fibrosis, polypoid growth, and inadequate ciliary action, hyperostosis (increased bone density on CT scan)
What are the symptoms?	Chronic nasal obstruction, postnasal drip, mucopurulent rhinorrhea, low-grade facial and periorbital pressure/pain
What are the causative organisms?	Usually anaerobes (such as *Bacteroides, Veillonella, Rhinobacterium*); also *H. influenzae, Streptococcus viridans, Staphylococcus aureus, Staphylococcus epidermidis*
What is the treatment?	Medical management with decongestants, mucolytics, topical steroids, and antibiotics; if this approach fails, proceed to endoscopic or external surgical intervention

What is FESS?	Functional Endoscopic Sinus Surgery
What are the complications of sinusitis?	Orbital cellulitis (if ethmoid sinusitis), meningitis, epidural or brain abscess (frontal sinus), cavernous sinus thrombosis (ethmoid or sphenoid), osteomyelitis (a.k.a. "Pott's puffy tumor" if frontal)

Cancer of the Nasal Cavity and Paranasal Sinuses

What are the usual locations?	Maxillary sinus (66%) Nasal cavity Ethmoid sinus Rarely in frontal or sphenoid sinuses
What are the associated cell types?	Squamous cell (80%) Adenocellular (15%) Uncommon: sarcoma, melanoma
What rare tumor arises from olfactory epithelium?	Esthesioneuroblastoma; usually arises high in the nose (cribriform plate) and is locally invasive
What are the signs/symptoms?	Early—nasal obstruction, blood-tinged mucus, epistaxis Late—localized pain, cranial nerve deficits, facial/palate asymmetry, loose teeth
How is the diagnosis made?	CT scan can adequately identify extent of the disease and local invasion; MRI is often also used to evaluate soft tissue disease
What is the treatment?	Surgery ± XRT
What is the prognosis?	5-year survival for T1 or T2 lesions approaches 70%

Juvenile Nasopharyngeal Angiofibroma

What is it?	Most commonly encountered vascular mass in the nasal cavity; locally aggressive but nonmetastasizing
What is the usual history?	Adolescent boys who present with nasal obstruction, recurrent massive epistaxis, possibly anosmia
What is the usual location?	Site of origin is the roof of the nasal cavity at the superior margin of sphenopalatine foramen
Into what can the mass transform?	Fibrosarcoma (rare cases reported)
How is the diagnosis made?	Carotid arteriography, CT scan; biopsy is contraindicated secondary to risk of uncontrollable hemorrhage

What are indications for biopsy?	**None!**
What is the treatment?	Surgery via lateral rhinotomy or sublabial maxillotomy with bleeding controlled by internal maxillary artery ligation or preoperative embolization, in the setting of hypotensive anesthesia; preoperative irradiation has also been used to shrink the tumor

ORAL CAVITY AND PHARYNX

Pharyngotonsillitis

What is the common site of referred throat pain?	EAR
What is it?	Acute or chronic infection of the nasopharynx or oropharynx and/or Waldeyer's ring of lymphoid tissue (consisting of palatine, lingual, and pharyngeal tonsils and the adenoids)
What is the etiology?	Acute attacks can be viral (adenovirus, enterovirus, coxsackievirus, Epstein–Barr virus in infectious mononucleosis) or bacterial (group A β-hemolytic streptococci are the leading bacterial agent); chronic tonsillitis often with mixed population, including streptococci, staphylococci, and *M. catarrhalis*
What are the symptoms?	Acute—Sore throat, fever, local lymphadenopathy, chills, headache, malaise Chronic—Noisy mouth breathing, speech and swallowing difficulties, apnea, halitosis
What are the signs?	Viral—Injected tonsils and pharyngeal mucosa; exudate may occur, but less often than with bacterial tonsillitis Bacterial—Swollen, inflamed tonsils with white-yellow exudate in crypts and on surface; cervical adenopathy
How is the diagnosis made?	CBC, throat culture, Monospot test
What are the possible complications?	Peritonsillar abscess (quinsy), retropharyngeal abscess (causing airway compromise), rheumatic fever, poststreptococcal glomerulonephritis (with β-hemolytic streptococci)

What is the treatment?	Viral—symptomatic → acetaminophen, warm saline gargles, anesthetic throat spray Bacterial—10 days PCN (erythromycin if PCN allergic)
What are the indications for tonsillectomy?	Sleep apnea/cor pulmonale secondary to airway obstruction, suspicion of malignancy, hypertrophy causing malocclusion, peritonsillar abscess, recurrent acute or chronic tonsillitis
What are the possible complications?	Acute or delayed hemorrhage

Peritonsillar Abscess

What is the clinical setting?	Inadequately treated recurrent acute or chronic tonsillitis
What is the associated microbiology?	Mixed aerobes and anaerobes (which may be PCN resistant)
What is the site of formation?	Begins at the superior pole of the tonsil
What are the symptoms?	Severe throat pain, drooling dysphagia, odynophagia, trismus, cervical adenopathy, fever, chills, malaise
What is the classic description of voice?	"Hot-potato" voice
What are the signs?	Bulging, erythematous, edematous tonsillar pillar; swelling of uvula and displacement to contralateral side
What is the treatment?	IV antibiotics and surgical evacuation by incision and drainage; most experts recommend tonsillectomy after resolution of inflammatory changes

Ludwig Angina

What is it?	Infection and inflammation of the floor of the mouth (sublingual and submandibular)
What is the source?	Dental infection
What is the treatment?	Antibiotics, emergency airway, I & D

Cancer of the Oral Cavity

What is the usual cell type?	Squamous cell (>90% of cases)
What are the most common sites?	**Lip,** tongue, floor of mouth, gingiva, cheek, and palate

What is the etiology?	Linked to smoking, alcohol, and smokeless tobacco products (alcohol and tobacco together greatly increase the risk), HPV (on the rise)
What is the frequency of the following conditions?	
Regional metastasis	≈30%
Second primary	≈25%
Nodal metastasis	Depends on size of tumor and ranges from 10% to 60%, usually to jugular and **jugulodigastric nodes, submandibular nodes**
Distant metastasis	Infrequent
How is the diagnosis made?	Full history and physical examination, dental assessment, Panorex or bone scan if mandible is thought to be involved, CT scan/MRI for extent of tumor and nodal disease, FNA (often U/S guided)
What is the treatment?	Radiation, surgery, or both for small lesions; localized lesions can usually be treated surgically; larger lesions require combination therapy, possible mandibulectomy, and neck dissection
What is the prognosis?	Depends on stage, site, and etiology:
	Most common cause of death in successfully treated head and neck cancer is development of a second primary (occurs in 20%–40% of cases)
	HPV+ tumors have better prognosis
	Tongue: 20% to 70% survival
	Floor of mouth: 30% to 80% survival

Salivary Gland Tumors

What is the frequency of gland involvement?	Parotid gland (80%) Submandibular gland (15%) Minor salivary glands (5%)
What is the potential for malignancy?	Greatest in **minor salivary gland** tumors (80% are malignant) and least in parotid gland tumors (80% are benign); **the smaller the gland, the greater the likelihood of malignancy**

How do benign and malignant tumors differ in terms of history and physical examination?	Benign—mobile, nontender, no node involvement or facial weakness Malignant—painful, fixed mass with evidence of local metastasis and facial paresis/paralysis
What is the diagnostic procedure?	FNA; **never** perform excisional biopsy of a parotid mass; superficial parotidectomy is the procedure of choice for benign lesions of the lateral lobe
What is the treatment?	Involves adequate surgical resection, sparing facial nerve if possible, neck dissection for node-positive necks
What are the indications for postop XRT?	Postoperative radiation therapy if high-grade cancer, recurrent cancer, residual disease, invasion of adjacent structures, any T3 or T4 parotid tumors
What is the most common benign salivary tumor?	**Pleomorphic adenoma** (benign mixed tumor) 66% (Think: **P**leomorphic = **P**opular)
What is the usual location?	Parotid gland
What is the clinical course?	They are well delineated and slow growing
What is the second most common benign salivary gland tumor?	Warthin's tumor (1% of all salivary gland tumors)
What is the usual location?	95% are found in parotid; 3% are bilateral
Describe the lesion?	Slow-growing, cystic mass is usually located in the tail of the superficial portion of the parotid; it rarely becomes malignant
What is the most common malignant salivary tumor?	**Mucoepidermoid carcinoma** (10% of all salivary gland neoplasms) (Think: **M**ucoepidermoid = **M**alignant) Most common parotid malignancy Second most common submandibular gland malignancy
What is the second most common malignant salivary tumor in adults?	Adenoid cystic carcinoma; most common malignancy in submandibular and minor salivary glands

Croup (Laryngotracheobronchitis)

What is it?	Viral infection of the larynx and trachea, generally affecting children (boys > girls)
What is the usual cause?	Parainfluenza virus (Think: crou**P** = **P**arainfluenza)

What age group is affected most?	Ages 6 months to 3 years
Is the condition considered seasonal?	Yes; outbreaks most often occur in autumn
What are the precipitating events?	Usually preceded by URI
What is the classic symptom?	Barking (seal-like), nonproductive cough
What are the other symptoms?	Respiratory distress, low-grade fever
What are the signs?	Tachypnea, inspiratory retractions, prolonged inspiration, inspiratory stridor, expiratory rhonchi/wheezes
What is the differential diagnosis?	Epiglottitis, bacterial tracheitis, foreign body, diphtheria, retropharyngeal abscess, peritonsillar abscess, asthma
How is the diagnosis made?	AP neck x-ray shows classic "steeple sign," indicating subglottic narrowing; ABG may show hypoxemia plus hypercapnia
What is the treatment?	**Keep child calm** (agitation only worsens obstruction); cool mist; steroids; aerosolized racemic EPI may be administered to reduce edema/airway obstruction
What are the indications for intubation?	If airway obstruction is severe or child becomes exhausted
What is the usual course?	Resolves in 3 to 4 days
What type of secondary infection occurs?	Secondary bacterial infection (streptococcal, staphylococcal)

Epiglottitis

What is it?	Severe, rapidly progressive infection of the epiglottis

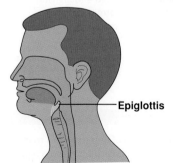 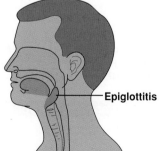

What is the usual causative agent?	*H. influenzae* type B
What age group is affected?	Children 2 to 5 years of age

What are the signs/symptoms?	Sudden onset, high fever (40°C); "hot-potato" voice; dysphagia (→ drooling); no cough; patient prefers to sit upright, lean forward; patient appears toxic and stridulous

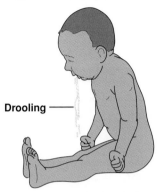

Drooling

How is the diagnosis made?	Can usually be made clinically and does not involve direct observation of the epiglottis (which may worsen obstruction by causing laryngospasm)
What is the treatment?	Involves immediate airway support in the O.R.: intubation or possibly tracheostomy, medical treatment is composed of steroids and IV antibiotics *against H. influenzae*

Malignant Lesions of the Larynx

What is the incidence?	Accounts for ≈2% of all malignancies, more often in males
What is the most common site?	Glottis (66%)
What is the second most common type?	Supraglottis (33%)
Which type has the worst prognosis?	Subglottic tumors (infrequent)
What are the risk factors?	Tobacco, alcohol
What is the pathology?	90% are squamous cell carcinoma
What are the symptoms?	Hoarseness, throat pain, dysphagia, odynophagia, neck mass, (referred) ear pain

Supraglottic Lesions

What is the usual location?	Laryngeal surface of epiglottis
What area is often involved?	Pre-epiglottic space

Extension?	Tend to remain confined to supraglottic region, though may extend to vallecula or base of tongue
What is the associated type of metastasis?	High propensity for nodal metastasis
What is the treatment?	Early stage = XRT Late stage = laryngectomy

Glottic Lesions

What is the usual location?	Anterior part of true cords
Extension?	May invade thyroid cartilage, cross midline to invade contralateral cord, or invade paraglottic space
What is the associated type of metastasis?	Rare nodal metastasis
What is the treatment?	Early stage = XRT Late stage = laryngectomy

Neck Mass

What is the usual etiology in infants?	Congenital (branchial cleft cysts, thyroglossal duct cysts)
What is the usual etiology in adolescents?	Inflammatory (cervical adenitis is #1), with congenital also possible
What is the usual etiology in adults?	Malignancy (squamous is #1), especially if painless and immobile
What is the "80% rule"?	In general, **80%** of neck masses are **benign** in children; **80%** are **malignant** in adults >40 years of age
What are the cardinal symptoms (7) of neck masses?	1. Dysphagia 2. Odynophagia 3. Hoarseness 4. Stridor (signifies upper airway obstruction) 5. Globus 6. Speech disorder 7. Referred ear pain (via CN V, IX, or X)
What comprises the workup?	Full head and neck examination, indirect laryngoscopy, CT scan and MRI, FNA for tissue diagnosis; biopsy contraindicated because it may adversely affect survival if malignant

What is the differential diagnosis?	Inflammatory: cervical lymphadenitis, cat-scratch disease, infectious mononucleosis, infection in neck spaces Congenital: thyroglossal duct cyst (midline, elevates with tongue protrusion), branchial cleft cysts (lateral), dermoid cysts (midline submental), hemangioma, cystic hygroma Neoplastic: primary or metastatic
What is the workup of node-positive squamous cell carcinoma and no primary site?	Triple endoscopy (laryngoscopy, esophagoscopy, bronchoscopy) and biopsies of likely sites, PET scan
What is the treatment?	Surgical excision for congenital or neoplastic; two most important procedures for cancer treatment are selective and modified neck dissection
What is the role of adjuvant treatment in head and neck cancer?	Postoperative chemotherapy/XRT

Radical Neck Dissection

What is involved?	Classically, removal of **nodes** from clavicle to mandible, sternocleidomastoid muscle, **submandibular gland,** tail of **parotid,** internal **jugular vein, digastric muscles, stylohyoid** and **omohyoid muscles, fascia** within the anterior and posterior triangles, CN XI, and cervical plexus sensory nerves

Modified Neck Dissection

What is involved?	Removal of lymph nodes in levels 1 to 5 with preservation of one of the three following structures: spinal accessory nerve, internal jugular vein, or sternocleidomastoid muscle
What are the contraindications?	1. Distant METS 2. Fixation of vital structures (e.g., carotid artery)

Selective Neck Dissection

What is involved?	One or more of the lymph node groups in levels 1 to 5 are preserved based on the location of the primary tumor
What are the advantages when compared to modified radical neck dissection?	Decision to perform a selective neck dissection is based on the location of the primary tumor and its likelihood to metastasize to a specific size

FACIAL FRACTURES

Mandible Fractures

What are the symptoms?

Gross disfigurement, pain, **malocclusion,** drooling

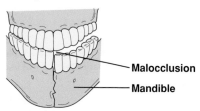

Malocclusion

Mandible

What are the signs?

Trismus, fragment mobility and lacerations of gingiva, hematoma in floor of mouth

What are the possible complications?

Malunion, nonunion, osteomyelitis, TMJ ankylosis

What is the treatment?

Open or closed reduction
MMF = **M**axillo**M**andibular **F**ixation (wire jaw shut)

Midface Fractures

How are they evaluated?

Careful physical examination and CT scan

Classification

Le Fort I?

Transverse maxillary fracture above the dental apices, which also traverses the pterygoid plate; palate is mobile, but nasal complex is stable

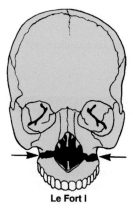

Le Fort I

Le Fort II?

Fracture through the frontal process of the maxilla, through the orbital floor and pterygoid plate; midface is mobile

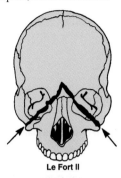

Le Fort II

Le Fort III?

Complete craniofacial separation; differs from II in that it extends through the nasofrontal suture and frontozygomatic sutures

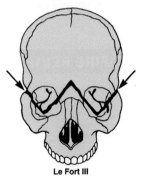

Le Fort III

What is a "tripod" fracture?

Fracture of the zygomatic complex; involves four fractures:

1. Frontozygomatic suture
2. Inferior orbital rim
3. Zygomaticomaxillary suture
4. Zygomaticotemporal suture

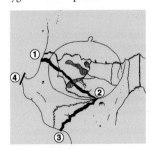

What is a "blowout" fracture?	Orbital fracture with "blowout" of supporting bony structural support of orbital floor; patient has enophthalmos (sunken-in eyeball)
What is "entrapment"?	Orbital fracture with "entrapment" of periorbital tissues within the fracture opening, including entrapment of extraocular muscles; loss of extraocular muscle mobility (e.g., lateral tracking) and diplopia (double vision)
What is a "step off"?	Fracture of the orbit with palpable "step off" of bony orbital rim (inferior or lateral)
Are mandibular fractures usually a single fracture?	No; because the mandible forms an anatomic ring, >95% of mandible fractures have more than one fracture site
What is the best x-ray study for mandibular fractures?	Panorex
What must be ruled out and treated with a broken nose (nasal fracture)?	Septal hematoma; must drain to remove chance of pressure-induced septal necrosis

RAPID-FIRE REVIEW

How can otitis externa be distinguished from otitis media on examination?	Otitis externa is characterized by severe pain upon manipulation of the auricle
What causes otitis media?	Most cases are caused by pneumococci and *Haemophilus influenzae*
What causes otitis externa?	*Pseudomonas aeruginosa*
What must be considered in unilateral serous otitis?	Nasopharyngeal carcinoma
What is the most common cause of facial paralysis?	**Bell's palsy,** which has an unidentified etiology
What is the single most important prognostic factor in Bell's palsy?	Whether the affected muscles are completely paralyzed (if not, prognosis is >95% complete recovery)
What is the most common cause of parotid swelling?	Mumps
What is Heerfordt's syndrome?	Sarcoidosis with parotid enlargement, facial nerve paralysis, and uveitis
Which systemic disease causes salivary gland stones?	Gout
What is the most common salivary gland site of stone formation?	Submandibular gland

What is Mikulicz's syndrome?	Any cause of bilateral enlargement of the parotid, lacrimal, and submandibular glands
What are the major functions (3) of the larynx?	1. Airway protection 2. Airway/respiration 3. Phonation
What is a cricothyroidotomy?	Emergent surgical airway by incising the cricothyroid membrane
What is the classic triad of Ménière's disease?	Hearing loss, tinnitus, vertigo (HTV)
What is the most common posterior fossa tumor, and where is it located?	Acoustic neuroma, usually occurring at the cerebellopontine angle
What is the most common site of sinus cancer?	Maxillary sinus
What tumor arises from olfactory epithelium?	Esthesioneuroblastoma
What cell type is most common in head and neck cancer?	Squamous cell
What are the most important predisposing factors to head and neck cancer?	Excessive alcohol use and **tobacco** abuse of any form—incidence of HPV-related cancer on the rise!
What is the most frequent site of salivary gland tumor?	Parotid gland
What is the most common salivary gland neoplasm?	
Benign	Pleomorphic adenoma
Malignant	Mucoepidermoid carcinoma
What is the classic feature of croup?	Barking, seal-like cough
What are the classic features of epiglottitis?	"Hot-potato" voice, sitting up, **drooling,** toxic appearance, high fever, **leaning forward**
What is the most common malignant neck mass in children, adolescents, and young adults?	Lymphoma
What is the most common primary malignant solid tumor of the head and neck in children?	Rhabdomyosarcoma
Most common causes of ENT infections?	
Croup	Parainfluenza virus
Otitis externa	*Pseudomonas*

Epiglottitis	*H. influenzae*
Malignant otitis externa	*Pseudomonas*
Parotitis	*Staphylococcus*
Acute suppurative otitis media	*S. pneumoniae* (33%)

What is the correct diagnosis?

"Hot potato" voice	Epiglottitis or peritonsillar abscess
Neck abscess with sulfur granules	*Actinomyces* infection

Name the most likely diagnosis:

28-year-old male with intermittent vertigo, intermittent hearing loss, tinnitus, and a subjective feeling of having ear swelling	Ménière's disease
16-year-old female with severe sore throat, lateral uvula displacement, bulging tonsillar pillar, + *Streptococcus pyogenes*	Quinsy's abscess (peritonsillar abscess)
61-year-old male develops acute onset of pain and "blurry" vision in the right eye; sees "rings" around lights; states that he feels a little nauseated	Open-angle glaucoma
23-year-old female while playing basketball gets hit in the left eye; has "blurry" vision in that eye; sees flashing lights and then sees things "floating" across	Detached retina
61-year-old female with history of left-sided headaches, left temporal tenderness with swelling, pain in the left side of her jaw when she eats, elevated ESR	Temporal arteritis
2-year-old male with a "lazy" left eye; left eye has decreased vision and lacks "red reflex" on exam	Retinoblastoma

Chapter 70 | Thoracic Surgery

THORACIC OUTLET SYNDROME (TOS)

What is thoracic outlet syndrome?

Compression of the neurovascular structures traversing the thoracic outlet, namely:
1. Subclavian artery ("arterial TOS")
2. Subclavian vein ("venous TOS")
3. Brachial plexus ("neurogenic TOS")

What is the pathophysiology of TOS?

Abnormal dynamics between the anterior scalene, middle scalene, and the first rib causing compression

What are the three causes of TOS?

1. Congenital anomalies, including cervical rib (an "extra first rib"), abnormal fascial bands to the first rib, or abnormal scalene muscles
2. Trauma—first rib or clavicle fracture, humeral head dislocation, or crush injury
3. Repetitive use/overuse (i.e., baseball pitchers)

What are the symptoms?

Paresthesias (neck, shoulder, arm, hand); 90% in ulnar nerve distribution
Weakness (neural/arterial)
Coolness of involved extremity (arterial)
Edema, venous distension, discoloration (venous)

What are the most common symptoms with TOS?

Neurogenic
Mixed neurogenic and arterial combined or pure neurogenic TOS accounts for 95% of TOS; pure arterial or venous TOS occurs 5% of the time

Which nerve is most often involved?

Ulnar nerve

What are the signs?

Paget–Schroetter syndrome—venous thrombosis (a.k.a. "effort thrombosis") leading to edema, arm discoloration, and distension of the superficial veins
Weak brachial and radial pulses in the involved arm
Hypesthesia/anesthesia
Atrophy in the distribution of the ulnar nerve
Positive Adson maneuver/Tinel's sign
Edema

What is the Adson maneuver?	**Evaluates for arterial compromise**
	Patient:
	    1. Extends neck (lifts head)
	    2. Takes a deep breath and holds
	    3. Turns head toward examined side
	Physician:
	    Monitors radial pulse on examined side
	    Test finding is positive if the radial
	        pulse decreases or disappears during
	        maneuver

What is Tinel's test?	Tapping of the supraclavicular fossa producing paresthesias

What is the treatment for neurogenic TOS?	1. 3 months of physical therapy
	2. Decompression of the thoracic outlet
	    Principles are: scalenectomy, brachial
	    plexus neurolysis, and first rib resection

What is the treatment for venous TOS (Paget–Schroetter disease?)	Thrombolytic and, soon after, surgery to decompress the thoracic outlet, including venolysis
What is the treatment for arterial TOS?	Surgery to decompress the thoracic outlet and, if necessary, repair/reconstruct the injured subclavian artery

CHEST WALL TUMORS

What are the most common benign chest wall tumors and their typical presentation?	1. Osteochondroma (30%–50%), painless mass on the rib metaphysis 2. Fibrous dysplasia (20%–30%), painful rib lesion or pathologic fracture 3. Chondroma (15%–20%), slowly enlarging, painless mess at the costochondral junction
What are the most common primary chest wall malignancies?	1. Chondrosarcoma 2. Osteosarcoma 3. Ewing's sarcoma and primitive neuroectodermal tumor or PNET (an aggressive form of Ewing's sarcoma) 4. Solitary plasmacytoma
Which chest wall tumor demonstrates a classic "onion-peel" appearance on x-ray?	Ewing's sarcoma
Which chest wall tumor demonstrates a classic "sunburst" appearance on x-ray?	Osteosarcoma
What is the treatment for malignant chest wall tumors?	Wide resection with 4- to 5-cm margins

DISEASES OF THE PLEURA

Pleural Effusion

What are the two types of pleural effusions and their etiologies?	1. Transudative—congestive heart failure, nephrotic syndrome, and cirrhosis 2. Exudative—infection, malignancy, trauma, and pancreatitis
What are Light's criteria, whereby if at least one of the criteria is met, the fluid is defined as exudative?	1. Pleural fluid-to-serum protein ratio >0.5 2. Pleural fluid-to-serum LDH ratio >0.6 3. Pleural fluid LDH >2/3 upper limit of laboratory's normal serum LDH
What is the diagnostic test of choice?	Thoracentesis (needle drainage) with pleural fluid studies, including cytology
What is the treatment?	1. Pigtail catheter or thoracostomy (chest tube) 2. Treat underlying condition 3. Consider sclerosis if malignant pleural effusion
What is an empyema?	Infected pleural effusion; must be drained, usually with chest tube(s) Decortication may be necessary if tube thoracostomy drainage is incomplete
What is a decortication?	Thoracotomy and removal of an infected fibrous rind from around the lung (think of it as taking off a fibrous "cortex" from the lung)

Spontaneous Pneumothorax

What are the causes?	Primary (idiopathic or no cause identified) or secondary (due to bleb disease/emphysema, rarely cancer)
What body habitus is associated with primary spontaneous pneumothorax?	Thin and tall
What is the treatment?	Chest tube or pigtail catheter
What are the options if refractory, recurrent, or bilateral?	Thoracoscopy with mechanical pleurodesis
Who might also need a pleurodesis after the first episode?	Those whose lifestyles place them at increased risk for pneumothorax (e.g., pilots, scuba divers)
What is a catamenial pneumothorax?	Pneumothorax due to intrathoracic endometriosis

DISEASES OF THE LUNGS

Lung Cancer

What is the number of annual deaths from lung cancer?	160,000; most common cancer death in the United States in men and women
What is the #1 risk factor?	Smoking
Does asbestos exposure increase the risk in patients who smoke?	Yes
What type of lung cancer arises in nonsmokers?	Adenocarcinoma
Cancer arises more often in which lung?	Right > left; upper lobes > lower lobes
What are the signs/symptoms?	Change in a chronic cough Hemoptysis, chest pain, dyspnea Pleural effusion (suggests chest wall involvement) Hoarseness (recurrent laryngeal nerve involvement) Superior vena cava syndrome Diaphragmatic paralysis (phrenic nerve involvement) Symptoms of metastasis/paraneoplastic syndrome Finger clubbing
What is a Pancoast (superior sulcus) tumor?	Tumor at the apex of the lung or superior sulcus that may involve the brachial plexus, sympathetic ganglia, and vertebral bodies, leading to pain, upper extremity weakness, and Horner's syndrome
What is Horner's syndrome?	Injury to the cervical sympathetic chain; think: **"MAP"** 1. **M**iosis (small pupil) 2. **A**nhidrosis of ipsilateral face 3. **P**tosis
What are the most common sites of extrathoracic metastases (5)?	1. Brain 2. Bone 3. Adrenals 4. Liver 5. Kidney
What are paraneoplastic syndromes?	Syndromes that are associated with tumors but may affect distant parts of the body; they may be caused by hormones released from endocrinologically active tumors or may be of uncertain etiology

What are the five general types of paraneoplastic syndromes?	1. Metabolic: Cushing's, SIADH, hypercalcemia 2. Neuromuscular: Eaton–Lambert, cerebellar ataxia 3. Skeletal: hypertrophic osteoarthropathy 4. Dermatologic: acanthosis nigricans 5. Vascular: thrombophlebitis
What are the associated radiographic tests?	CXR, CT scan, PET scan
How is the tumor diagnosed?	1. Needle biopsy (CT or fluoro guidance) 2. Bronchoscopy with brushings, biopsies, or both 3. ± Mediastinoscopy, mediastinotomy, scalene node biopsy, or thoracoscopic/open lung biopsy for definitive diagnosis
How is small cell carcinoma treated?	Chemotherapy ± XRT and prophylactic whole-brain irradiation (very small isolated lesions can be surgically resected)
What are the contraindications to surgery for lung cancer?	Think: **"SSSTOP IT"**: **S**uperior vena cava syndrome **S**upraclavicular node metastasis **S**calene node metastasis **T**racheal carina involvement **O**at cell carcinoma (treat with chemotherapy ± radiation) **P**ulmonary function tests show FEV_1 <0.8 L **I**nfarction (myocardial); a.k.a. "cardiac cripple" **T**umor elsewhere (metastatic disease)
What postoperative FEV_1 must you have?	FEV_1 ≥800 cc; thus, a preoperative FEV_1 ≥2 L is usually needed for a pneumonectomy If FEV_1 is <2 L, a ventilation perfusion scan should be performed
What is hypertrophic pulmonary osteoarthropathy?	Periosteal proliferation and new bone formation at the end of long bones and in the bones of the hand (seen in 10% of patients with lung cancer)

Solitary Pulmonary Nodules (Coin Lesions)

What is a solitary pulmonary nodule (SPN)?	Intraparenchymal pulmonary lesion that is <3 cm (considered a "mass" at 3 cm); causes can be benign (60%) or malignant (40%)

What is the risk of malignancy based on size?	Size (mm)	Risk (%)
	<3	0.2
	4–7	0.9
	8–20	18
	>20	50

How is the diagnosis made?

CXR, chest CT scan

What is the characteristic appearance of hamartoma on CXR?

"Popcorn" calcification

What are the common benign etiologies of SPN?

1. Infectious granuloma (80% of benign SPN)
2. Hamartoma (10% of benign SPN)

What percentage is malignant?

Overall, 5% to 10% (but >50% are malignant in smokers >50 years)

Is there a gender risk?

Yes; the incidence of coin lesions is 3 to 9× higher and malignancy is nearly twice as common in men as in women

What are the risk factors for malignancy?

1. Size: lesions >1 cm have a significant chance of malignancy; those >4 cm are very likely to be malignant
2. Indistinct margins (corona radiata)
3. Documented growth on follow-up x-ray (if no change in 2 years, most likely benign)
4. Increasing age

What are the diagnostic modalities available for tissue diagnosis?

1. CT-guided percutaneous biopsy (excellent accuracy if ≥1 cm)
2. Navigational bronchoscopy (employs CT scan and electromagnetic guidance to target the bronchus associated with pulmonary nodule for biopsy; also can place markers to aid in thoracoscopic identification for wedge resection)
3. Thoracoscopic (better tolerated) or open thoracotomy with wedge resection

What if the patient has an SPN and pulmonary hypertrophic osteoarthropathy?

>75% chance of carcinoma

What is its incidence?

≈7% of patients with lung cancer (2%–12%)

What are the signs?

Associated with finger clubbing; diagnosed by x-ray of long bones, revealing periosteal bone hypertrophy

Carcinoid Tumor

What is it?	**APUD** (**A**mine-**P**recursor **U**ptake and **D**ecarboxylation) cell tumor of the bronchus
What is its natural course in the lung?	Slow growing (but may be malignant)
What are the primary local findings?	Wheezing and atelectasis caused by bronchial obstruction/stenosis
What condition can it be confused with?	Asthma
How is the diagnosis made?	Bronchoscopy reveals round red-yellow-purple mass covered by epithelium that protrudes into bronchial lumen
What is the treatment?	Surgical resection (lobectomy with lymph node dissection) Sleeve resection is also an option for proximal bronchial lesions
What is a sleeve resection?	Resection of a ring segment of bronchus (with tumor inside) and then end-to-end anastomosis of the remaining ends, allowing salvage of lower lobe
What is the most common benign lung tumor?	Hamartoma (normal cells in a weird configuration)

Pulmonary Sequestration

What is it?	Abnormal benign lung tissue with separate blood supply that **DOES NOT** communicate with the normal tracheobronchial airway; have **systemic arterial blood supply** (usually off thoracic aorta)
Define the following terms and venous drainage:	
Interlobar	Sequestration in normal lung tissue covered by normal visceral pleura; **pulmonary venous drainage** (and usually found in adults)
Extralobar	Sequestration not in normal lung covered by its own pleura; **systemic venous drainage** (and usually found in children)

Lung Abscess

What are the signs/symptoms?	Fever, productive cough, sepsis, fatigue
What are the associated diagnostic studies?	CXR: air–fluid level CT scan to define position and to differentiate from an empyema Bronchoscopy (looking for cancer/culture)
What is the treatment?	1. Antibiotics and bronchoscopy for culture and drainage 2. Percutaneous drainage 3. Surgical resection if nonoperative management fails or underlying cancer
What is middle lobe syndrome?	Recurrent right middle lobe pneumonia caused most commonly by intermittent extrinsic bronchial obstruction

Hemoptysis

What is it?	Bleeding into the bronchial tree
What are the causes?	1. Bronchitis (50%) 2. Tumor mass (20%) 3. TB (8%) 4. Other causes: bronchiectasis, pulmonary catheters, trauma
What defines massive hemoptysis?	>600 cc/24 hr
What comprises the workup?	CXR Bronchoscopy CT arteriogram
What is the usual cause of death?	Asphyxia (not hemorrhagic shock)
Which arterial system is most often the source of massive hemoptysis?	Bronchial (not pulmonary) arteries
What is the acute management of massive hemoptysis?	1. Protect the nonbleeding lung by positioning the patient "bleeding side down" 2. Establish an airway with at least #8 endotracheal tube or ETT (for bronchoscopy and intervention)—either single-lumen ETT into nonbleeding lung ± fiberoptic bronchoscopic guidance or double-lumen ETT with bronchial cuff inflated to protect good lung from bleeding lung 3. Reverse any coagulopathies 4. Stop the bleeding

What are the options for controlling the bleeding?	1. Bronchoscopy with 4-Fr Fogarty balloon occlusion 2. Arteriography and selective bronchial artery embolization

DISEASES OF THE MEDIASTINUM

Primary Mediastinal Tumors

Thymoma

Where are they found in the mediastinum?	Anterior
How is the diagnosis made?	CT scan
What percentage of patients with thymoma has myasthenia gravis?	30% to 45%
What percentage of myasthenia gravis patients has thymoma?	10% to 15%
Should myasthenia gravis patients undergo thymectomy?	Yes, and counterintuitively, myasthenia patients **without thymoma have better symptomatic improvement** after thymectomy than patients with thymoma

Teratomas

What are they?	Tumors of branchial cleft cells; the tumors contain ectoderm, endoderm, and mesoderm
What is a dermoid cyst?	Teratoma made up of ectodermal derivatives (e.g., teeth, skin, hair)
Which age group is affected?	Usually adolescents, but can occur at any age
Where in the mediastinum do they occur?	Anterior
What are the characteristic x-ray findings?	Calcifications or teeth; tumors may be cystic
What percentage is malignant?	≈15%
What is the treatment of benign dermoid cysts?	Surgical excision
What is the treatment of malignant teratoma?	Preoperative chemotherapy until tumor markers are normal, then surgical resection
Which tumor markers are associated with malignant teratomas?	AFP, CEA

Neurogenic Tumors

What is the incidence?	**Most common** mediastinal tumors in all age groups
Where in the mediastinum do they occur?	Posterior, in the paravertebral gutters
What percentage is malignant?	50% in children 10% in adults

Lymphoma

Where in the mediastinum does it occur?	Anywhere, but most often in the anterosuperior mediastinum or hilum in the middle mediastinum
What percentage of lymphomas involves mediastinal nodes?	≈50%
What are the symptoms?	Cough, fever, chest pain, weight loss, SVC syndrome, chylothorax
How is the diagnosis made?	1. CXR, CT scan 2. Mediastinoscopy or mediastinotomy with node biopsy
What is the treatment?	Nonsurgical (chemotherapy, radiation, or both)

Mediastinitis

Acute Mediastinitis

What is it?	Acute suppurative mediastinal infection
What are the etiologies (6)?	1. Esophageal perforation (Boerhaave's syndrome) 2. Postoperative wound infection 3. Head and neck infections 4. Lung or pleural infections 5. Rib or vertebral osteomyelitis 6. Distant infections
What are the clinical features?	Fever, chest pain, dysphagia (especially with esophageal perforation), respiratory distress, leukocytosis
What is the treatment?	1. Wide drainage (via right thoracoscopy or thoracotomy or transcervical mediastinal drainage) 2. Treatment of primary cause 3. Antibiotics

Chronic Mediastinitis

What is it?	Mediastinal fibrosis secondary to *chronic* granulomatous infection
What is the most common etiology?	Histoplasma capsulatum
What are the clinical features?	50% are asymptomatic; symptoms are related to compression of adjacent structures: SVC syndrome, bronchial and esophageal strictures, constrictive pericarditis
How is the diagnosis made?	CXR or CT scan may be helpful, but surgery/biopsy often makes the diagnosis
What is the treatment?	Antibiotics; surgical removal of the granulomas is rarely helpful

Superior Vena Cava Syndrome

What is it?	Obstruction of the superior vena cava, usually by extrinsic compression
What is the #1 cause?	Malignant tumors cause ≈90% of cases; lung cancer is by far the most common; other tumors include thymoma, lymphoma, and Hodgkin's disease
What are the clinical manifestations?	1. Blue discoloration and puffiness of the face, arms, and shoulders 2. CNS manifestations may include headache, nausea, vomiting, visual distortion, stupor, and convulsions. 3. Cough, hoarseness, and dyspnea

What is the treatment?	The goals are to relieve symptoms and attempt to cure any malignant process:
	  1. Elevation of the head and supplemental oxygen
	  2. Steroids and diuretics for laryngeal or cerebral edema is controversial
	  3. Prompt radiation therapy ± chemotherapy for any causative cancer (symptoms improve, but overall prognosis is poor)

DISEASES OF THE ESOPHAGUS

Anatomic Considerations

Identify the esophageal muscle type:

Proximal 1/3 — Skeletal muscle

Middle 1/3 — Smooth muscle > skeletal muscle

Distal 1/3 — Smooth muscle

Why is the esophagus notorious for anastomotic leaks? — Esophagus has no serosa (same as the distal rectum)

What nerve runs with the esophagus? — Vagus nerve

Zenker's Diverticulum

What is it? — Pharyngoesophageal diverticulum; a false diverticulum containing mucosa and submucosa at the UES at the pharyngoesophageal junction through Killian's triangle

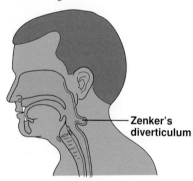

Zenker's diverticulum

What are the signs/symptoms? — Dysphagia, neck mass, halitosis, food regurgitation, heartburn

How is the diagnosis made? — Barium swallow

What is the treatment? —
1. One stage cricopharyngeal myotomy and diverticulectomy
2. Other options are cricopharyngeal myotomy and diverticulopexy to the prevertebral fascia or transoral stapling of the common wall between the diverticulum and the esophagus with diverticulum ≥3 cm (to fit the stapler)

Achalasia

What is it?	1. Failure of the LES to relax during swallowing 2. Aperistalsis of the esophageal body
What are the proposed etiologies?	1. Neurologic (ganglionic degeneration of Auerbach's plexus, vagus nerve, or both); possibly infectious in nature 2. Chagas' disease in South America
What are the associated long-term conditions?	Esophageal carcinoma secondary to Barrett's esophagus from food stasis
What are the symptoms?	Dysphagia for both solids and liquids, followed by regurgitation; dysphagia for liquids is worse

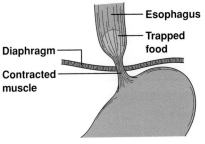

What are the diagnostic findings?	Radiographic contrast studies reveal dilated esophageal body with narrowing inferiorly **Manometry:** Motility studies reveal failure of the LES to relax during swallowing and aperistalsis of the esophageal body
What are the treatment options?	1. Upper endoscopy and balloon dilation of the LES 2. Laparoscopic Heller myotomy of the lower esophagus and LES (6 cm) and 2 cm onto the stomach

Diffuse Esophageal Spasm

What is it?	Strong, nonperistaltic contractions of the esophageal body; sphincter function is usually normal
What is the associated condition?	Gastroesophageal reflux
What are the symptoms?	Spontaneous chest pain that radiates to the back, ears, neck, jaw, or arms

What is the differential diagnosis?	Angina pectoris Psychoneurosis Nutcracker esophagus
What are the associated diagnostic tests?	**Esophageal manometry:** Motility studies reveal repetitive, high-amplitude contractions with normal sphincter response Upper GI may be normal, but 50% show segmented spasms or corkscrew esophagus Endoscopy
What is the classic finding on esophageal contrast study (UGI)?	"Corkscrew esophagus"
What is the treatment?	Medical (antireflux measures, calcium channel blockers, nitrates) Long esophagomyotomy in refractory cases

Nutcracker Esophagus

What is it also known as?	Hypertensive peristalsis
What is it?	Very strong peristaltic waves
What are the symptoms?	Spontaneous chest pain that radiates to the back, ears, neck, jaw, or arms
What is the differential diagnosis?	Angina pectoris Psychoneurosis Diffuse esophageal spasm
What are the associated diagnostic tests?	1. Esophageal manometry: Motility studies reveal repetitive, high-amplitude contractions with normal sphincter response 2. Results of UGI may be normal (rule out mass) 3. Endoscopy
What is the treatment?	Medical (antireflux measures, calcium channel blockers, nitrates) Long esophagomyotomy in refractory cases

ESOPHAGEAL REFLUX

What is it?	Reflux of gastric contents into the lower esophagus resulting from the decreased function of the LES

What are the causes?	1. Decreased LES tone 2. Decreased esophageal motility 3. Hiatal hernia 4. Gastric outlet obstruction 5. NGT
What are four associated conditions/factors?	1. Sliding hiatal hernia 2. Tobacco and alcohol 3. Scleroderma 4. Decreased endogenous gastrin production
What are the symptoms?	Substernal pain, heartburn, regurgitation; symptoms are worse when the patient is supine and after meals
How is the diagnosis made?	Bravo pH study (wireless capsule pH monitoring) of the lower esophagus reveals acid reflux; allows for 48-hour (vs. >24-hour) monitoring and better tolerated compared to traditional catheter-based "pH probe"
What is the initial treatment?	Medical: H_2-blockers, antacids, metoclopramide, omeprazole Elevation of the head of the bed; small, multiple meals
Which four complications require surgery?	1. Failure of medical therapy 2. Esophageal strictures 3. Progressive pulmonary insufficiency secondary to documented nocturnal aspiration 4. Barrett's esophagus
Describe each of the following types of surgery:	
Nissen	60° fundoplication: wrap fundus of stomach all the way around the esophagus
Belsey Mark IV	Left thoracic approach: 270° fundoplication (wrap fundus of stomach to recreate LES)
Hill	Tighten arcuate ligament around esophagus and tack stomach to diaphragm
Laparoscope Nissen	360° fundoplication (Nissen) via laparoscope
Laparoscopic Toupet	Laparoscopic fundoplication posteriorly with less than 220° to 250° wrap used with decreased esophageal motility; disadvantage is more postoperative reflux
What is Barrett's esophagus?	Replacement of the lower esophageal squamous epithelium with columnar epithelium secondary to reflux

Why is it significant?	This lesion is premalignant
What is the treatment?	People with significant reflux should be followed with regular surveillance, EGDs with biopsies, proton pump inhibitor (PPI), and antireflux precautions
	Patients with severe dysplasia should undergo endoscopic mucosal resection (EMR) of dysplastic areas or nodules plus radiofrequency ablation of all Barrett's
	Any invasive cancer identified should undergo staging and treatment with esophagectomy

Caustic Esophageal Strictures

Which agents may cause strictures if ingested?	Lye, oven cleaners, drain cleaners, batteries, sodium hydroxide tablets (Clinitest)
How is the diagnosis made?	History; EGD is clearly indicated early on to assess the extent of damage (<24 hours); scope to level of severe injury (deep ulcer) only, water-soluble contrast study for deep ulcers to rule out perforation
What is the initial treatment?	1. NPO/IVF/H$_2$-blocker 2. Do **not** induce emesis 3. Corticosteroids (controversial—probably best for shallow/moderate ulcers), antibiotics (penicillin/gentamicin) for moderate ulcers 4. Antibiotic for deep ulcers 5. Upper GI at 10 to 14 days
What is the long-term follow-up?	Because of increased risk of esophageal squamous cancer (especially with ulceration), **endoscopies every other year**

Esophageal Carcinoma

What are the two main types?	1. Adenocarcinoma at the GE junction 2. Squamous cell carcinoma in most of the esophagus
What is the most common histology?	**Worldwide:** squamous cell carcinoma (95%) **United States:** adenocarcinoma

What is the age and gender distribution?	Most common in the sixth decade of life, and men predominate
What are the etiologic factors (5)?	1. Tobacco 2. Alcohol 3. GE reflux 4. Barrett's esophagus 5. Radiation
What are the symptoms?	Dysphagia, weight loss Other symptoms include chest pain, back pain, hoarseness, symptoms of metastasis
What comprises the workup?	1. UGI 2. EGD 3. Endoscopic (endoesophageal) ultrasound (EUS) 4. PET-CT scan
What is the differential diagnosis?	Leiomyoma, metastatic tumor, lymphomas, benign stricture, achalasia, diffuse esophageal spasm, GERD
How is the diagnosis made?	1. Upper GI localizes tumor 2. EGD obtains biopsy and assesses resectability 3. Full metastatic workup (CXR, PET-CT scan, LFTs)
Describe the stages of adenocarcinoma esophageal cancer:	
Stage I	Tumor: invades lamina propria, muscularis mucosae, or submucosa (T1) Nodes: negative
Stage IIa	Tumor: invades muscularis propria (T2) Nodes: negative (N0)
Stage IIb	1. Tumor: invades muscularis propria (T2) Nodes: positive regional nodes (N1) 2. **Invades** adventitia with negative nodes (T3N0)
Stage III	1. Tumor: invades adventitia (T3) 2. Nodes: positive regional nodes (N1) 3. Invades adjacent structures (T4anyN)
Stage IV	Distant metastasis
What is the treatment by stage?	Esophagectomy with gastric pull-up

What is the operative mortality rate?	10% overall
What is the postop complication rate?	≈33% (mainly due to anastomotic leak, pulmonary complications, and atrial fibrillation)

RAPID-FIRE REVIEW

Name the most likely diagnosis:

54-year-old female with dysphagia (to both liquid and solids) and intermittent chest pain; food "comes up" after falling asleep at night; manometry reveals high LES pressures that do not decrease with swallowing; absent esophageal peristalsis	Achalasia
Recurrent pneumonias, infiltrate on chest x-ray, no bronchus leading to area of infiltrate	Pulmonary sequestration
58-year-old male smoker with oat cell cancer of the lung and hyponatremia	SIADH
45-year-old male with hypertension and Marfan's syndrome describes abrupt onset of severe chest pain "tearing to my back"	Aortic dissection
30-year-old male seat belted involved in high-speed head-on MVC presents with massive subcutaneous air over entire chest, chest tube placed for massive pneumothorax on right reveals massive air leak	Bronchial tear
45-year-old male back from a visit to South America who was exposed to *Trypanosoma cruzi* now presents with dysphagia	Chagas' disease

What is the treatment?

57-year-old s/p a fall with a right-sided tension pneumothorax	Right-sided chest tube; if delay in placing chest tube, then needle decompression can temporize until the chest tube is placed

Chapter 71 | Cardiovascular Surgery

What do the following abbreviations stand for?

AI	Aortic Insufficiency/regurgitation
AS	Aortic Stenosis
ASD	Atrial Septal Defect
CABG	Coronary Artery Bypass Grafting
CAD	Coronary Artery Disease
CPB	CardioPulmonary Bypass
IABP	Intra-Aortic Balloon Pump
LAD	Left Anterior Descending coronary artery
IMA	Internal Mammary Artery
MR	Mitral Regurgitation
PTCA	Percutaneous Transluminal Coronary Angioplasty (balloon angioplasty)
VAD	Ventricular Assist Device
VSD	Ventricular Septal Defect

Define the following terms:

Stroke volume (SV)	mL of blood pumped per heartbeat (SV = CO/HR)
Cardiac output (CO)	Amount of blood pumped by the heart each minute: heart rate × SV
Cardiac index (CI)	CO/BSA (body surface area)
Ejection fraction	Percentage of blood pumped out of the left ventricle: SV ÷ end-diastolic volume (nl 55%–70%)
Compliance	Change in volume ÷ change in pressure

SVR	Systemic Vascular Resistance = $$\frac{MAP - CVP}{CO \times 80}$$
Preload	Left ventricular end-diastolic pressure or volume
Afterload	Arterial resistance the heart pumps against
PVR	Pulmonary Vascular Resistance = $PA_{(mean)} - PCWP/CO \times 80$
MAP	Mean Arterial Pressure = diastolic BP + 1/3 (systolic BP − diastolic BP)
What is a normal CO?	4 to 8 L/min
What is a normal CI?	2.5 to 4 L/min
When does most of the coronary blood flow take place?	During diastole (66%)
What are the three major coronary arteries?	1. Left Anterior Descending (**LAD**) 2. Circumflex 3. Right coronary
What are the three main "cardiac electrolytes"?	1. Calcium (inotropic) 2. Potassium (dysrhythmias) 3. Magnesium (dysrhythmias)

ACQUIRED HEART DISEASE

Coronary Artery Disease (CAD)

What is it?	Atherosclerotic occlusive lesions of the coronary arteries; segmental nature makes CABG possible
What is the incidence?	CAD is the #1 killer in the Western world; >50% of cases are triple vessel diseases involving the LAD, circumflex, and right coronary arteries
Who classically gets "silent" MIs?	Patients with diabetes (autonomic dysfunction)
What is the treatment?	Medical therapy (β-blockers, aspirin, nitrates, HTN medications), angioplasty (PTCA), ± stents, surgical therapy: CABG

CABG

What is it?	Coronary **A**rtery **B**ypass **G**rafting

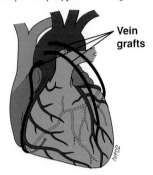

What are the indications?	Left main disease ≥2-vessel disease (especially diabetics) Unstable or disabling angina unresponsive to medical therapy/PTCA Postinfarct angina Coronary artery rupture, dissection, thrombosis after PTCA
CABG versus PTCA ± stents?	CABG = Survival improvement for diabetics and ≥2-vessel disease, ↑ short-term morbidity PTCA = ↓ short-term morbidity, ↓ cost, ↓ hospital stay, ↑ reintervention, ↑ postprocedure angina
What procedures are most often used in the treatment?	Coronary arteries grafted (usually 3–6): internal mammary pedicle graft and saphenous vein free graft are most often used (IMA 95% 10-year patency vs. 50% with saphenous)
What medications should almost every patient be given after CABG?	Aspirin, β-blocker
Can a CABG be performed off cardiopulmonary bypass?	Yes, today they are performed with or without bypass

Postpericardiotomy Syndrome

What is it?	Pericarditis after pericardiotomy (unknown etiology), occurs weeks to 3 months postoperatively
What are the signs/symptoms?	Fever Chest pain, atrial fibrillation Malaise Pericardial friction rub Pericardial effusion/pleural effusion

What is the treatment?	NSAIDs, ± steroids
What is pericarditis after an MI called?	Dressler's syndrome

Cardiopulmonary Bypass (CPB)

What is it?

Pump and oxygenation apparatus remove blood from SVC and IVC and return it to the aorta, bypassing the heart and lungs and allowing cardiac arrest for open-heart procedures, heart transplant, lung transplant, or heart–lung transplant as well as procedures on the proximal great vessels

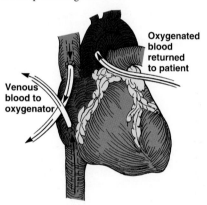

Oxygenated blood returned to patient

Venous blood to oxygenator

Is anticoagulation necessary?

Yes, just before and during the procedure, with heparin

How is anticoagulation reversed?

Protamine

What are the ways to manipulate CO after CPB?

Rate, rhythm, afterload, preload, inotropes, mechanical (IABP and VAD)

What mechanical problems can decrease CO after CPB?

Cardiac tamponade, pneumothorax

What is "tamponade physiology"?

↓ CO, ↑ heart rate, hypotension, ↑ **CVP** = ↑ **wedge pressure**

What are the possible complications?

Trauma to formed blood elements (especially thrombocytopenia and platelet dysfunction)
Pancreatitis (low flow)
Heparin rebound
CVA
Failure to wean from bypass
Technical complications (operative technique)
MI

What are the options for treating postop CABG mediastinal bleeding?	Protamine, ↑ PEEP, FFP, platelets, aminocaproic acid
What is "heparin rebound"?	Increased anticoagulation after CPB from increased heparin levels, as increase in peripheral blood flow after CPB returns heparin residual that was in the peripheral tissues
What are the options if a patient cannot be weaned from CPB?	Inotropes (e.g., epinephrine) VAD, IABP
What is the workup of a postoperative patient with AFib?	Rule out PTX (ABG, CT scan), acidosis (ABG), electrolyte abnormality (LABS), and ischemia (EKG), CXR
What is a MIDCAB?	**M**inimally **I**nvasive **D**irect **C**oronary **A**rtery **B**ypass—LIMA to LAD bypass without CPB and through a small thoracotomy
What is TMR?	**T**rans**M**yocardial laser **R**evascularization: Laser through groin catheter makes small holes (intramyocardial sinusoids) in cardiac muscle to allow blood to nourish the muscle
What is OPCAB?	**O**ff-**P**ump **C**oronary **A**rtery **B**ypass—median sternotomy but no bypass pump

Aortic Stenosis (AS)

What is it?	Destruction and calcification of valve leaflets, resulting in obstruction of left ventricular outflow

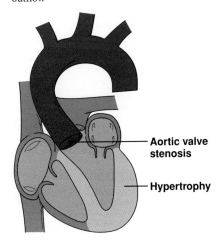

Aortic valve stenosis

Hypertrophy

What are the causes?	Calcification of bicuspid aortic valve Rheumatic fever Acquired calcific AS (7th–8th decades)
What are the symptoms?	Angina (5 years life expectancy if left untreated) Syncope (3 years life expectancy if left untreated) CHF (2 years life expectancy if left untreated) Often asymptomatic until late
What is the memory aid for the AS complications?	**A**ortic **S**tenosis **C**omplications = **A**ngina **S**yncope **CHF**—5, 3, 2
What are the signs?	Murmur: crescendo-decrescendo systolic second right intercostal space with radiation to the carotids Left ventricular heave or lift from left ventricular hypertrophy
What tests should be performed?	CXR, ECG, echocardiography Cardiac catheterization—needed to plan operation
What is the surgical treatment?	Valve replacement with tissue or mechanical prosthesis
What are the indications for surgical repair?	If patient is symptomatic or valve cross-sectional area is <0.75 cm^2 (nl 2.5–3.5 cm^2) and/or gradient >50 mm Hg
What are the pros/cons of mechanical valve?	Mechanical valve is more durable, but requires lifetime anticoagulation
What is the treatment option in poor surgical candidates?	Balloon aortic "valvuloplasty" (percutaneous)
Why is a loud murmur often a good sign?	Implies a high gradient, which indicates preserved LV function
Why might an AS murmur diminish over time?	It may imply a decreasing gradient from a decline in LV function

Aortic Insufficiency (AI)

What is it?	Incompetency of the aortic valve (regurgitant flow)
What are the causes?	Bacterial endocarditis (*Staphylococcus aureus, Streptococcus viridans*) Rheumatic fever (rare) Annular ectasia from collagen vascular disease (especially Marfan's syndrome)

What are the predisposing conditions?	Bicuspid aortic valve, connective tissue disease
What are the symptoms?	Palpitations from dysrhythmias and dilated left ventricle Dyspnea/orthopnea from left ventricular failure Excess fatigue Angina from ↓ diastolic BP and coronary flow (***Note:*** Most coronary blood flow occurs during diastole and aorta rebound) Musset sign (bobble-head)
What are the signs?	↑ Diastolic BP Murmur: blowing, decrescendo diastolic at left sternal border Austin-Flint murmur: reverberation of regurgitant flow Increased pulse pressure: "pistol shots," "water-hammer" pulse palpated over peripheral arteries Quincke's sign (capillary pulsations of uvula)
Which diagnostic tests should be performed?	1. CXR: Increasing heart size can be used to follow progression 2. Echocardiogram 3. Catheterization (definitive) 4. TEE
What is the treatment?	Aortic valve replacement
What are the indications for surgical treatment?	Symptomatic patients (CHF, PND, etc.), left ventricle dilatation, decreasing LV function, decreasing EF, acute AI onset

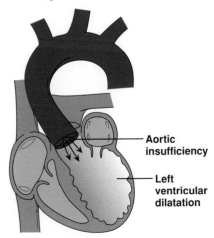

Aortic insufficiency

Left ventricular dilatation

What is the prognosis?	Surgery gives symptomatic improvement and may improve longevity; low operative risk

Mitral Stenosis (MS)

What is it?	Calcific degeneration and narrowing of the mitral valve resulting from rheumatic fever in most cases

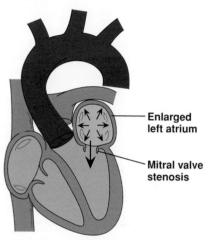

Enlarged left atrium

Mitral valve stenosis

What are the symptoms?	1. Dyspnea from increased left atrial pressure, causing pulmonary edema (i.e., CHF) 2. Hemoptysis (rarely life-threatening) 3. Hoarseness from dilated left atrium impinging on the recurrent laryngeal nerve 4. Palpations (AFib)
What are the signs?	Murmur: crescendo diastolic rumble at apex Irregular pulse from AFib caused by dilated left atrium Stroke caused by systemic emboli from left atrium (AFib and obstructed valve allow blood to pool in the left atrium and can lead to thrombus formation)
Which diagnostic tests should be performed?	Echocardiogram Catheterization

What are the indications for intervention?	1. Symptoms (severe) 2. Pulmonary HTN and mitral valve area $<1 \text{ cm}^2/\text{m}^2$ 3. Recurrent thromboembolism
What are the treatment options?	1. Open commissurotomy (open heart operation) 2. Balloon valvuloplasty: percutaneous 3. Valve replacement
What is the medical treatment for mild symptomatic patients?	Diuretics
What is the prognosis?	>80% of patients are well at 10 years with successful operation

Mitral Regurgitation (MR)

What is it?	Incompetence of the mitral valve
What are the causes?	Severe mitral valve prolapse (some prolapse is found in 5% of the population, with women $\geq$ men) Rheumatic fever Post-MI from papillary muscle dysfunction/rupture Ruptured chordae
What are the most common causes?	Rheumatic fever (#1 worldwide), ruptured chordae/papillary muscle dysfunction
What are the symptoms?	Often insidious and late: dyspnea, palpitations, fatigue
What are the signs?	Murmur: holosystolic, apical radiating to the axilla
What are the indications for treatment?	1. Symptoms 2. LV >45 mm end-systolic dimension (left ventricular dilation)
What is the treatment?	1. Valve replacement 2. Annuloplasty: Suture a prosthetic ring to the dilated valve annulus

Artificial Valve Placement

What is it?	Replacement of damaged valves with tissue or mechanical prosthesis
What are the types of artificial valves?	Tissue and mechanical

What are the pros and cons?

Tissue	NO anticoagulation but shorter duration (20%–40% need replacement in 10 years); good for elderly
Mechanical	Last longer (>15 years) but require ANTICOAGULATION
Contraindications for tissue valve	Dialysis (calcify), youth
Contraindications for mechanical valve	Pregnancy (or going to be pregnant due to anticoagulation), bleeding risk (alcoholic, PUD)

What is the operative mortality? From 1% to 5% in most series

What must patients with an artificial valve receive before dental procedures? Antibiotics

What is the Ross procedure? Aortic valve replacement with a pulmonary **auto**graft (i.e., patient's own valve!)

Infectious Endocarditis

What is it? Microbial infection of heart valves

What are the predisposing conditions? Pre-existing valvular lesion, procedures that lead to bacteremia, IV drug use

What are the common causative agents?
Streptococcus viridans: associated with abnormal valves
Staphylococcus aureus: associated with IV drug use
Staphylococcus epidermidis: associated with prosthetic valves

What are the signs/symptoms?
Murmur (new or changing)
Petechiae
Splinter hemorrhage (fingernails)
Roth spots (on retina)
Osler nodes (raised, **painful** on soles and palms; **O**sler = **O**uch!)
Janeway lesions (similar to Osler nodes, but flat and **painless**) (Jane **WAY** = pain a**WAY**)

Which diagnostic tests should be performed?
Echocardiogram, TEE
Serial blood cultures (definitive)

What is the treatment? Prolonged IV therapy with bactericidal antibiotics to which infecting organisms are sensitive

What is the prognosis?	Infection can progress, requiring valve replacement

CONGENITAL HEART DISEASE

Ventricular Septal Defect (VSD)

What is its claim to fame?	Most common congenital heart defect
What is it?	Failure of ventricular septum to completely close; **80% of cases involve the membranous portion of the septum,** resulting in left-to-right shunt, increased pulmonary blood flow, and CHF if pulmonary to systemic flow is >2:1

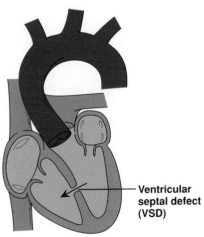

Ventricular septal defect (VSD)

What is pulmonary vascular obstructive disease?	Pulmonary artery hyperplasia from increased pulmonary pressure caused by a left-to-right shunt (e.g., VSD)
What is Eisenmenger's syndrome?	Irreversible pulmonary HTN from chronic changes in pulmonary arterioles and increased right heart pressures; cyanosis develops when the shunt reverses (becomes right to left across the VSD)
What is the treatment of Eisenmenger's syndrome?	Only option is heart–lung transplant; otherwise, the disease is untreatable
What is the incidence of VSD?	30% of heart defects (most common defect)

Patent Ductus Arteriosus (PDA)

What is it?	Physiologic right-to-left shunt in fetal circulation connecting the pulmonary artery to the aorta bypassing fetal lungs; often, this shunt persists in the neonate

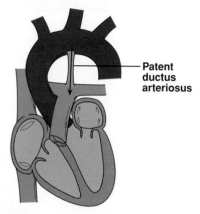

Patent ductus arteriosus

What are the factors preventing closure?	Hypoxia, increased prostaglandins, prematurity
What are the symptoms?	Often asymptomatic Poor feeding Respiratory distress CHF with respiratory infections
What are the signs?	Acyanotic, unless other cardiac lesions are present; continuous "machinery" murmur
Which diagnostic tests should be performed?	Physical examination Echocardiogram (to rule out associated defects) Catheter (seldom required)
What is the medical treatment?	Indomethacin is an NSAID: prostaglandin (PG) inhibitor (PG keeps PDA open)
What is the surgical treatment?	Surgical ligation or cardiac catheterization closure at 6 months to 2 years of age

Tetralogy of Fallot (TOF)

What is it?	Misalignment of the infundibular septum in early development, leading to the characteristic tetrad: 1. Pulmonary stenosis/obstruction of right ventricular outflow 2. Overriding aorta 3. Right ventricular hypertrophy 4. VSD

What are the symptoms?	Hypoxic spells (squatting behavior increases SVR and increases pulmonary blood flow)
What are the signs?	Cyanosis Clubbing Murmur: SEM at left third intercostal space
Which diagnostic tests should be performed?	CXR: small, "boot-shaped" heart and decreased pulmonary blood flow Echocardiography
What is the prognosis?	95% survival at specialized centers

IHSS

What is IHSS?	**I**diopathic **H**ypertrophic **S**ubaortic **S**tenosis
What is it?	Aortic outflow obstruction from septal tissue
What is the usual presentation?	Similar to AS

Coarctation of the Aorta

What is it?	Narrowing of the thoracic aorta, with or without intraluminal "shelf" (infolding of the media); usually found near ductus/ligamentum arteriosum

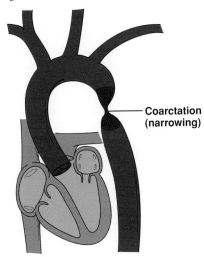

Coarctation (narrowing)

What are the three types?	1. Preductal (fatal in infancy if untreated) 2. Juxtaductal 3. Postductal
What percentage is associated with other cardiac defects?	60% (bicuspid aortic valve is most common)

What is the major route of collateral circulation?	Subclavian artery to the IMA to the intercostals to the descending aorta
What are the risk factors?	Turner's syndrome, male > female
What are the symptoms?	Headache Epistaxis Lower extremity fatigue → claudication

What are the signs?	Pulses: decreased lower extremity pulses
	Murmurs:
	   1. Systolic—from turbulence across coarctation, often radiating to infrascapular region
	   2. Continuous—from dilated collaterals

Which diagnostic tests should be performed?	CXR: "3" sign is aortic knob, coarctation, and dilated poststenotic aorta; rib notching is bony erosion from dilated intercostal collaterals Echocardiogram Cardiac catheterization if cardiac defects

What is the treatment?	Surgery:
	   Resection with end-to-end anastomosis
	   Subclavian artery flap
	   Patch graft (rare)
	   Interposition graft
	   Endovascular repair an option in adults

What are the indications for surgery?	Symptomatic patient Asymptomatic patient >3 to 4 years
What are the possible postoperative complications?	Paraplegia "Paradoxic" HTN Mesenteric necrotizing panarteritis (GI bleeding), Horner's syndrome, injury to recurrent laryngeal nerve

Transposition of the Great Vessels

What is it?	Aorta originates from the right ventricle and the pulmonary artery from the left ventricle; fatal without PDA, ASD, or VSD—to allow communication between the left and right circulations
What is the incidence?	From 5% to 8% of defects
What are the signs/symptoms?	Most common lesion that presents with cyanosis and CHF in neonatal period (>90% by day 1)
Which diagnostic tests should be performed?	CXR: "egg-shaped" heart contour Catheterization (definitive)

What is the treatment?	Arterial switch operation—aorta and pulmonary artery are moved to the correct ventricle and the coronaries are reimplanted

Ebstein's Anomaly

What is it?	Tricuspid valve is placed abnormally low in the right ventricle, forming a large right atrium and a small right ventricle, leading to tricuspid regurgitation and decreased right ventricular output
What are the signs/symptoms?	Cyanosis
What are the risk factors?	400× the risk if the mother has taken lithium

Vascular Rings

What are they?	Many types; represent an anomalous development of the aorta/pulmonary artery from the embryonic aortic arch that surrounds and obstructs the trachea/esophagus
How are they diagnosed?	Barium swallow, MRI
What are the signs/symptoms?	Most prominent is stridor from tracheal compression

Cyanotic Heart Disease

What are the causes?	**"Five T's"** of cyanotic heart disease: 1. Tetralogy of Fallot 2. Truncus arteriosus 3. Totally anomalous pulmonary venous return (TAPVR) 4. Tricuspid atresia 5. Transposition of the great vessels

CARDIAC TUMORS

What is the most common benign lesion?	Myxoma in adults
What is the most common location?	Left atrium with pedunculated morphology
What are the signs/symptoms?	Dyspnea, emboli
What is the most common malignant tumor in children?	Rhabdomyosarcoma

DISEASES OF THE GREAT VESSELS

Thoracic Aortic Aneurysm

What is the cause?	Vast majority result from atherosclerosis, connective tissue disease
What is the major differential diagnosis?	Aortic dissection
What percentage of patients has aneurysms of the aorta at a different site?	≈33%! (Rule out AAA)
What are the signs/symptoms?	Most are asymptomatic Chest pain, stridor, hemoptysis (rare), recurrent laryngeal nerve compression
How is it most commonly discovered?	Routine CXR
Which diagnostic tests should be performed?	CXR, CT scan, MRI, aortography
What are the indications for treatment?	>6 cm in diameter Symptoms Rapid increase in diameter Rupture
What is the treatment?	Replace with graft, open or endovascular stent
What are the dreaded complications after treatment of a thoracic aortic aneurysm?	Paraplegia (up to 20%) Anterior spinal syndrome
What is anterior spinal syndrome?	Syndrome characterized by: Paraplegia Incontinence (bowel/bladder) Pain and temperature sensation loss
What is the cause?	Occlusion of the great radicular artery of **Adamkiewicz**, which is one of the intercostal/lumbar arteries from T8 to L4

Aortic Dissection

What is it?	Separation of the walls of the aorta from an intimal tear and disease of the tunica media; a false lumen is formed and a "reentry" tear may occur, resulting in "double-barrel" aorta
What are the aortic dissection classifications?	DeBakey classification Stanford classification

Define the Stanford classifications:

Type A

Ascending aorta (requires surgery)
± Descending aorta (includes DeBakey
    types I and II)

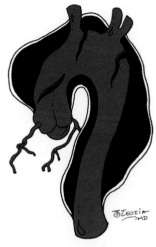

Type B

Descending aorta only (nonoperative, except
for complications) (same as DeBakey type III)

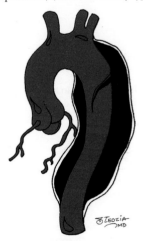

What is the etiology?

HTN (most common)
Marfan's syndrome
Bicuspid aortic valve
Coarctation of the aorta
Cystic medial necrosis
Proximal aortic aneurysm

What are the signs/symptoms?	**Abrupt onset of severe chest pain, most often radiating/"tearing" to the back;** onset is typically more abrupt than that of MI; the pain can migrate as the dissection progresses; patient describes a **"tearing pain"**
What are three other sequelae?	1. Cardiac tamponade; Beck's triad—distant heart sounds, ↑ CVP with JVD, ↓ BP 2. AI—diastolic murmur 3. Aortic arterial branch occlusion/shearing, leading to ischemia in the involved circulation (i.e., unequal pulses, CVA, paraplegia, renal insufficiency, bowel ischemia, claudication)

Which diagnostic tests are indicated?	CXR:
	    1. Widened mediastinum
	    2. Pleural effusion
	TEE
	CTA (CT angiography)

What is the treatment of the various types?	

Stanford type A	Surgical because of risk of:
	    1. AI
	    2. Compromise of cerebral and coronary circulation
	    3. Tamponade
	    4. Rupture

Stanford type B	Medical (control BP), unless complicated by rupture or significant occlusions
How is the surgery for an aortic dissection (Stanford A) done?	Open the aorta at the proximal extent of dissection, and then sew—graft to—intimal flap and adventitia circumferentially (endovascular an option)
What is the preoperative treatment?	Control BP with sodium nitroprusside and β-blockers (e.g., esmolol); β-blockers decrease shear stress
What is the postoperative treatment?	Lifetime control of BP and monitoring of aortic size
What is the possible cause of MI in a patient with aortic dissection?	Dissection involves the coronary arteries or underlying LAD
What is a dissecting aortic aneurysm?	Misnomer! Not an aneurysm!

What are the EKG signs of the following disorders?

Atrial fibrillation

Irregularly irregular

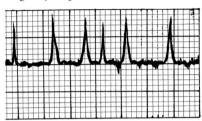

PVC

Premature **V**entricular **C**omplex: Wide QRS

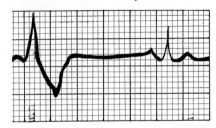

Ventricular aneurysm

ST elevation

Ischemia

ST elevation/ST depression/flipped T waves

Infarction

Q waves

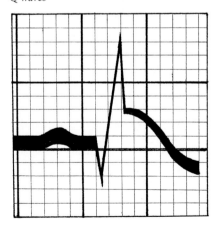

Pericarditis

ST elevation throughout leads

RBBB

Right **B**undle **B**ranch **B**lock: wide QRS and "rabbit ears" or R-R in V1 or V2

LBBB	Left Bundle Branch Block: wide QRS and "rabbit ears" or R-R in V5 or V6
Wolff–Parkinson–White	Delta wave = slurred upswing on QRS
First-degree AV block	Prolonged PR interval (0.2 second)
Second-degree AV block	Dropped QRS; not all P waves transmit to produce ventricular contraction
Wenckebach phenomenon	Second-degree block with progressive delay in PR interval prior to dropped beat
Third-degree AV block	Complete AV dissociation; random P wave and QRS

MISCELLANEOUS

What is Mondor's disease?	Thrombophlebitis of the thoracoepigastric veins
What is a VAD?	Ventricular Assist Device
How does an IABP work?	Intra-Aortic Balloon Pump has a balloon tip resting in the aorta Balloon inflates in diastole, increasing diastolic BP and coronary blood flow; in systole the balloon deflates, creating a negative pressure, lowering afterload, and increasing systolic BP

RAPID-FIRE REVIEW

What is the correct diagnosis?

| Chest pain "tearing" to the back | Aortic dissection |
| Chest pain described as "an elephant sitting on my chest" | Myocardial infarction |

Name the most likely diagnosis:

45-year-old female with CHF, diastolic murmur, atrial fibrillation, atrial hypertrophy	Mitral stenosis
15-year-old male with hypertension, lower extremity fatigue, and notching ("scalloping") of ribs on chest x-ray	Aortic coarctation
20-year-old male presents with ice pick to his left chest, hypotension, JVD, decreased muffled heart sounds	Cardiac tamponade

Chapter 72 | Transplant Surgery

Define the following terms:

Autograft	Same individual is both donor and recipient
Isograft	Donor and recipient are genetically identical (identical twins)
Allograft	Donor and recipient are genetically dissimilar, but of the same species (e.g., human to human)
Orthotopic	Donor organ is placed in normal anatomic position (liver, heart)
Heterotopic	Donor organ is placed in a different site than the normal anatomic position (kidney, pancreas)
Paratopic	Donor organ is placed close to original organ
Chimerism	Sharing cells between the graft and donor (thus, immunosuppression is minimal or not required)

BASIC IMMUNOLOGY

What are histocompatibility antigens?	Distinct (genetically inherited) cell surface proteins of the human leukocyte antigen (HLA) system
Why are they important?	They are targets (class I antigens) and initiators (class II antigens) of immune response to donor tissue (i.e., distinguishing self from nonself)
Which cells have class I antigens?	All nucleated cells (Think: class **I = ALL** cells and thus "**ONE** for **ALL**")
Which cells have class II antigens?	Macrophages, monocytes, B cells, activated T cells, endothelial cells
What are the gene products of MHC called in humans?	**HLA** (**H**uman **L**eukocyte **A**ntigen)

IMMUNOSUPPRESSION

What are the major drugs used for immunosuppression?	Triple therapy: corticosteroids, azathioprine, cyclosporine/tacrolimus
What are the other drugs?	OKT3, ATGAM, mycophenolate
What is the advantage of "triple therapy"?	Employs three immunosuppressive drugs; therefore, a lower dose of each can be used, decreasing the toxic side effects of each
What is "induction therapy"?	High doses of immunosuppressive drugs to "induce" immunosuppression

Corticosteroids

Which is most commonly used in transplants?	Prednisone
How does it function?	Primarily blocks production of IL-1 by macrophage and stabilizes lysosomal membrane of macrophage
What is the associated toxicity?	"Cushingoid," alopecia, striae, HTN, diabetes, pancreatitis, ulcer disease, osteomalacia, aseptic necrosis (especially of the femoral head)

What is the relative potency of the following corticosteroids?

Cortisol	1
Prednisone	4
Methylprednisolone	5
Dexamethasone	25

Azathioprine (AZA [Imuran®])

How does it function?	Prodrug that is cleaved into mercaptopurine; inhibits synthesis of DNA and RNA, leading to decreased cellular (T/B cells) production
What is the associated toxicity?	Toxic to bone marrow (leukopenia + thrombocytopenia), hepatotoxic, associated with pancreatitis
When should a lower dose of AZA be administered?	When WBC is <4
What is the associated drug interaction?	Decrease dose if patient is also on allopurinol, because allopurinol inhibits the enzyme xanthine oxidase, which is necessary for the breakdown of azathioprine

Cyclosporine (CSA)

What is its function?	"Calcineurin inhibitor" inhibits production of IL-2 by Th cells
What is the associated toxicity?	Toxicity for cyclosporine includes the **"11 Hs and 3 Ns": H**epatitis, **H**ypertrichosis, gingival **H**yperplasia, **H**yperlipidemia (worse than FK), **H**yperglycemia, **H**ypertension (worse than FK), **H**emolytic uremic syndrome, **H**yperkalemia, **H**ypercalcemia, **H**ypomagnesemia, **H**yperuricemia, **N**ephrotoxicity, **N**eurotoxicity (headache, tremor), **N**eoplasia (lymphoma, KS, squamous cell skin cancers)

What drugs decrease CSA levels?	By inducing the P450 system: Dilantin®, Tegretol®, rifampin, isoniazid, barbiturates
What are the drugs of choice for HTN from CSA?	Clonidine, calcium channel blockers

Atgam/Antithymocyte Globulin

How does it function?	Antibody against thymocytes, lymphocytes (polyclonal)
When is it typically used?	For induction
What is the associated toxicity?	Thrombocytopenia, leukopenia, serum sickness, rigors, fever, anaphylaxis, increased risk of viral infection, arthralgia

OKT3

How does it work?	MONOclonal antibody that binds CD3 receptor (on T cells)
What is a major problem with multiple doses?	Blocking antibodies develop, and OKT3 is less effective each time it is used
What are basiliximab and daclizumab?	Anti-CD25 monoclonal antibodies

Tacrolimus

What is tacrolimus also known as?	Prograf® (FK506)
How does it work?	Similar to CSA—"calcineurin inhibitor," blocks IL-2 receptor expression, inhibits T cells
What is its potency compared to CSA?	$100\times$ more potent than CSA
What are its side effects?	Nephrotoxicity and CNS toxicity (tremor, seizure, paresthesia, coma), hyperkalemia, alopecia, diabetes

Sirolimus

What is sirolimus also known as?	Rapamycin, Rapamune®
How does it work?	Like CSA and tacrolimus, it does not bind to and inhibit calcineurin; rather, it blocks T-cell signaling
Toxicity?	Hypertriglyceridemia, thrombocytopenia, wound/healing problems, anemia, oral ulcers

Mycophenolate Mofetil (MMF)

What is MMF also known as? CellCept®

How does it work? Inhibitor of inosine monophosphate dehydrogenase required for de novo purine synthesis, which expanding T and B cells depend on; also inhibits adhesion molecule and antibody production

OVERVIEW OF IMMUNOSUPPRESSION MECHANISMS

What drug acts at the following sites?

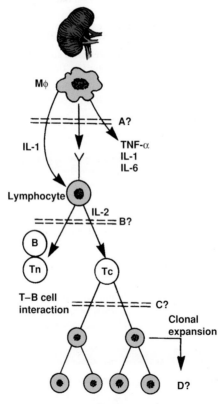

A	Corticosteroids
B	CSA/tacrolimus
C	AZA/MMF
D	OKT3/ATGAM

MATCHING OF DONOR AND RECIPIENT

How is ABO crossmatching performed?	Same procedure as in blood typing
What is the purpose of lymphocytotoxic crossmatching?	Tests for HLA antibodies in serum; most important in kidney and pancreas transplants
How is the test performed?	Mix recipient serum with donor lymphocyte and rabbit complement
Is HLA crossmatching important?	Yes, for kidney and pancreas transplants

REJECTION

How many methods of rejection are there?	2: humoral and cell mediated
Name the four types of rejection and their associated time courses:	1. Hyperacute—immediate in O.R. 2. Accelerated acute—7 to 10 days posttransplant 3. Acute—weeks to months posttransplant 4. Chronic—months to years posttransplant
What happens in hyperacute rejection?	Antigraft antibodies in recipient recognize foreign antigen immediately after blood perfuses transplanted organ
What happens in acute rejection?	T cell–mediated rejection
What type of rejection is responsible for chronic rejection?	Cellular, antibody (humoral), or both
What is the treatment of hyperacute rejection?	Remove transplanted organ
What is the treatment of acute rejection?	High-dose steroids/OKT3
What is the treatment of chronic rejection?	Not much (irreversible) or retransplant

ORGAN PRESERVATION

What is the optimal storage temperature of an organ?	4°C—keep on ice in a cooler

Why should it be kept cold?	Cold decreases the rate of chemical reactions; decreased energy use minimizes effects of hypoxia and ischemia
What is UW solution?	University of Wisconsin solution; used to perfuse an organ prior to removal from the donor
What is in it?	Potassium phosphate, buffers, starch, steroids, insulin, electrolytes, adenosine
Why should it be used?	Lengthens organ preservation time
What is the maximum time between harvest and transplant of organs?	
Heart	6 hours
Lungs	6 hours
Pancreas	24 hours
Liver	24 hours
Kidney	Up to 72 hours

KIDNEY TRANSPLANT

In what year was the first transplant performed in man?	1954
By whom?	Joseph E. Murray—1990 Nobel Prize winner in Medicine
What is the most common cause for kidney transplant?	**Diabetes** (25%)

Statistics

What are the sources of donor kidneys?	Deceased donor (70%) Living related donor (LRD; 30%)
What survival rate is associated with deceased donor source?	90% at 1 year if HLA matched; 80% at 1 year if not HLA matched; 75% graft survival at 3 years
What survival rate is associated with LRD?	95% patient survival at 1 year; 75% to 85% graft survival at 3 years
What are the tests for compatibility?	ABO, HLA typing

If a choice of left or right donor kidney is available, which is preferred?

Left—longer renal vein allows for easier anastomosis

Should the placement of the kidney be hetero- or orthotopic?

Heterotopic—retroperitoneal in the RLQ or LLQ above the inguinal ligament

Why?

Preserves native kidneys, allows easy access to iliac vessels, places ureter close to the bladder, easy to biopsy kidney

Define anastomoses of a heterotopic kidney transplant:

1. Renal artery to iliac artery
2. Renal vein to iliac vein
3. Ureter to bladder

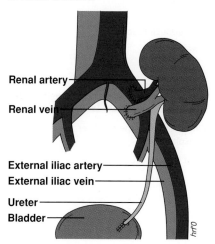

Renal artery
Renal vein
External iliac artery
External iliac vein
Ureter
Bladder

What is the correct placement of the ureter?

Submucosally through the bladder wall—decreases reflux

What is the differential diagnosis of postrenal transplant fluid collection?

"HAUL":
  Hematoma
  Abscess
  Urinoma
  Lymphocele

Why keep native kidneys?

Increased morbidity if they are removed

What is the indication for removal of native kidneys?

Uncontrollable HTN, ongoing renal sepsis

Rejection

What is the red flag that indicates rejection?	↑ Creatinine
What is the differential diagnosis of increased creatinine?	Remember: "-**TION**"–obstruc**TION,** dehydra**TION,** infec**TION,** intoxica**TION** (CSA); plus lymphocele, ATN
What are the signs/symptoms?	Fever, malaise, HTN, ipsilateral leg edema, pain at transplant site, oliguria

What is the workup for the following tests?

U/S with Doppler	Look for fluid collection around the kidney, hydronephrosis, flow in vessels
Radionuclide scan	Look at flow and function
Biopsy	Distinguish between rejection and cyclosporine toxicity

LIVER TRANSPLANT

Who performed the first liver transplant?	Thomas Starzl (1963)
What is the MELD score?	"**M**odel for **E**nd Stage **L**iver **D**isease" is the formula currently used to assign points for prioritizing position on the waiting list for deceased donor liver transplant; based on INR, bilirubin, and creatinine with extra points given for the presence of liver cancer
What is the test for compatibility?	ABO typing
What is the placement?	Orthotopic
What are the options for biliary drainage?	1. Donor common bile to recipient common bile duct end to end 2. Roux-en-Y choledochojejunostomy
What is the "piggyback" technique?	Recipient vena cava is left in place; the donor infrahepatic IVC is oversewn; the donor superior IVC is anastomosed onto a cuff made from the recipient hepatic veins (allows for greater hemodynamic stability of the recipient during OLT)

How does Living Donor Liver Transplantation (LDLT) work?

Adult donates a left lateral segment to a child or an adult donates a right lobe to another adult

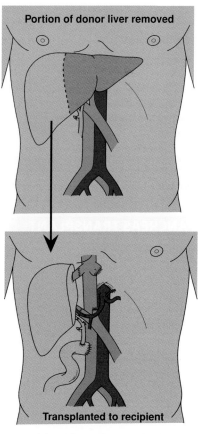

Portion of donor liver removed

Transplanted to recipient

What is a split liver transplant?

Deceased donor liver is harvested and divided into two "halves" for two recipients

Rejection

What are the red flags indicating rejection?

Decreased bile drainage, increased serum bilirubin, increased LFTs

What is the site of rejection?

Rejection involves the biliary epithelium first, and later, the vascular endothelium

What is the workup with the following tests?

U/S with Doppler	Look at flow in portal vein, hepatic artery; rule out thrombosis, leaky anastomosis, infection (abscess)
Cholangiogram	Look at bile ducts
Biopsy	Especially important 3 to 6 weeks postoperatively, when CMV is of greatest concern

Does hepatorenal syndrome renal function improve after liver transplant? — Yes

Survival Statistics

What is the 1-year survival rate? — ≈80% to 85%

PANCREAS TRANSPLANT

What are the indications? — Type I (juvenile) diabetes mellitus associated with severe complications (renal failure, blindness, neuropathy) or very poor glucose control

What are the tests for compatibility? — ABO, DR matching (class II)

What is the placement? — Heterotopic, in iliac fossa, or paratopic

Where is anastomosis of the exocrine duct in heterotopic placement? — To the bladder

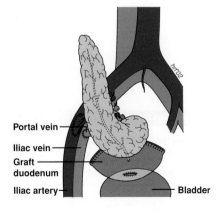

Portal vein

Iliac vein

Graft duodenum

Iliac artery

Bladder

Why?	Measures the amount of amylase in urine, gives an indication of pancreatic function (i.e., high urine amylase indicates good pancreatic function)
What is the associated electrolyte complication?	Loss of bicarbonate
What are the most common complications after pancreas transplant?	Thrombosis (#1), rejection
Where is anastomosis of the exocrine duct in paratopic placement?	To the jejunum
Why?	It is close by and physiologic
What is the advantage of paratopic placement?	Endocrine function drains to the portal vein directly to the liver, and pancreatic contents stay within the GI tract (no need to replace bicarbonate)
What are the red flags indicating rejection?	Hyperamylasemia, hyperglycemia, hypoamylasuria, graft tenderness
Why should the kidney and pancreas be transplanted together?	Kidney function is a better indicator of rejection; also better survival of graft is associated with kidney-pancreas transplant than pancreas alone
Why is hyperglycemia not a good indicator for rejection surveillance?	Hyperglycemia appears relatively late with pancreatic rejection

HEART TRANSPLANT

Who performed the first heart transplant?	Christiaan Barnard (1967)
What are the indications?	Age birth to 65 years with terminal acquired heart disease—class IV of New York Heart Association classification (inability to do any physical activity without discomfort = 10% chance of surviving 6 months)
What are the contraindications?	Active infection Poor pulmonary function Increased pulmonary artery resistance
What are the tests for compatibility?	ABO, size
What is the placement?	Orthotopic anastomosis of atria, aorta, pulmonary artery

What is sewn together in a heart transplant?	Donor heart atriums, pulmonary artery, and aorta are sewn to the recipient heart atriums, pulmonary artery, and aorta

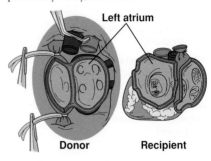

What are the red flags of rejection?	Fever, hypotension or hypertension, increased T4/T8 ratio
What is coronary artery vasculopathy?	Small vessel occlusion from chronic rejection—often requires retransplant
What are the tests for rejection?	Endomyocardial biopsy—much more important than clinical signs/symptoms; patient undergoes routine biopsy
What are survival statistics?	
1 year	85%
5 years	65%

INTESTINAL TRANSPLANTATION

What is it?	Transplantation of the small bowel
What types of donors are there?	Living donor, deceased donor
Anastomosis?	
Living donor	Ileocolic artery and vein
Deceased donor	SMA, SMV
What are indications?	Short-gut syndrome, motility disorders, and inability to sustain TPN (liver failure, lack of venous access, etc.)
What is a common postoperative problem other than rejection?	**GVHD** (**G**raft-**V**ersus-**H**ost **D**isease) from large lymphoid tissue in transplanted intestines
CMV status of donor?	Must be CMV negative if recipient is CMV negative

What is the most common cause of death postoperatively?	Sepsis
How is rejection surveillance conducted?	Endoscopic biopsies
What is the clinical clue to rejection?	Watery diarrhea

LUNG TRANSPLANT

Who performed the first lung transplant?	James Hardy (1963)
What are necessary anastomoses?	Bronchi, PA, pulmonary veins (bronchial artery is not necessary)

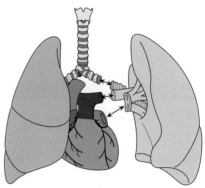

What are the postop complications?	Bronchial necrosis/stricture, reperfusion, pulmonary edema, rejection
What are the four red flags of rejection?	1. Decreased arterial O_2 tension 2. Fever 3. Increased fatigability 4. Infiltrate on x-ray
What is chronic lung rejection called?	**O**bliterative **B**ronchiolitis (**OB**)

TRANSPLANT COMPLICATIONS

What are four major complications?	1. Infection 2. Rejection 3. Posttransplant lymphoproliferative disease (PTLD) 4. Complications of steroids

Infection

What are the usual agents?	DNA viruses, especially CMV, HSV, VZV
When should CMV infection be suspected?	>21 days posttransplant
What is the time of peak incidence of CMV infections?	4 to 6 weeks posttransplant
What are the signs/symptoms of CMV?	Fever, neutropenia, signs of rejection of transplant; also can present as viral pneumonitis, hepatitis, colitis
How is CMV diagnosed?	Biopsy of transplant to differentiate rejection, cultures of blood, urine
What is the treatment of CMV?	Ganciclovir, with or without immunoglobulin; foscarnet
What are the signs/symptoms of HSV?	Herpetic lesions, shingles, fever, neutropenia, rejection of transplant
What is the treatment of HSV?	Acyclovir until patient is asymptomatic

Malignancy

What are the most common types?	Skin/lip cancer (40%), B-cell cancer, cervical cancer in women, T-cell lymphoma, Kaposi's sarcoma
Which epithelial cancers are important after transplant?	Skin/lip cancer, especially basal cell and squamous cell
What is posttransplant lymphoma associated with?	Multiple doses of OKT3 EBV Young > elderly
What is the treatment for PTLD?	1. Drastically reduce immunosuppression 2. ± Radiation 3. ± Chemotherapy

RAPID-FIRE REVIEW

48-year-old female undergoes second renal transplant; when the clamp is removed to allow arterial inflow, the kidney immediately swells and all the vessels thrombose	Hyperacute rejection

Chapter 73 | Orthopedic Surgery

ORTHOPEDIC TERMS

Define the following terms:

Supination	Palm up
Pronation	Palm down
Plantarflexion	Foot down at ankle joint (**PLANT** foot in ground)
Foot dorsiflexion	Foot up at ankle joint
Adduction	Movement toward the body (**ADD**uction = **ADD** to the body)
Abduction	Movement away from the body
Inversion	Foot sole faces midline
Eversion	Foot sole faces laterally
Volarflexion	Hand flexes at wrist joint toward flexor tendons
Wrist dorsiflexion	Hand flexes at wrist joint toward extensor tendons
Allograft bone	Bone from human donor other than patient
Reduction	Maneuver to restore proper alignment to fracture or joint
Closed reduction	Reduction done without surgery (e.g., casts, splints)
Open reduction	Surgical reduction
Fixation	Stabilization of a fracture after reduction by means of surgical placement of hardware that can be external or internal (e.g., pins, plates, screws)

Tibial pin

Pin placed in the tibia for treating femur or pelvic fractures by applying skeletal traction

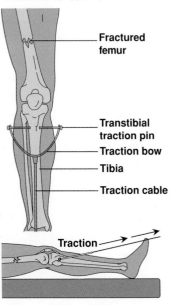

Fractured femur

Transtibial traction pin

Traction bow

Tibia

Traction cable

Traction

Unstable fracture or dislocation

Fracture or dislocation in which further deformation will occur if reduction is **not** performed

Varus

Extremity abnormality with apex of defect pointed away from midline (e.g., genu varum = bowlegged; with valgus, this term can also be used to describe fracture displacement)

(Think: Knees are very **varied** apart)

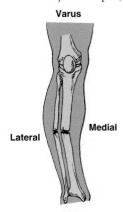

Varus

Lateral

Medial

Valgus	Extremity abnormality with apex of defect pointed toward the midline (e.g., genu valgus = knock-kneed)

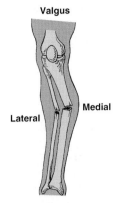

Valgus

Lateral   **Medial**

Dislocation	Total loss of congruity and contact between articular surfaces of a joint
Subluxation	Loss of congruity between articular surfaces of a joint; articular contact remains
Arthroplasty	Total joint replacement
Arthrodesis	Joint fusion with removal of articular surfaces
Osteotomy	Cutting bone (usually wedge resection) to help realigning of joint surfaces
Nonunion	Failure of fractured bone ends to fuse
Define each of the following:	
Diaphysis	Main shaft of long bone
Metaphysis	Flared end of long bone
Physis	Growth plate, found only in immature bone

TRAUMA GENERAL PRINCIPLES

Define extremity examination in fractured extremities:	1. Observe entire extremity (e.g., open, angulation, joint disruption) 2. Neurologic (sensation, movement) 3. Vascular (e.g., pulses, cap refill)
Which x-rays should be obtained?	Two views (also joint above and below fracture)
How are fractures described?	1. Skin status (open or closed) 2. Bone (by thirds: proximal/middle/distal) 3. Pattern of fracture (e.g., comminuted) 4. Alignment (displacement, angulation, rotation)

How do you define the degree of angulation, displacement, or both?

Define lateral/medial/anterior/posterior displacement and angulation of the distal fragment(s) in relation to the proximal bone

Identify each numbered structure:

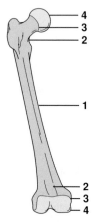

1. Diaphysis
2. Metaphysis
3. Physis
4. Epiphysis

FRACTURES

Define the following patterns of fracture:

Closed fracture

Intact skin over fracture/hematoma

Open fracture

Wound overlying fracture, through which fracture fragments are in continuity with outside environment; high risk of infection (***Note:*** Called "compound fracture" in the past)

Simple fracture

One fracture line, two bone fragments

Comminuted fracture

Results in more than two bone fragments (a.k.a. "fragmentation")

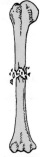

Comminuted fracture

Segmental fracture

Two complete fractures with a "segment" in between

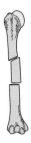

Oblique fracture

Fracture line creates an oblique angle with long axis of bone

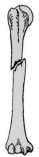

Oblique fracture

Spiral fracture

Severe oblique fracture in which fracture plane rotates along the long axis of bone; caused by a twisting injury

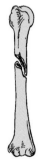

Spiral fracture

Impacted fracture

Fracture resulting from compressive force; end of bone is driven into contiguous metaphyseal region without displacement

Pathologic fracture

Fracture through abnormal bone (e.g., tumor-laden or osteoporotic bone)

Stress fracture	Fracture in normal bone from cyclic loading on bone
Greenstick fracture	Incomplete fracture in which cortex on **only one side** is disrupted; seen in children

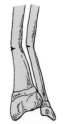

Greenstick fracture

Torus fracture	Impaction injury in children in which cortex is buckled but not disrupted (a.k.a. "buckle fracture")

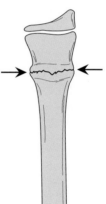

Torus fracture

Avulsion fracture	Fracture in which tendon is pulled from bone, carrying with it a bone chip

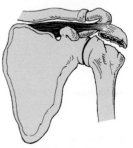

Avulsion fracture

Periarticular fracture	Fracture close to but not involving the joint
Intra-articular fracture	Fracture through the articular surface of a bone (usually requires ORIF)

Define the following specific fractures:

Colles' fracture	**Distal radius** fracture with dorsal displacement and angulation, usually from falling on an outstretched hand

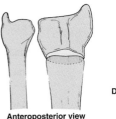 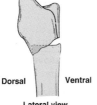

Dorsal   Ventral

Anteroposterior view   **Lateral view**

Smith's fracture	"Reverse Colles' fracture"—distal radial fracture with volar displacement and angulation, usually from falling on the **dorsum** of the hand (uncommon)
Jones' fracture	Fracture at the base of the fifth metatarsal diaphysis
Bennett's fracture	Fracture–dislocation of the base of the first metacarpal (thumb) with disruption of the carpometacarpal joint

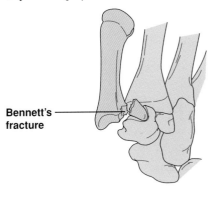

Bennett's fracture

Boxer's fracture	Fracture of the metacarpal neck, "classically" of the small finger

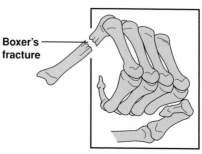

Boxer's fracture

Nightstick fracture	Ulnar fracture
Clay shoveler's avulsion fracture	Fracture of spinous process of C6–7
Hangman's fracture	Fracture of the pedicles of C2
Transcervical fracture	Fracture through the neck of the femur
Tibial plateau fracture	Intra-articular fracture of the proximal tibia (the plateau is the flared proximal end)
Monteggia fracture	Fracture of the proximal third of the ulna with dislocation of the radial head
Galeazzi fracture	Fracture of the radius at the junction of the middle and distal thirds accompanied by disruption of the distal radioulnar joint
Tibial "plateau" fracture	Proximal tibial fracture

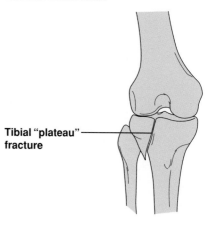

Tibial "plateau" fracture

"Pilon" fracture	Distal tibial fracture

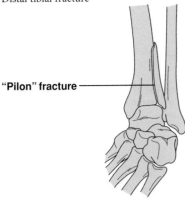

Pott's fracture	Fracture of distal fibula
Pott's disease	Tuberculosis of the spine

ORTHOPEDIC TRAUMA

What are the major orthopedic emergencies?

1. Open fractures/dislocations
2. Vascular injuries (e.g., knee dislocation)
3. Compartment syndromes
4. Neural compromise, especially spinal injury
5. Osteomyelitis/septic arthritis; acute, that is, when aspiration is indicated
6. Hip dislocations—require immediate reduction or patient will develop avascular necrosis; "reduce on the x-ray table"
7. Exsanguinating pelvic fracture (binder, external fixator)

What is the main risk when dealing with an open fracture?

Infection

Which fracture has the highest mortality?

Pelvic fracture (up to 50% with open pelvic fractures)

Define open fractures by Gustilo-Anderson classification:

Grade I

<1-cm laceration

Grade II

>1 cm, minimal soft tissue damage

Grade IIIA

Open fracture with massive tissue devitalization/loss, contamination

Grade IIIB	Open fracture with massive tissue devitalization/loss and extensive periosteal stripping, contamination, inadequate tissue coverage
Grade IIIC	Open fracture with major vascular injury requiring repair
What are the five steps in the initial treatment of an open fracture?	1. Prophylactic antibiotics to include IV gram-positive ± anaerobic coverage: Grade I—cefazolin (Ancef®) Grade II or III—cefoxitin/gentamicin 2. Surgical débridement 3. Inoculation against tetanus 4. Lavage wound <6 hours postincident with sterile irrigation 5. Open reduction of fracture and stabilization (e.g., use of external fixation)
What structures are at risk with a humeral fracture?	Radial nerve, brachial artery
What are the advantages?	Nearly immediate mobility with decreased morbidity/mortality
What is the chief concern following tibial fractures?	Recognition of associated compartment syndrome
What is suggested by pain in the anatomic snuffbox?	Fracture of scaphoid bone (a.k.a. "navicular fracture")
What is the most common cause of a "pathologic" fracture in adults?	Osteoporosis

Compartment Syndrome

What is acute compartment syndrome?	Increased pressure within an osteofascial compartment that can lead to ischemic necrosis
How is it diagnosed?	Clinically, using intracompartmental pressures is also helpful (especially in unresponsive patients); fasciotomy is clearly indicated if pressure in the compartment is >40 mm Hg (30–40 mm Hg is a gray area)
What are the causes?	Fractures, vascular compromise, reperfusion injury, compressive dressings; can occur after any musculoskeletal injury
What are common causes of forearm compartment syndrome?	Supracondylar humerus fracture, brachial artery injury, radius/ulna fracture, crush injury
What is Volkmann's contracture?	Final sequela of forearm compartment syndrome; **contracture** of the forearm flexors from replacement of dead muscle with fibrous tissue

What is the most common site of compartment syndrome?	Calf (four compartments: anterior, lateral, deep posterior, superficial posterior compartments)
What four situations should immediately alert one to be on the lookout for a developing compartment syndrome?	1. Supracondylar elbow fractures in children 2. Proximal/midshaft tibial fractures 3. Electrical burns 4. Arterial/venous disruption
What are the symptoms of compartment syndrome?	Pain, paresthesias, paralysis
What are the signs of compartment syndrome?	Pain on passive movement (out of proportion to injury), cyanosis or pallor, hypoesthesia (decreased sensation, decreased 2-point discrimination), firm compartment
Complication of missed anterior compartment, compartment syndrome?	Foot drop due to superficial peroneal nerve injury
Can a patient have a compartment syndrome with a palpable or Doppler-detectable distal pulse?	YES!
What are the possible complications of compartment syndrome?	Muscle necrosis, nerve damage, contractures, myoglobinuria
What is the initial treatment of the orthopedic patient developing compartment syndrome?	Bivalve and split casts, remove constricting clothes/dressings, place extremity at heart level
What is the definitive treatment of compartment syndrome?	Fasciotomy within 4 hours (6–8 hours maximum) if at all possible

Miscellaneous Trauma Injuries and Complications

Name the motor and sensation tests used to assess the following peripheral nerves:	
Radial	Wrist extension; dorsal web space; sensation: between thumb and index finger
Ulnar	Little finger abduction; sensation: little finger-distal ulnar aspect
Median	Thumb opposition or thumb pinch sensation: index finger-distal radial aspect
Axillary	Arm abduction; sensation: deltoid patch on lateral aspect of upper arm
Musculocutaneous	Elbow (biceps) flexion; lateral forearm sensation
How is a peripheral nerve injury treated?	Controversial, although clean lacerations may be repaired primarily; most injuries are followed for 6 to 8 weeks (EMG)

What fracture is associated with a calcaneus fracture?	L-spine fracture (usually from a fall)
Name the nerves of the brachial plexus	Think: "morning rum" or **"A.M. RUM"** = **A**xillary, **M**edian, then **R**adial, **U**lnar, and **M**usculocutaneous nerves
What are the two indications for operative exploration with a peripheral nerve injury?	1. Loss of nerve function *after* reduction of fracture 2. No EMG signs of nerve regeneration after 8 weeks (nerve graft)

DISLOCATIONS

Shoulder

What is the most common type?	95% are anterior (posterior is associated with seizures or electrical shock)
Which two structures are at risk?	1. Axillary nerve 2. Axillary artery
How is it diagnosed?	Indentation of soft tissue beneath acromion
What are the three treatment steps?	1. Reduction via gradual traction 2. Immobilization for 3 weeks in internal rotation 3. ROM exercises

Elbow

What is the most common type?	Posterior
Which three structures are at risk?	1. Brachial artery 2. Ulnar nerve 3. Median nerve
What is the treatment?	Reduce and splint for 7 to 10 days

Hip

When should hip dislocations be reduced?	Immediately, to decrease risk of avascular necrosis; "reduce on the x-ray table!"
What is the most common cause of a hip dislocation?	High-velocity trauma (e.g., MVC)
What is the most common type?	Posterior—"dashboard dislocation"—often involves fracture of posterior lip of acetabulum
Which structures are at risk?	Sciatic nerve; blood supply to femoral head—avascular necrosis (AVN)
What is the treatment?	Closed or open reduction

Knee

What are the common types?

Anterior or posterior

Which structures are at risk?

Popliteal artery and vein, peroneal nerve—especially with posterior dislocation, ACL, PCL (*Note:* need arteriogram)

What is the treatment?

Immediate attempt at relocation, arterial repair, and then ligamentous repair (delayed or primary)

THE KNEE

What are the five ligaments of the knee?

1. **A**nterior **C**ruciate **L**igament (**ACL**)
2. **P**osterior **C**ruciate **L**igament (**PCL**)
3. **M**edial **C**ollateral **L**igament (**MCL**)
4. **L**ateral **C**ollateral **L**igament (**LCL**)
5. Patellar ligament

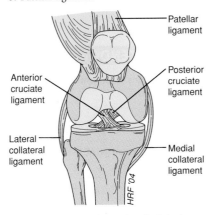

What is the Lachman test for a torn ACL?

Thigh is secured with one hand while the other hand pulls the tibia anteriorly

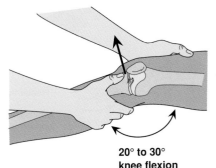

20° to 30° knee flexion

What is the meniscus of the knee?	Cartilage surface of the tibia plateau (lateral and medial meniscus); tears are repaired usually by arthroscopy with removal of torn cartilage fragments
What is McMurray's sign?	Seen with a medial meniscus tear: medial tenderness of knee with flexion and internal rotation of the knee
What is the "unhappy triad"?	Lateral knee injury resulting in: 1. ACL tear 2. MCL tear 3. Medial meniscus injury
What is a "locked knee"?	Meniscal tear that displaces and interferes with the knee joint and prevents complete extension
What is a "bucket-handle tear"?	Meniscal tear longitudinally along contour of normal "C" shape of the meniscus
In collateral ligament and menisci injuries, which are more common, the medial or the lateral?	Medial

ACHILLES TENDON RUPTURE

What are the signs of an Achilles tendon rupture?	Severe calf pain, also bruised swollen calf, two ends of ruptured tendon may be felt, patient will have weak plantar flexion from great toe flexors that should be intact; patient often hears a "pop"
What is the test for an INTACT Achilles tendon?	**Thompson's test:** A squeeze of the gastrocnemius muscle results in plantar flexion of the foot (with Achilles tendon rupture = **no** plantar flexion)

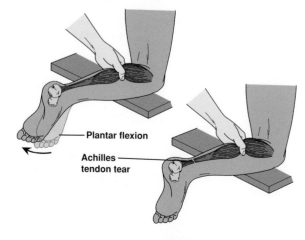

Plantar flexion

Achilles tendon tear

What is the treatment for an Achilles tendon rupture?	Young = surgical repair Elderly = many can be treated with progressive splints

ROTATOR CUFF

What four muscles form the rotator cuff?	Think: **"SITS"**: 1. **S**upraspinatus, etc. 2. **I**nfraspinatus 3. **T**eres minor 4. **S**ubscapularis
When do tears usually occur?	Fifth decade
What is the usual history?	Intermittent shoulder pain especially with **overhead** activity, followed by an episode of acute pain corresponding to a tendon tear; weak abduction
What is the treatment?	Most tears: symptomatic pain relief Later: if poor muscular function persists, surgical repair is indicated

MISCELLANEOUS

Define the following terms:

Dupuytren's contracture	Thickening and contracture of palmar fascia; incidence increases with age
Charcot's joint	Joint arthritis from peripheral neuropathy
Tennis elbow	Tendonitis of the lateral epicondyle of the humerus; classically seen in tennis players
Turf toe	Hyperextension of the great toe (tear of the tendon of the flexor hallucis brevis); classically seen in football players
Shin splints	Exercise-induced anterior compartment hypertension (compartment syndrome); seen in runners
Heel spur	Plantar fasciitis with abnormal bone growth in the plantar fascia; classically seen in runners and walkers
Nightstick fracture	Ulnar fracture
Kienbock's disease	Avascular necrosis of the lunate
What is traumatic myositis?	Abnormal bone deposit in a muscle after blunt trauma deep muscle contusion (benign)

How does a "cast saw" cut the cast but not the underlying skin?	It is an "oscillating" saw (designed by Dr. Homer Stryker in 1947) that goes back and forth cutting anything hard while moving the skin back and forth without injuring it

ORTHOPEDIC INFECTIONS

Osteomyelitis

What is osteomyelitis?	Inflammation/infection of bone marrow and adjacent bone
What is the most common organism isolated in osteomyelitis in the general adult population?	*Staphylococcus aureus*
What is the most common isolated organism in patients with sickle cell disease?	*Salmonella*
What is seen on physical examination?	Tenderness, decreased movement, swelling
What are the diagnostic steps?	History and physical examination, needle aspirate, blood cultures, CBC, ESR, bone scan
What are the treatment options?	Antibiotics with or without surgical drainage
What is a Marjolin's ulcer?	Squamous cell carcinoma that arises in a chronic sinus from osteomyelitis

Septic Arthritis

What is it?	Inflammation of a joint beginning as synovitis and ending with destruction of articular cartilage if left untreated
What are the causative agents?	Same as in osteomyelitis, except that gonococcus is a common agent in the adult population
What are the findings on physical examination?	Joint pain, decreased motion, joint swelling, joint warm to the touch
What are the diagnostic steps?	Needle aspirate (look for pus; culture plus Gram stain), x-ray, blood cultures, ESR
What is the treatment?	Decompression of the joint via needle aspiration and IV antibiotics; hip, shoulder, and spine must be surgically incised, debrided, and drained

ORTHOPEDIC TUMORS

What is the most common type in adults?	Metastatic!
What are the common sources?	Breast, lung, prostate, kidney, thyroid, and multiple myeloma
What is the usual presentation?	Bone pain or as a pathologic fracture
What is the most common primary malignant bone tumor?	Multiple myeloma (45%)
What is the differential diagnosis of a possible bone tumor?	Metastatic disease Primary bone tumors Metabolic disorders (e.g., hyperparathyroidism) Infection

Compare benign and malignant bone tumors in terms of:

Size	Benign—small; <1 cm Malignant—>1 cm
Bone reaction	Benign—sclerotic bone reaction Malignant—little reaction
Margins	Benign—sharp Malignant—poorly defined
Invasive	Benign—confined to bone Malignant—often extends to surrounding tissues

Are most pediatric bone tumors benign or malignant?	80% are benign (most common is osteochondroma)
Are most adult bone tumors benign or malignant?	66% are malignant (most commonly metastatic)
What are the four diagnostic steps?	1. PE/lab tests 2. Radiographs 3. CT scan, technetium scan, or both 4. Biopsy
What are the radiographic signs of malignant tumors?	Large size Aggressive bone destruction, poorly defined margins Ineffective bone reaction to tumor Extension to soft tissues
What are the radiographic signs of benign tumors?	Small Well-circumscribed, sharp margins Effective bone reaction to the tumor (sclerotic periostitis) No extension—confined to bone

What are some specific radiographic findings of the following?	
Osteosarcoma	"Sunburst" pattern
Fibrous dysplasia	Bubbly lytic lesion, "ground glass"
Ewing's sarcoma	"Onion skinning"
What is the mainstay of treatment for bone tumors?	Surgery (excision plus débridement) for both malignant and benign lesions; radiation therapy and chemotherapy as adjuvant therapy for many malignant tumors

Osteosarcoma

What is the usual age at presentation?	10 to 20 years
What is the gender distribution?	Male > female
What is the most common location?	≈66% in the distal femur, proximal tibia
What is the radiographic sine qua non?	Bone formation somewhere within tumor
What is the treatment?	Resection (limb sparing if possible) plus chemotherapy
What is the most common site of metastasis?	Lungs
What is the most common benign bone tumor?	**Osteochondroma;** it is cartilaginous in origin and may undergo malignant degeneration
What is a chondrosarcoma?	Malignant tumor of cartilaginous origin; presents in middle-aged and older patients and is unresponsive to chemotherapy and radiotherapy

Ewing's Sarcoma

What is the usual presentation?	Pain, swelling in involved area
What is the most common location?	Around the knee (distal femur, proximal tibia)
What is the usual age at presentation?	Evenly spread among those <20 years of age

What are the associated radiographic findings?	Lytic lesion with periosteal reaction termed "onion skinning," which is calcified layering Central areas of tumor can undergo liquefaction necrosis, which may be confused with purulent infection (particularly in a child with fever, leukocytosis, and bone pain)
What is a memory aid for Ewing's sarcoma?	"**TKO** Ewing": **T**wenty years old or younger **K**nee joint "**O**nion skinning"
What is the 5-year survival rate?	50%
How can Ewing's sarcoma mimic the appearance of osteomyelitis?	Bone cysts
What is a unicameral bone cyst?	Fluid-filled cyst most commonly found in the proximal humerus in children 5 to 15 years of age
What is the usual presentation?	Asymptomatic until pathologic fracture
What is the treatment?	Steroid injections
What is an aneurysmal bone cyst?	Hemorrhagic lesion that is locally destructive by expansile growth, but does not metastasize
What is the usual presentation?	Pain and swelling; pathologic fractures are rare
What is the treatment?	Curettage and bone grafting

ARTHRITIS

Which arthritides are classified as degenerative?	Osteoarthritis Posttraumatic arthritis
What signs characterize osteoarthritis?	Heberden's nodes/Bouchard's nodes **Symmetric** destruction, usually of the hip, knee, or spine
What are Bouchard's nodes?	Enlarged PIP joints of the hand from cartilage/bone growth
What are Heberden's nodes?	Enlarged DIP joints of the hand from cartilage/bone growth
What is posttraumatic arthritis?	Usually involves one joint of past trauma
What are the three treatment options for degenerative arthritis?	1. NSAIDs for acute flare-ups, **not** for long-term management 2. Local corticosteroid injections 3. Surgery

What are the characteristics of rheumatoid arthritis?	Autoimmune reaction in which invasive pannus attacks hyaline articular cartilage; rheumatoid factor (anti-IgG/IgM) in 80% of patients; 3× more common in females; skin nodules (e.g., rheumatoid nodule)
What is pannus?	Inflammatory exudate overlying synovial cells inside the joint
What are the classic hand findings with rheumatoid arthritis?	Wrist: radial deviation Fingers: ulnar deviation
What are the three surgical management options for joint/bone diseases?	1. Arthroplasty 2. Arthrodesis (fusion) 3. Osteotomy
What is the major difference between gout and pseudogout?	Gout: caused by urate deposition, negative birefringent, needle crystal Pseudogout: caused by calcium pyrophosphate–positive birefringent square crystals (Think: **P**ositive **S**quare crystals = **PS**eudogout)
What is a Charcot's joint?	Arthritic joint from peripheral neuropathy

PEDIATRIC ORTHOPEDICS

What types of fractures are unique to children?	Greenstick fracture Torus fracture Fracture through physis

Salter–Harris Classification

What does it describe?	Fractures in children involving physis
What does it indicate high risk of?	Potential growth arrest
Define the following terms:	
Salter I	Through physeal plate only
Salter II	Involves metaphysis and physis
Salter III	Involves physis and epiphysis
Salter IV	Extends from metaphysis through physis, into epiphysis
Salter V	Axial force crushes physeal plate
What acronym can help you remember the Salter classifications?	"SALTR": **S**eparated = type I **A**bove = type II **L**ower = type III **T**hrough = type IV **R**uined = type V

What is the simple numerical method for remembering the Salter–Harris classification? (N = normal)

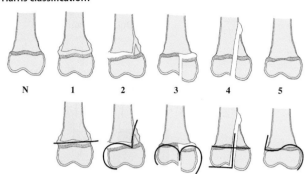

Why is the growth plate of concern in childhood fractures?

Growth plate represents the "weak link" in the child's musculoskeletal system; fractures involving the growth plate of long bones may compromise normal growth, so special attention should be given to them

What is a chief concern when oblique/spiral fractures of long bones are seen in children?

Child abuse is a possibility; other signs of abuse should be investigated

What is usually done during reduction of a femoral fracture?

Small amount of overlap is allowed because increased vascularity from injury may make the affected limb longer if overlap is not present; treatment after reduction is a spica cast

What is unique about ligamentous injury in children?

Most "ligamentous" injuries are actually fractures involving the growth plate!

What two fractures have a high incidence of associated compartment syndrome?

1. Tibial fractures
2. Supracondylar fractures of humerus (Volkmann's contracture)

Congenital Hip Dislocation

What is the epidemiology?

Female > male, firstborn children, breech Presentation, 1 in 1,000 births

What percentage is bilateral?

10%

How is the diagnosis made?

Barlow's maneuver, Ortolani's sign Radiographic confirmation is required

What is Barlow's maneuver?

Detects unstable hip: Patient is placed in the supine position and attempt is made to push femurs posteriorly with knees at 90°/hip flexed and hip will dislocate (Think: push **B**ack = **B**arlow)

What is Ortolani's sign?

"Clunk" produced by relocation of a dislocated femoral head when the examiner abducts the flexed hip and lifts the greater trochanter anteriorly; detects a dislocated hip (Think: **O**ut = **O**rtolani's)

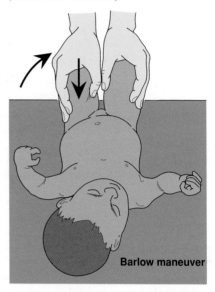

Barlow maneuver

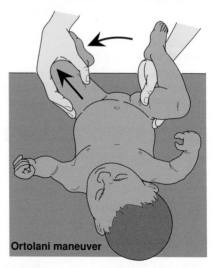

Ortolani maneuver

What is the treatment?

Pavlik harness—maintains hip reduction with hips flexed at 100° to 110°

Scoliosis

What is the definition?

Lateral curvature of a portion of the spine

Nonstructural: corrects with positional change

Structural: does not correct

What are three treatment options?

1. Observation
2. Braces (Milwaukee brace)
3. Surgery

What are the indications for surgery for scoliosis?

Respiratory compromise

Rapid progression

Curves >40°

Failure of brace

MISCELLANEOUS

Define the following terms:

Legg–Calvé–Perthes disease

Idiopathic avascular necrosis of femoral head in children

Slipped capital femoral epiphysis

Migration of proximal femoral epiphysis on the metaphysis in children; the proximal femoral epiphysis externally rotates and displaces anteriorly from the capital femoral epiphysis, which stays reduced in the acetabulum

(**Note:** Hip pain in children often presents as knee pain)

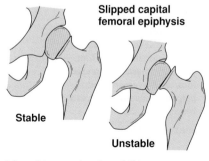

Slipped capital femoral epiphysis

Stable

Unstable

Blount's disease

Idiopathic varus bowing of tibia

Nursemaid's elbow

Dislocation of radial head (from pulling toddler's arm)

Little League elbow

Medial epicondylitis

Osgood–Schlatter's disease	Apophysitis of the tibial tubercle resulting from repeated powerful contractions of the quadriceps; seen in adolescents with an open physis
	Treatment of mild cases: activity restriction
	Treatment of severe cases: cast
What is the most common pediatric bone tumor?	Osteochondroma (Remember, 80% of bone tumors are benign in children)

RAPID-FIRE REVIEW

What is the correct diagnosis?

Bone tumor with "onion skinning" histology	Ewing's sarcoma
25-year-old s/p MVC with seatbelt sign and severe lower back pain	Chance fracture of lumbar spine
8-year-old s/p fall from a swing with a humerus fracture; weeks later he develops contraction of the forearm flexors	Volkmann's contracture
55-year-old male develops acute severe calf pain during an aerobics class; x-rays negative for fracture; on exam, there is no plantar flexion with squeeze of gastrocnemius muscle	Achilles' tendon rupture
28-year-old male with traumatic superficial femoral arterial occlusion for 7 hours develops severe calf pain with passive dorsiflexion of foot, foot paresthesias, decreased foot/toe movement, and palpable pulse after successful bypass procedure	Calf compartment syndrome

Name the most likely diagnosis:

| 30-year-old female with thoracic back pain, destruction of thoracic vertebral bodies on x-ray, + PPD | Pott's disease (tuberculosis of the spine) |
| 16-year-old male with right knee pain and fevers; x-ray reveals a distal femur lesion with "sunburst" pattern with a triangle of elevated periosteum | Osteosarcoma |

Femur fracture, dyspnea, mental status changes, tachycardia, petechiae	Fat embolism syndrome
Elderly male with shortened and inverted LE	Hip dislocation
35-year-old female trips and lands on her right hand; x-rays are negative for fracture; severe pain on palpating over the anatomical "snuff box"	Scaphoid fracture
What is the treatment?	
18-year-old male s/p motorbike jump crash with closed rib fib fracture; good distal pulses but severe pain on passive foot extension	Fasciotomy for compartment syndrome
45-year-old male s/p fall with severe pain with breathing due to multiple rib fractures	Epidural catheter for pain control

Chapter 74 | Neurosurgery

HEAD TRAUMA

What percentage of trauma deaths results from head trauma?	50%

Identify the dermatomes:

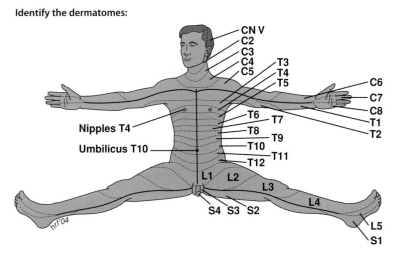

What is the Glasgow Coma Scale (GCS)?	GCS is an objective assessment of the level of consciousness after trauma

GCS Scoring System

Eyes?	Eye Opening (E)
	(Think: "**4 eyes**")
	    4—opens spontaneously
	    3—opens to voice (command)
	    2—opens to painful stimulus
	    1—does not open eyes

Motor?	Motor Response (M)
	(Think: **6**-cylinder **motor**)
	    6—obeys commands
	    5—localizes painful stimulus
	    4—withdraws from pain
	    3—decorticate posture
	    2—decerebrate posture
	    1—no movement

Verbal?	Verbal Response (V)
	(Think: Jackson **5** = **verbal 5**)
	    5—appropriate and oriented
	    4—confused
	    3—inappropriate words
	    2—incomprehensible sounds
	    1—no sounds

What indicates coma by GCS score?	<8 (Think: "less than eight—it may be too late")
What does unilateral, dilated, nonreactive pupil suggest?	Focal mass lesion with ipsilateral herniation and compression of CN III
What do bilateral fixed and dilated pupils suggest?	Diffusely increased ICP
What are the four signs of basilar skull fracture?	1. **Raccoon eyes**—periorbital ecchymoses 2. **Battle's sign**—postauricular ecchymoses 3. **Hemotympanum** 4. **CSF** rhinorrhea/otorrhea
What is the initial radiographic neuroimaging in trauma?	1. Head CT scan (if LOC or GCS <15) 2. C-spine CT scan 3. T/L spine AP and lateral
Should the trauma head CT scan be with or without IV contrast?	**Without!**
What is normal ICP?	5 to 15 mm H_2O
What is the worrisome ICP?	>20 mm H_2O

What determines ICP (Monro–Kellie hypothesis)?	1. Volume of brain 2. Volume of blood 3. Volume of CSF
What is the CPP?	**C**erebral **P**erfusion **P**ressure = mean arterial pressure − ICP (normal CPP is >70)

What is Cushing's reflex?	Physiologic response to increased ICP:
	  1. Hypertension
	  2. Bradycardia
	  3. Decreased RR

What are the three general indications to monitor ICP after trauma?	1. GCS <9 2. Altered level of consciousness or unconsciousness with multiple system trauma 3. Decreased consciousness with focal neurologic examination abnormality
What is Kocher's point?	Landmark for placement of ICP monitor bolt:

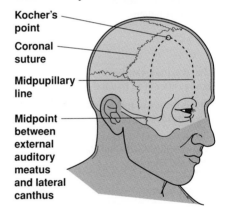

Kocher's point
Coronal suture
Midpupillary line
Midpoint between external auditory meatus and lateral canthus

What nonoperative techniques are used to decrease ICP?	1. **Elevate** head of bed (HOB) 30° (if spine cleared) 2. Osmotic therapy: 3% hypertonic saline (HTS) (or mannitol) 3. Limit fluid intake ±Lasix© 4. Intubation (keep Pco_2 normal) 5. Sedation 6. Pharmacologic paralysis 7. Ventriculostomy (CSF drainage)
How does hyperventilation ↓ ICP?	By ↓ Pco_2 resulting in cerebral vasoconstriction (and thus less intracranial volume)—RARELY USED, most commonly for short periods of time to temporize uncal herniation

What is the acronym for the treatment of elevated ICP?	**"ICP HEAD":** Intubate Calm (sedate) Place drain (ventriculostomy)/Paralysis Hyperventilate to $Pco_2 \approx 35$ Elevate head Adequate blood pressure (CPP >70) Diuretic (e.g., Lasix©, mannitol, or 3% HTS)
Can a tight c-collar increase the ICP?	Yes (it blocks venous drainage from brain!)
Why is prolonged hyperventilation dangerous?	It may result in severe vasoconstriction and ischemic brain necrosis!
What is a Kjellberg? (pronounced "shellberg")	Decompressive bifrontal craniectomy with removal of frontal bone frozen for possible later replacement
How does cranial nerve examination localize the injury in a comatose patient?	CNs proceed caudally in the brainstem as numbered: Presence of corneal reflex (CN 5 + 7) indicates intact pons; intact gag reflex (CN 9 + 10) shows functioning upper medulla (*Note:* CN 6 palsy is often a false localizing sign)
What is acute treatment of seizures after head trauma?	Benzodiazepines (Ativan or Keppra®)
What is seizure prophylaxis after severe head injury?	Give phenytoin for 7 days
What is the significance of hyponatremia (low sodium level) after head injury?	SIADH must be ruled out; remember, **SIADH = Sodium Is Always Down Here**

Epidural Hematoma

What is an epidural hematoma?	Collection of blood between the skull and dura
What causes it?	Usually occurs in association with a skull fracture as bone fragments lacerate meningeal arteries
Which artery is associated with epidural hematomas?	Middle meningeal artery
What is the most common sign of an epidural hematoma?	>50% have ipsilateral blown pupil
What is the classic history with an epidural hematoma?	LOC followed by a "lucid interval" followed by neurologic deterioration

What are the classic CT scan findings with an epidural hematoma?

Lenticular (lens)-shaped hematoma (Think: Epidural = LEnticular)

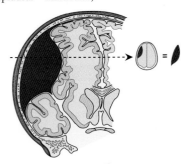

What is the surgical treatment for an epidural hematoma with significant mass effect?

Surgical evacuation and drain placement

Subdural Hematoma

What is it?

Blood collection under the dura

What causes it?

Tearing of "bridging" veins that pass through the space between the cortical surface and the dural venous sinuses or injury to the brain surface with resultant bleeding from cortical vessels

What are the three types of subdurals?

1. Acute—symptoms within 48 hours of injury
2. Subacute—symptoms within 3 to 14 days
3. Chronic—symptoms after 2 weeks or longer

What is the treatment of subdural hematomas?

If significant mass effect, craniotomy with clot evacuation is usually required

What is mass effect?

Midline shift; if ≥5 mm of midline shift, most will need an operation

What classic findings appear on head CT scan for a subdural hematoma?

Curved, crescent-shaped hematoma (Think: sUbdural = cUrved)

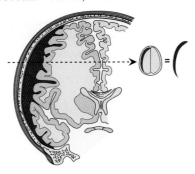

Traumatic Subarachnoid Hemorrhage

What is it?	Head trauma resulting in blood below the arachnoid membrane and above the pia
What is the treatment?	Anticonvulsants and observation

Cerebral Contusion

What is it?	Hemorrhagic contusion of brain parenchyma
What are coup and contrecoup injuries?	Coup—injury at the site of impact Contrecoup—injury at the site opposite the point of impact
What is DAI?	**D**iffuse **A**xonal **I**njury (shear injury to brain parenchyma) from rapid deceleration injury
What is the best diagnostic test for DAI?	MRI
What can present after blunt trauma with neurologic deficits and a normal brain CT scan?	DAI, carotid artery injury

Skull Fracture

What is a depressed skull fracture?	Fracture in which one or more fragments of the skull are forced below the inner table of the skull
What are the indications for surgery?	1. Contaminated wound requiring cleaning and débridement 2. Severe deformity 3. Impingement on cortex 4. Open fracture 5. CSF leak
What is the treatment for open skull fractures?	1. Antibiotics 2. Seizure prophylaxis 3. Surgical therapy

SPINAL CORD TRAUMA

What are the two general types of injury?	1. Complete—no motor/sensory function below the level of injury 2. Incomplete—residual function below the level of injury
What is "spinal shock"?	Loss of all reflexes and motor function
What is "sacral sparing"?	Sparing of sacral nerve level: anal sphincter intact, toe flexion, perianal sensation

What are the diagnostic studies?	CT scan, MRI
What are the indications for emergent surgery with spinal cord injury?	Unstable vertebral fracture Incomplete injury with extrinsic compression Spinal epidural or subdural hematoma

Describe the following conditions:

Anterior cord syndrome

Affects corticospinal and lateral spinothalamic tracts, paraplegia, loss of pain/temperature sensation, preserved touch/vibration/proprioception

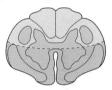

Central cord syndrome

Preservation of some lower extremity motor and sensory ability with upper extremity weakness

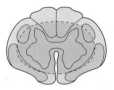

Brown-Séquard syndrome

Hemisection of cord resulting in ipsilateral motor touch/proprioception loss with contralateral pain/temperature loss

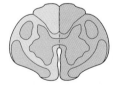

Posterior cord syndrome

Injury to posterior spinal cord with loss of proprioception distally

How can the findings associated with Brown-Séquard syndrome be remembered?

Think: **CAPTAIN** Brown-Séquard = **"CPT"**:
  Contralateral
  Pain
  Temperature loss

Define the following terms:

Jefferson's fracture

Fracture through **C1** arches from axial loading (unstable fracture)

Hangman's fracture	Fracture through the pedicles of **C2** from hyperextension; usually stable
	Think: A hangman (C2) is below stature of President T. Jefferson (C1)
Odontoid fracture	Fracture of the odontoid process of C2 (view with open-mouth odontoid x-ray)
Priapism	Penile erection seen with spinal cord injury
Chance fracture	Transverse vertebral fracture
Clay-shoveler's fracture	Fracture of spinous process of C7
Odontoid fractures	A: Type I—fracture through tip of dens
	B: Type II—fracture through base of dens
	C: Type III—fracture through body of C2

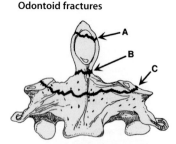

TUMORS

General

What is the incidence of CNS tumors?	≈1% of all cancers; third leading cause of cancer deaths in people 15 to 34 years of age; second leading cause of cancer deaths in children
What is the usual location of primary tumors in adults/children?	In adults, ≈66% of tumors are supratentorial, ≈33% are infratentorial; the reverse is true in children (i.e., ≈66% infratentorial)
What is the differential diagnosis of a ring-enhancing brain lesion?	Metastatic carcinoma, abscess, GBM, lymphoma
What are the signs/symptoms of brain tumors?	1. Neurologic deficit (66%)
	2. Headache (50%)
	3. Seizures (25%)
	4. Vomiting (classically in the morning)
How is the diagnosis made?	CT scan or MRI is the standard diagnostic study
What are the surgical indications?	1. Establishing a tissue diagnosis
	2. Relief of increased ICP
	3. Relief of neurologic dysfunction caused by tissue compression
	4. Attempt to cure in the setting of localized tumor

What are the most common intracranial tumors in adults?	Metastatic neoplasms are most common; among primaries, gliomas are #1 (50%) and meningiomas are #2 (25%)
What are the three most common tumors in children?	1. Medulloblastomas (33%) 2. Astrocytomas (33%) 3. Ependymomas (10%)

Gliomas

What is a glioma?	General name for several tumors of neuroglial origin (e.g., astrocytes, ependymal, oligodendrocytes)
What are the characteristics of a LOW-grade astrocytoma?	Nuclear atypia, high mitotic rate, high signal on T2-weighted images, nonenhancing with contrast CT scan
What is the most common primary brain tumor in adults?	Glioblastoma multiforme (GBM) (Think: **GBM** = **G**reatest **B**rain **M**alignancy)
What are its characteristics?	Poorly defined, highly aggressive tumors occurring in the white matter of the cerebral hemispheres; spread extremely rapidly
What is the average age of onset?	Fifth decade
What is the treatment?	Surgical debulking followed by radiation
What is the prognosis?	Without treatment, >90% of patients die within 3 months of diagnosis; with treatment, 90% die within 2 years

Meningiomas

What is the layer of origination?	Arachnoid cap cells
What are the risk factors?	Radiation exposure Neurofibromatosis type 2 Female gender
What are the associated histologic findings?	Psammoma bodies (concentric calcifications), whorl formations ("onion skin" pattern)
What is the histologic malignancy determination?	Brain parenchymal invasion
What is the peak age of occurrence?	40 to 50 years
What is the gender ratio?	Females predominate almost 2:1
What is the clinical presentation?	Variable depending on location; lateral cerebral convexity tumors can cause focal deficits or headache; sphenoid tumors can present with seizures; posterior fossa tumors with CN deficits; olfactory groove tumors with anosmia

What is the treatment?	± Preoperative embolization and surgical resection

Cerebellar Astrocytomas

What is the peak age of occurrence?	5 to 9 years
What is the usual location?	Usually in the cerebellar hemispheres; less frequently in the vermis
What are the signs/symptoms?	Usually lateral cerebellar signs occur: ipsilateral incoordination or dysmetria (patient tends to fall to side of tumor) as well as nystagmus and ataxia; CN deficits are also frequently present, especially in CNs VI and VII

Medulloblastoma

What is the peak age of occurrence?	First decade (3–7 years)
What is the most common location?	Cerebellar vermis in children; cerebellar hemispheres of adolescents and adults

Pituitary Tumors

What is the most common pituitary tumor?	Prolactinoma
What is the most common presentation of a prolactinoma?	Bitemporal hemianopsia (lateral visual fields blind)

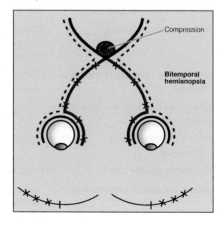

What are the blood prolactin levels with a prolactinoma?	>300 mg/L is diagnostic for prolactinoma (>100 mg/L is abnormal)
Medical treatment of a prolactinoma?	Bromocriptine
Surgical treatment for a prolactinoma?	Transsphenoidal resection of the pituitary tumor (in cases refractory to bromocriptine)
What is the treatment of a recurrent prolactinoma after surgical resection?	Radiation therapy

VASCULAR NEUROSURGERY

Subarachnoid Hemorrhage (SAH)

What are the usual causes?	Most cases are due to **trauma;** of nontraumatic SAH, the leading cause is ruptured **berry aneurysm,** followed by arteriovenous malformations
What is a berry aneurysm?	Saccular outpouching of vessels in the circle of Willis, usually at bifurcations
What is the usual location of a berry aneurysm?	Anterior communicating artery is #1 (30%), followed by posterior communicating artery and middle cerebral artery
What medical diseases increase the risk of berry aneurysms?	Polycystic kidney disease and connective tissue disorders (e.g., Marfan's syndrome)
What are the signs/symptoms of SAH?	Classic symptom is **"the worst headache of my life";** meningismus is documented by neck pain and positive Kernig's and Brudzinski's signs; occasionally LOC, vomiting, nausea, photophobia
What comprises the workup of SAH?	If SAH is suspected, head CT scan should be the first test ordered
What are the possible complications of SAH?	1. Brain edema leading to increased ICP 2. Rebleeding (most common in the first 24–48 hours post hemorrhage) 3. **Vasospasm** (most common cause of morbidity and mortality)
What is the treatment for vasospasm?	Nimodipine (calcium channel blocker)

What is the treatment of aneurysms?	Surgical treatment by placing a metal clip on the aneurysm is the mainstay of therapy; alternatives include balloon occlusion or coil embolization

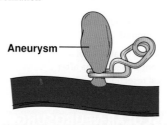

What is the treatment of arteriovenous malformations (AVMs)?	Many are on the brain surface and accessible operatively; preoperative embolization can reduce the size of the AVM; for surgically inaccessible lesions, radiosurgery (gamma knife) has been effective in treating AVMs <3 cm in diameter

SPINE

Lumbar Disc Herniation

What is it?	Extrusion of the inner portion of the intervertebral disc (nucleus pulposus) through the outer annulus fibrosis, causing impingement on nerve roots exiting the spinal canal
Which nerve is affected?	Nerve exiting at the level below (e.g., an L4–5 disc impinges on the L5 nerve exiting between L5 and S1)
What are the most common sites?	L5–S1 (45%) L4–5 (40%)
What is the treatment?	Conservative—bed rest and analgesics Surgical—partial hemilaminectomy and discectomy (removal of herniated disc)
What are the indications for emergent surgery?	1. Cauda equina syndrome 2. Progressive motor deficits
What is cauda equina syndrome?	Herniated disc compressing multiple S1, S2, S3, S4 nerve roots, resulting in bowel/bladder incontinence, "saddle anesthesia" over buttocks/perineum, low back pain, sciatica

Cervical Disc Disease

What are the most common sites?	C6–7 (70%) C5–6 (20%)
What is Spurling's sign?	Reproduction of radicular pain by having the patient turn his head to the affected side and applying axial pressure to the top of the head

Spinal Epidural Abscess

What is the etiology?	Hematogenous spread from skin infections is most common; also, distant abscesses/infections, UTIs, postoperative infections, spinal surgery, epidural anesthesia
What is the most common organism?	*Staphylococcus aureus*
What are the signs/symptoms?	Fever; severe pain over affected area and with flexion/extension of spine; weakness can develop, ultimately leading to paraplegia; 15% of patients have a back furuncle
What is the treatment?	Surgical drainage and appropriate antibiotic coverage
What is the prognosis?	Depends on preop condition; severe neurologic deficits (e.g., paraplegia) show little recovery; 15% to 20% of cases are fatal

PEDIATRIC NEUROSURGERY

Hydrocephalus

What is it?	Abnormal condition consisting of an increased volume of CSF along with distension of CSF spaces
What are the signs/symptoms?	Signs of increased ICP: HA, nausea, vomiting, ataxia, increasing head circumference exceeding norms for age
What is the treatment?	1. Remove obvious offenders 2. Perform bypass obstruction with ventriculoperitoneal shunt or ventriculoatrial shunt
What is a "shunt series"?	Series of x-rays covering the entire shunt length—looking for shunt disruption/kinking to explain malfunction of shunt

Spinal Dysraphism/Neural Tube Defects

What is spina bifida occulta?	Defect in the development of the posterior portion of the vertebrae
What is the treatment?	With open myelomeningoceles, patients are operated on immediately to prevent infection
Which vitamin is thought to lower the rate of neural tube defects in utero?	Folic acid

Craniosynostosis

What is it?	Premature closure of one or more of the sutures between the skull plates
What is the timing of surgery?	Usually 3 to 4 months of age; earlier surgery increases the risk of anesthesia; later surgeries are more difficult because of the worsening deformities and decreasing malleability of the skull

Miscellaneous

What is syringomyelia?	Central pathologic cavitations of the spinal cord

RAPID-FIRE REVIEW

Name the GCS:

18-year-old female s/p MVC in a "coma"	= 8
40-year-old male brought in dead after an MVC by the rescue paramedics	3: eyes = 1, motor = 1, verbal = 1
20-year-old female s/p motorcycle collision with open eyes, grunting only, and withdrawals to pain	10: eyes = 4, motor = 4, verbal = 2
29-year-old female s/p skiing accident into a tree who is intubated; eyes closed even to pain, decorticate posturing only	5T: eyes = 1, intubated = IT, motor = 3

Name the most likely diagnosis:

28-year-old male involved in high-speed MVC with lower back spine fracture, bladder/bowel incontinence, decreased lower extremity sensation, and decreased lower extremity strength	Cauda equina syndrome
24-year-old female with spine fracture; paraplegia but with touch and proprioception intact	Anterior spinal cord syndrome
29-year-old male s/p 45-feet fall with left-sided loss of temperature and pain sensation; right-sided paresis and loss of right-sided proprioception	Brown-Séquard syndrome
18-year-old female with a cervical spinal fracture after diving into a shallow pool; she can't move her upper extremities but has some movement in her legs	Central cord syndrome
50-year-old female with painless proptosis and a brain tumor stuck to the dura	Meningioma
19-year-old female involved in a high-speed MVC and was thrown unrestrained into the windshield; she has a GCS of 15 at the scene and initially upon admission to the ER; she then becomes comatose with a GCS of 3	Epidural hematoma and "lucid interval"
Patient with head trauma and a peripheral "crescent"-shaped hematoma on CT scan	Subdural hematoma
Patient with head trauma and a peripheral "lenticular" (lens-like) hematoma on CT scan	Epidural hematoma
Hypoxia after brain injury without lung injury, no fractures, no DVTs	Neurogenic pulmonary edema
Coagulopathy after isolated brain injury	Brain thromboplastin
40-year-old s/p fall from a balcony, GCS of 3, heart rate 40, SBP of 190/90, blown right pupil	Elevated ICP with brain herniation

22-year-old female s/p MVC, GCS of 3, nl brain CT scan	Cervical vascular injury (e.g., carotid or vertebral artery dissection, thrombosis, ± embolus)
21-year-old male s/p MVC with hypotension, bradycardia, nl CXR, nl FAST exam, nl pelvic x-ray	Spinal cord injury with neurologic shock
39-year-old female lifting weights has onset of lower back pain, cannot urinate, and is passing flatus that she cannot control; on exam, the bladder is distended, poor rectal tone, and perineal skin numbness (anesthesia)	Cauda equina syndrome
29-year-old patient with diabetes with chronic bacterial sinusitis, new-onset seizures, fever, and right-sided weakness	Brain abscess
40-year-old male with chronic low back pain lifts a refrigerator and experiences severe pain shooting down his right leg out his right big toe	Herniated disc at L4–5

Name the diagnostic modality:

18-year-old female with fall from horse with loss of consciousness	Brain CT scan without contrast
39-year-old female librarian with acute loss of hearing in her left ear	MRI to rule out acoustic nerve neuroma

What is the treatment?

28-year-old male s/p motorcycle collision, presents with eyes closed, not making any verbal sounds, decorticate posturing to painful stimuli	GCS of 5 and in a "coma"; must be intubated
34-year-old female with small prolactinoma	Bromocriptine (transsphenoidal resection if refractory)

Name the radiographic test for localizing the following:

Pituitary adenoma	Gadolinium-enhanced MRI

Chapter 75 | Urology

Define the following terms:

Hydrocele	Clear fluid in the processus vaginalis membrane
Communicating hydrocele	Hydrocele that communicates with peritoneal cavity and, thus, gets smaller and larger as fluid drains and then reaccumulates

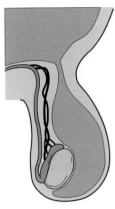

Noncommunicating hydrocele	Hydrocele that does not communicate with the peritoneal cavity; hydrocele remains the same size

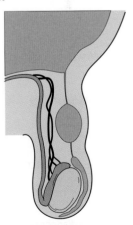

Varicocele	Abnormal dilation of the pampiniform plexus to the spermatic vein in the spermatic cord; described as a "bag of worms"

UROLOGIC DIFFERENTIAL DIAGNOSIS

What is the differential diagnosis of scrotal mass?	Cancer, torsion, epididymitis, hydrocele, spermatocele, varicocele, inguinal hernia, testicular appendage, swollen testicle after trauma, nontesticular tumor (paratesticular tumor: e.g., rhabdomyosarcoma, leiomyosarcoma, liposarcoma)
What are the causes of hematuria?	Bladder cancer, trauma, UTI, cystitis from chemotherapy or radiation, stones, kidney lesion, BPH
What is the most common cause of severe gross hematuria without trauma or chemotherapy/radiation?	Bladder cancer
What is the differential diagnosis for bladder outlet obstruction?	BPH, stone, foreign body, urethral stricture, urethral valve
What is the differential diagnosis for ureteral obstruction?	Stone, tumor, iatrogenic (suture), stricture, gravid uterus, radiation injury, retroperitoneal fibrosis
What is the differential diagnosis for kidney tumor?	Renal cell carcinoma, sarcoma, adenoma, angiomyolipoma, hemangiopericytoma, oncocytoma

RENAL CELL CARCINOMA (RCC)

What is it?	Most common solid renal tumor (90%); originates from proximal renal tubular epithelium
What is the epidemiology?	Primarily a tumor of adults 40 to 60 years of age with a 3:1 male-to-female ratio; 5% of cancers overall in adults
What are the risk factors?	Male sex, tobacco, von Hippel–Lindau syndrome, polycystic kidney
What are the symptoms?	Pain (40%), hematuria (35%), weight loss (35%), flank mass (25%), HTN (20%)
What is the classic TRIAD of RCC?	1. Flank pain 2. Hematuria 3. Palpable mass (**Triad** occurs in only 10%–15% of cases)
How are most cases diagnosed these days?	Found incidentally on an imaging study (CT scan, MRI, U/S) for another reason
What radiologic tests are performed?	1. IVP 2. Abdominal CT scan with contrast

What is the metastatic workup?	CXR, IVP, CT scan, LFTs, calcium
What are the sites of metastases?	Lung, liver, brain, bone; tumor thrombus entering renal vein or IVC is not uncommon
What is the unique route of spread?	Tumor thrombus into **IVC lumen**
What is the treatment of RCC?	Radical nephrectomy (excision of the kidney and adrenal, including Gerota's fascia) for stages I through IV
What gland is removed with a radical nephrectomy?	Adrenal gland
What is the unique treatment for metastatic spread?	1. α-Interferon 2. **LAK** cells (**L**ymphokine-**A**ctivated **K**iller) and IL-2 (interleukin-2)
What is a syndrome of RCC and liver disease?	Stauffer's syndrome
What is the concern in an adult with new-onset left varicocele?	Left RCC—the left gonadal vein drains into the left renal vein

BLADDER CANCER

What is the incidence?	Second most common urologic malignancy Male-to-female ratio of 3:1 White patients are more commonly affected than African American patients
What is the most common histology?	**T**ransitional **C**ell **C**arcinoma (**TCC**)—90%; remaining cases are squamous or adenocarcinomas
What are the risk factors?	**Smoking,** industrial carcinogens (aromatic amines), schistosomiasis, truck drivers, petroleum workers, cyclophosphamide
What are the symptoms?	**Hematuria,** with or without irritative symptoms (e.g., dysuria), frequency
What is the classic presentation of bladder cancer?	"Painless hematuria"
What tests are included in the workup?	Urinalysis and culture, IVP, cystoscopy with cytology and biopsy
What is the treatment according to stage?	
Stage 0	TURB and intravesical chemotherapy
Stage I	TURB

Stages II and III	Radical cystectomy, lymph node dissection, removal of prostate/uterus/ovaries/anterior vaginal wall, and urinary diversion (e.g., ileal conduit) ± chemo
Stage IV	± Cystectomy and systemic chemotherapy
What are the indications for a partial cystectomy?	Superficial, isolated tumor, apical with 3-cm margin from any orifices
What is TURB?	**T**rans**U**rethral **R**esection of the **B**ladder
If after a TURB the tumor recurs, then what?	Repeat TURB and intravesical chemotherapy (mitomycin C) or BCG
What is and how does bacillus Calmette-Guérin work?	Attenuated TB vaccine—thought to work by immune response

PROSTATE CANCER

What is the incidence?	**Most common** GU cancer (>100,000 new cases per year in the United States); most common carcinoma in US males; second most common cause of death in US males
What is the epidemiology?	"Disease of elderly men" present in 33% of men 70 to 79 years of age and in 66% of males 80 to 89 years of age at autopsy; African American patients have a 50% higher incidence than white patients
What is the histology?	Adenocarcinoma (95%)
What are the symptoms?	Often asymptomatic; usually presents as a nodule found on routine rectal examination; in 70% of cases cancer begins in the **periphery** of the gland and moves centrally; thus, obstructive symptoms occur late
What percentage of patients has metastasis at diagnosis?	40% of patients have metastatic disease at presentation, with symptoms of bone pain and weight loss
What are the common sites of metastasis?	Osteoblastic bony lesions, lung, liver, adrenal
What provides lymphatic drainage?	Obturator and hypogastric nodes
What is the significance of Batson's plexus?	Spinal cord venous plexus; route of isolated skull/brain metastasis
What are the steps in early detection?	1. Prostate-specific antigen (PSA)—most sensitive and specific marker 2. Digital rectal examination (DRE)

When should men get a PSA-level check?	Controversial: 1. All males >50 years old 2. >40 years old if first-degree family history or African American patient
What percentage of patients with prostate cancer will have an elevated PSA?	≈60%
What is the imaging test for prostate cancer?	TransRectal UltraSound (**TRUS**)
How is the diagnosis made?	Transrectal biopsy
What is the Gleason score?	Histologic grades 2 to 10: Low score = well differentiated High score = poorly differentiated
What are the indications for transrectal biopsy with normal rectal examination?	PSA >10 or abnormal transrectal ultrasound
What does a "radical prostatectomy" remove?	1. Prostate gland 2. Seminal vesicles 3. Ampullae of the vasa deferentia
What is "androgen ablation" therapy?	1. Bilateral orchiectomy or 2. Luteinizing Hormone–Releasing Hormone (**LHRH**) agonists
What are the generalized treatment options according to stage?	
Stage I	Radical prostatectomy
Stage II	Radical prostatectomy, ± lymph node dissection
Stage III	Radiation therapy, ± androgen ablation
Stage IV	Androgen ablation, radiation therapy
What is the medical treatment for systemic metastatic disease?	Androgen ablation
What is the option for treatment in the early-stage prostate cancer patient >70 years old with comorbidity?	XRT

BENIGN PROSTATIC HYPERPLASIA

What is it also known as?	BPH
What is it?	Disease of elderly males (average age is 60–65 years); prostate gradually enlarges, creating symptoms of urinary outflow obstruction

What is the size of a normal prostate?	20 to 25 g
Where does BPH occur?	Periurethrally (*Note:* Prostate cancer occurs in the periphery of the gland)
What are the symptoms?	Obstructive-type symptoms: hesitancy, weak stream, nocturia, intermittency, UTI, urinary retention
How is the diagnosis made?	History, DRE, elevated **P**ost**V**oid **R**esidual (**PVR**), urinalysis, cystoscopy, U/S
What lab tests should be performed?	Urinalysis, PSA, BUN, CR
What is the differential diagnosis?	**Prostate cancer** (e.g., nodular)—biopsy Neurogenic bladder—history of neurologic disease Acute prostatitis—hot, tender gland Urethral stricture—RUG, history of STD Stone UTI
What are the treatment options?	Pharmacologic—α-1 blockade Hormonal—antiandrogens Surgical—TURP, TUIP, open prostate resection Transurethral balloon dilation
Why do α-adrenergic blockers work?	1. Relax sphincter 2. Relax prostate capsule
What is Proscar®?	Finasteride: 5-α-reductase inhibitor; blocks transformation of testosterone to dihydrotestosterone; may shrink and slow progression of BPH
What is Hytrin®?	Terazosin: α-blocker; may increase urine outflow by relaxing prostatic smooth muscles

What are the indications for surgery in BPH?	Because of obstruction:
	    Urinary retention
	    Hydronephrosis
	    UTIs
	    Severe symptoms

What is TURP?	**T**rans**U**rethral **R**esection of **P**rostate: resection of prostate tissue via a scope
What is TUIP?	**T**rans**U**rethral **I**ncision of **P**rostate
What percentage of tissue removed for BPH will have malignant tissue on histology?	Up to 10%!

What are the possible complications of TURP?	Immediate:
	    Failure to void
	    Bleeding
	    Clot retention
	    UTI
	    Incontinence

TESTICULAR CANCER

What is the incidence?	Rare; 2 to 3 new cases per 100,000 males per year in the United States
What is its claim to fame?	Most common solid tumor of young adult males (20–40 years)
What are the risk factors?	Cryptorchidism (6% of testicular tumors develop in patients with a history of cryptorchidism)
What is cryptorchidism?	Failure of the testicle to descend into the scrotum
Does orchiopexy as an adult remove the risk of testicular cancer?	NO
What are the symptoms?	Most patients present with a painless lump, swelling, or firmness of the testicle; they often notice it after incidental trauma to the groin
What percentage of patients presents with an acute hydrocele?	10%
What percentage presents with symptoms of metastatic disease (back pain, anorexia)?	≈10%
What is the major classification based on therapy?	Seminomatous and nonseminomatous tumors
What are the tumor markers for testicular tumors?	1. β-Human chorionic gonadotropin (β-HCG) 2. α-Fetoprotein (AFP)
What are the tumor markers by tumor type?	β-HCG—↑ in choriocarcinoma (100%), embryonal carcinoma (50%), and rarely in pure seminomas (10%); nonseminomatous tumors (50%) AFP—↑ in embryonal carcinoma and yolk sac tumors; nonseminomatous tumors (50%)
What is the difference between seminomatous and NONseminomatous germ cell testicular tumor markers?	NONseminomatous **common** = 90% have a positive AFP and/or β-HCG Seminomatous **rare** = **only** 10% are AFP positive

In which tumor is β-HCG almost always found elevated?	Choriocarcinoma
What other tumor markers may be elevated and useful for recurrence surveillance?	LDH, CEA, **H**uman **C**horionic **S**omatomammotropin (**HCS**), γ-**G**lutamyl **T**ranspeptidase (**GGT**), **PL**acental **P**hosphate (**PLAP**)
What are the steps in workup?	PE, scrotal U/S, check tumor markers, CXR, CT scan (chest/pelvis/abd)
Define the stages according to TMN staging (AJCC):	
Stage I	Any tumor size, no nodes, no metastases
Stage II	**Positive** nodes, no metastases, any tumor
Stage III	Distant **metastases** (any nodal status, any size tumor)
What is the initial treatment for all testicular tumors?	**Inguinal** orchiectomy (removal of testicle through a groin incision)
What is the treatment of SEMIMOMA at the various stages?	
Stages I and II	Inguinal orchiectomy and **radiation** to retroperitoneal nodal basins
Stage III	Orchiectomy and chemotherapy
What is the treatment of NONseminomatous disease at the various stages?	
Stages I and II	Orchiectomy and retroperitoneal lymph node **dissection** versus close follow-up for retroperitoneal nodal involvement
Stage III	Orchiectomy and chemotherapy
What percentage of stage I seminomas is cured after treatment?	95%
Which type is most radiosensitive?	Seminoma (Think: **S**eminoma = **S**ensitive to radiation)
Why not remove testis with cancer through a scrotal incision?	It could result in tumor seeding of the scrotum
What is the major side effect of retroperitoneal lymph node dissection?	Erectile dysfunction

TESTICULAR TORSION

What is it?	Torsion (twist) of the spermatic cord, resulting in venous outflow obstruction, and subsequent arterial occlusion → infarction of the testicle
What is the classic history?	Acute onset of scrotal pain usually after vigorous activity or minor trauma
What is a "bell clapper" deformity?	Bilateral nonattachment of the testicles by the gubernaculum to the scrotum (free like the clappers of a bell)

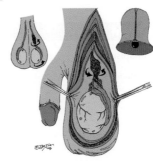

What are the symptoms?	Pain in the scrotum, suprapubic pain
What are the signs?	Very tender, swollen, elevated testicle; nonillumination; absence of cremasteric reflex
What is the differential diagnosis?	Testicular trauma, inguinal hernia, epididymitis, appendage torsion
How is the diagnosis made?	Surgical exploration, U/S (solid mass), and Doppler flow study
What is the treatment?	Surgical detorsion and bilateral orchiopexy to the scrotum
How much time is available from the onset of symptoms to detorse the testicle?	<6 hours will bring about the best results
What are the chances of testicle salvage after 24 hours?	<10%

EPIDIDYMITIS

What is it?	Infection of the epididymis
What are the signs/symptoms?	Swollen, tender testicle; dysuria; scrotal ache/pain; fever; chills; scrotal mass
What is the cause?	Bacteria from the urethra

What are the common bugs in the following types of patients?	
Elderly patients/children	*Escherichia coli*
Young males	STD bacteria: gonorrhea, chlamydia
What is the major differential diagnosis?	Testicular torsion
What is the workup?	U/A, urine culture, swab if STD suspected, ± U/S with Doppler or nuclear study to rule out torsion
What is the treatment?	Antibiotics

PRIAPISM

What is priapism?	Persistent penile erection
What are its causes?	Low flow: leukemia, drugs (e.g., prazosin), sickle cell disease, erectile dysfunction treatment gone wrong High flow: pudendal artery fistula, usually from trauma
What is first-line treatment?	1. Aspiration of blood from corpus cavernosum 2. α-Adrenergic agent

ERECTILE DYSFUNCTION

What is it?	Inability to achieve an erection
What are the six major causes?	1. **Vascular:** decreased blood flow or leak of blood from the corpus cavernosum (most common cause) 2. **Endocrine:** low testosterone 3. **Anatomic:** structural abnormality of the erectile apparatus (e.g., Peyronie's disease) 4. **Neurologic:** damage to nerves (e.g., postoperative, IDDM) 5. **Medications** (e.g., clonidine) 6. **Psychological:** performance anxiety, etc. (very rare)
What lab tests should be performed?	Fasting GLC (rule out diabetes and thus diabetic neuropathy) Serum testosterone Serum prolactin

CALCULUS DISEASE

What is the incidence?	1 in 10 people will have stones
What are the risk factors?	Poor fluid intake, IBD, hypercalcemia ("CHIMPANZEES"), renal tubular acidosis, small bowel bypass
What are the four types of stones?	1. Calcium oxalate/calcium PO_4 (75%)—secondary to hypercalciuria ($\uparrow$ intestinal absorption, $\downarrow$ renal reabsorption, $\uparrow$ bone reabsorption)
	2. Struvite (MgAmPh) (15%)—infection stones; seen in UTI with urea-splitting bacteria (*Proteus*); may cause staghorn calculi; high urine pH
	3. Uric acid (7%)—stones are radiolucent (Think: **U**ric = **U**nseen); seen in gout, Lesch–Nyhan syndrome, chronic diarrhea, cancer; low urine pH
	4. Cystine (1%)—genetic predisposition
What type of stones is not seen on AXR?	Uric acid (Think: **U**ric = **U**nseen)
What stone is associated with UTIs?	Struvite stones (Think: **S**truvite = **S**epsis)
What stones are seen in IBD/bowel bypass?	Calcium oxalate
What are the symptoms of calculus disease?	Severe pain; patient cannot sit still: renal colic (typically pain in the kidney/ureter that radiates to the testis or penis), hematuria (remember, patients with peritoneal signs are motionless)
What are the classic findings/symptoms?	Flank pain, stone on AXR, hematuria
Diagnosis?	KUB (90% radiopaque), IVP, urinalysis and culture, BUN/Cr, CBC
What is the significance of hematuria and pyuria?	Stone with concomitant infection
Treatment?	Narcotics for pain, vigorous hydration, observation
	Further options: ESWL (lithotripsy), ureteroscopy, percutaneous lithotripsy, open surgery; metabolic workup for recurrence
What are the indications for intervention?	Urinary tract obstruction
	Persistent infection
	Impaired renal function

What are the contraindications of outpatient treatment?	Pregnancy, diabetes, obstruction, severe dehydration, severe pain, urosepsis/fever, pyelonephritis, previous urologic surgery, only one functioning kidney
What are the three common sites of obstruction?	1. Uretero**P**elvic **J**unction (**UPJ**) 2. Uretero**V**esicular junction (**UVJ**) 3. Intersection of the ureter and the iliac vessels

INCONTINENCE

What are the common types of incontinence?	Stress incontinence, overflow incontinence, urge incontinence
Define the following terms:	
Stress incontinence	Loss of urine associated with coughing, lifting, exercise, etc.; seen most often in females, secondary to relaxation of pelvic floor following multiple deliveries
Overflow incontinence	Failure of the bladder to empty properly; may be caused by bladder outlet obstruction (BPH or stricture) or detrusor hypotonicity
Urge incontinence	Loss of urine secondary to detrusor instability in patients with stroke, dementia, Parkinson's disease, etc.
Mixed incontinence	Stress **and** urge incontinence combined
Enuresis	Bedwetting in children
How is the diagnosis made?	History (including meds), physical examination (including pelvic/rectal examination), urinalysis, **P**ost**V**oid **R**esidual (**PVR**), urodynamics, cystoscopy/**V**esico**C**ysto**U**rethro**G**ram (VCUG) may be necessary
What is the "Marshall test"?	Female with urinary stress incontinence placed in the lithotomy position with a full bladder leaks urine when asked to cough
What is the treatment of the following disorders?	
Stress incontinence	Bladder neck suspension
Urge incontinence	Pharmacotherapy (anticholinergics, α-agonists)
Overflow incontinence	Self-catheterization, surgical relief of obstruction, α-blockers

URINARY TRACT INFECTION (UTI)

What is the etiology?	Ascending infection, instrumentation, coitus in females
What are the three common organisms?	1. *E. coli (90%)* 2. *Proteus* 3. *Klebsiella*
What are the predisposing factors?	Stones, obstruction, reflux, diabetes mellitus, pregnancy, indwelling catheter/stent
What are the symptoms?	Lower UTI—frequency, urgency, dysuria, nocturia Upper UTI—back/flank pain, fever, chills
How is the diagnosis made?	Symptoms, urinalysis (>10 WBCs/HPF, >10^5 CFU)
When should workup be performed?	After the first infection in male patients (unless Foley is in place) After the first pyelonephritis in prepubescent female patients
What is the treatment?	Lower: 1 to 4 days of oral antibiotics Upper: 3 to 7 days of IV antibiotics

MISCELLANEOUS UROLOGY QUESTIONS

What is the most common intraoperative bladder tumor?	Foley catheter—don't fall victim!
What provides drainage of the left gonadal (e.g., testicular) vein?	Left renal vein
What provides drainage of the right gonadal vein?	IVC
What are the signs of urethral injury in the trauma patient?	"High-riding, ballottable" prostate, blood at the urethral meatus, severe pelvic fracture, ecchymosis of scrotum
What is the evaluation for urethral injury in the trauma patient?	**RUG** (**R**etrograde **U**rethro**G**ram)
What is the evaluation for a transected ureter intraoperatively?	IV indigo carmine and then look for leak of blue urine in the operative field
What aid is used to help identify the ureters in a previously radiated retroperitoneum?	Ureteral stents
How can a small traumatic EXTRAperitoneal bladder rupture be treated?	Foley catheter

How should a traumatic INTRAperitoneal bladder rupture be treated?

Operative repair

What is the classic history for papillary necrosis?

Patient with diabetes taking NSAIDs or patient with sickle cell trait

What is Fournier's gangrene?

Necrotizing fasciitis of perineum, polymicrobial, diabetes = major risk factor

What unique bleeding problem can be seen with prostate surgery?

Release of TPA and urokinase (treat with ε-aminocaproic acid)

What is the scrotal "blue dot" sign?

Torsed appendix testis

What is Peyronie's disease?

Curved penile orientation with erection due to fibrosis of corpora cavernosa

What is a "three-way" irrigating Foley catheter?

Foley catheter that irrigates and then drain

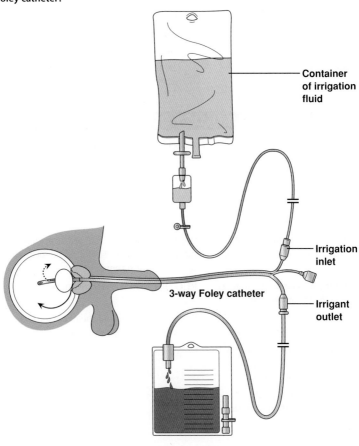

Container of irrigation fluid

Irrigation inlet

3-way Foley catheter

Irrigant outlet

RAPID-FIRE REVIEW

What is the correct diagnosis?

Abdominal pain, flank mass, hematuria	Renal cell carcinoma
Acute varicocele and hematuria	Left renal tumor
56-year-old male presents with right sided flank pain; cannot sit still, blood in his urine, and fever; x-ray nl; no mass palpated on exam	Nephrolithiasis due to uric acid stone with obstructive urinary infection
60-year-old white male smoker who works at a refinery develops hematuria; no pain or other symptoms	Bladder cancer ("painless hematuria")

Name the most likely diagnosis:

70-year-old male retired leather worker, cigarette smoker; presents with painless gross hematuria	Bladder transitional cell carcinoma
22-year-old male who develops a right scrotal hydrocele with elevated serum β-HCG	Testicular cancer
55-year-old female with diabetes, recurrent pyelonephritis, increased creatinine, increased BUN; IVP reveals radiolucent defects in the kidney collecting system	Papillary necrosis
31-year-old male with right flank pain radiating into scrotum, gross hematuria, right-sided hydronephrosis, and normal abdominal x-ray	Uric acid kidney stone
18-year-old female with fever; costovertebral tenderness; flank mass; and WBCs, RBCs, and gram-negative rods in the urine	Kidney (renal) abscess

65-year-old male with groin pain who goes into septic shock after a rectal prostatic exam	Bacterial prostatitis
19-year-old male status post (s/p) spinal anesthetic for a groin hernia repair returns to clinic with back pain, fever, and decreased left lower extremity sensation and movement	Epidural abscess

Name the diagnostic modality:

80-year-old male with history of intermittent hematuria; CT scan is normal	Cystoscopy to rule out bladder cancer
27-year-old male s/p MVC with pelvic fracture and blood at the urethral meatus	Retrograde urethrogram (RUG) to rule out urethral injury
30-year-old female with a pelvic fracture and free fluid in the pelvis	CT scan with CT cystogram to rule out bladder injury

Three-Dimensional Surgical Vignette Chess for the Shelf Examination

HOW TO USE SURGICAL VIGNETTE CHESS

1. Cover the three columns under the vignette, then read the vignette.
2. Uncover and read the additional vignette information in column 1 (far left).
3. Next, uncover and read the question and answer choices in column 2. Choose your answer.
4. Finally, uncover and reveal the answer in column 3.
5. Repeat until you have mastered all of the information.

A 28-year-old female goes to the ER with the c/o chronic RUQ pain that got progressively worse today. The pain previously had been described as constant and not associated with food. Ultrasound 2 weeks ago revealed no gallstones.

Her only medication is birth control pills. A STAT CT reveals a liver mass.	The most likely diagnosis is: A. Hepatocellular carcinoma B. AV fistula C. Fibrolamellar carcinoma D. Hepatic adenoma	**Answer: D** (see p. 244)
The patient has normal vital signs and normal labs.	The initial treatment is: A. Testosterone patch B. Stop birth control pills C. Prolactin D. Bromocriptine PO	**Answer: B** (see p. 244)
Two weeks later, she returns to the ER. The patient becomes hypotensive and then is unresponsive in front of the triage nurse.	What is the most likely cause of the hypotension? A. Hemorrhagic shock B. Vasovagal C. Cytokine release from necrotic tumor center D. Acute compression of the IVC	**Answer: A** (see p. 160)
The patient responds to blood transfusion. Her SBP is now 95/55.	What is the source of blood loss? A. Gastritis B. Tumor hemorrhage into peritoneal cavity C. Hemobilia D. Bilhemia	**Answer: B** (see p. 163)

| The patient's SBP again drops to 55/palp. | What is the safest thing to do?

A. Blood, FFP IV, and O.R. stat for ex lap and packing
B. Call in interventional radiology to consider angio
C. 1:1:1 massive transfusion and tranexamic acid and observe
D. Kcentra | **Answer: A**
(see p. 163) |

A 36-year-old male restrained driver is involved in a high-speed, head-on motor vehicle collision. His SBP is 95 in the field with a HR of 120. He denies LOC but states he is short of breath.

In the ER, his SBP drops to 80/palp.	Causes of hypotension acutely after blunt trauma include all EXCEPT: A. Tension pneumothorax B. High spinal cord transection C. Open book pelvic fx D. Succus peritonitis E. Bilateral femur fx F. Spleen/liver laceration	**Answer: D** (see p. 151)
The patient has a pelvis x-ray that reveals an open book fx.	In addition to massive blood transfusion to treat the hypotension, the patients need an immediate: A. Bladder decompression B. NGT tube C. Pelvic binder D. Buck's traction	**Answer: C** (see p. 161)
The patient receives a chest x-ray that reveals no lung markings on the left with tracheal deviation to the right.	Immediate treatment includes: A. Left-sided chest tube B. Right-sided needle decompression (2nd intercostal/midclavicular line) C. STAT intubation D. NGT E. Incentive spirometry	**Answer: A** (see p. 57)
A patient has a FAST examination with positive fluid seen in the Morrison's pouch in the RUQ view. Despite 2 units of PRBCs and FFP, his BP is now 70/palp.	The next move for this patient is: A. STAT CT scan of the abdomen B. O.R. for exploratory laparotomy C. Massive transfusion including IV calcium, saline bolus D. STAT angiography and embolization	**Answer: B** (see p. 136)

The hemorrhage has been stopped, and on examination after the patient awakens, it is noted that he cannot move any of his extremities and has no sensation below his neck.	The hypotension could be caused by: A. Spinal shock B. Transfusion-related autoimmune reaction C. Neurogenic shock D. Anaphylactic shock	**Answer: C** (see p. 109)
The patient receives a CT scan of the entire torso that reveals no hemorrhage but a severely displaced spinal column fx. He is hypotensive after fluid challenge.	The next step to treat the hypotension is: A. IV calcium B. Narcan IV C. Vasopressors (e.g., norepinephrine) D. Thyroxine IV E. Stress-dose steroids (e.g., hydrocortisone 100 mg IV)	**Answer: C** (see p. 102)

A 33-year-old female is involved in a house fire.

She has 47% total body surface area full-thickness burns.	The best test to confirm inhalation injury is: A. PET scan B. Xenon-131 inhalation extraction C. Chest x-ray D. CT scan E. Bronchoscopy	**Answer: E** (see p. 171)
Her entire right arm is burned from axilla to fingertips.	This represents what percentage of total surface area? A. 5% B. 9% C. 18% D. 22% E. 25%	**Answer: B** (see p. 171)
She receives tetanus immunization in the ER.	She should also receive: A. IV antibiotics B. Steroids C. DDAVP D. Lactated Ringer's IV	**Answer: D** (see p. 173)
She has elevated carboxyhemoglobin.	The best treatment for this is: A. Steroids B. DDAVP C. 100% oxygen D. Xenon-132	**Answer: C** (see p. 173)

After 24 hours, she stabilizes.	At this time, the IV fluid management should change to add:	**Answer: A** (see p. 171)
	A. Colloid albumin	
	B. Steroids	
	C. DDAVP	
	D. Fat emulsion	
	E. Magnesium	

She has circumferential burns around her chest. Her peak airway pressures are going up.	The best treatment at this time is:	**Answer: D** (see p. 172)
	A. 100% FiO_2	
	B. Steroids IV	
	C. Fasciotomy of the chest	
	D. Escharotomy of the chest	
	E. Increase tidal volume	

She develops a duodenal ulcer.	This ulcer associated with burn injury is called a:	**Answer: B** (see p. 173)
	A. Cushing's ulcer	
	B. Curling's ulcer	
	C. Marjolin's ulcer	
	D. Decubitus ulcer	
	E. Pyro ulcer	

Her right arm with total circumferential burn loses the radial pulse.	The best treatment option at this time is:	**Answer: C** (see p. 170)
	A. Increase intravascular volume	
	B. Steroids IV	
	C. Escharotomy of the entire right arm	
	D. Fasciotomy of the entire right arm	
	E. DDAVP	

On hospital day#5, she undergoes split-thickness skin grafts.	The skin grafts live for the first 24 hours by a process called:	**Answer: B** (see p. 173)
	A. Osmosis	
	B. Imbibition	
	C. Capillary ingrowth	
	D. Deceased donor nutrition	

A 34-year-old male presents to his PCP with c/o face redness and heat as well as chronic diarrhea. He is afebrile at the visit.

He develops lower extremity edema, and echo reveals right-sided heart failure.	This classic triad is c/w what diagnosis?	**Answer: C** (see p. 206)
	A. Pheochromocytoma	
	B. Glucagonoma	
	C. Carcinoid syndrome	
	D. Cushing's triad	
	E. Nesidioma	

| The PCP orders a urine screen. | Which lab urine test would help confirm the diagnosis? | Answer: D (see p. 207) |

A. Epinephrine
B. Norepinephrine
C. Dopamine
D. Urine 5-HIAA
E. Sodium

| The PCP also orders a serum test. | Which serum lab will support the diagnosis? | Answer: E (see p. 207) |

A. Epinephrine
B. Norepinephrine
C. Dopamine
D. 5-HIAA
E. Serotonin

| The PCP orders a liver ultrasound. | It will show: | Answer: D (see p. 243) |

A. Gallstones
B. Choledocholithiasis
C. AV fistula
D. Multiple metastatic disease
E. Multiple cysts

| The PCP starts a medication for diarrhea and refers the patient to a specialist. | What is the first medication used to treat this patient's diarrhea? | Answer: D (see p. 206) |

A. Amlodipine
B. Vasopressin
C. Lisinopril
D. Zofran

| The patient develops emesis and SBO. | The most likely site of GI involvement with this disease is: | Answer: F (see p. 208) |

A. Stomach
B. Esophagus
C. Rectum
D. Jejunum
E. Ileum
F. Appendix

| The patient sees a specialist who orders an IV medication to treat the "syndrome" associated with this diagnosis. | What medication can treat the syndrome? | Answer: E (see p. 208) |

A. Amlodipine
B. Vasopressin
C. Lisinopril
D. Zofran
E. Octreotide

A 44-year-old male presents with a 2-day history of emesis and "abd getting really big." He has never had an operation, has no fever or diarrhea, and there is no sickness in the family.

Abdominal x-ray reveals dilated bowel and "air–fluid levels."	These x-ray findings can be seen with all of the following EXCEPT: A. Rapid replacement of hyponatremia B. Partial and complete bowel obstruction C. Colon obstruction D. Hypokalemia E. Ileus	**Answer: A** (see p. 73)
The patient continues to vomit. He is hydrated IV, electrolytes are corrected, and the stomach is decompressed with an NGT.	The best way to tell if this partial versus complete obstruction is to order: A. Gastrografin enema B. EGD C. Abd/pelvis CT scan with PO contrast D. Colonoscopy E. Repeat abdominal x-rays to follow air–fluid level size	**Answer: C** (see p. 200)
The diagnosis of complete small bowel obstruction is made, and he now has a fever, leukocytosis, and intense abdominal pain without peritoneal signs.	What is the best thing to do? A. ICU for an arterial line and blood pressure monitoring B. IV antibiotics with Gm– and anaerobic coverage and serial clinical examinations C. Emergent angio of the mesenteric vessels D. Emergent ex lap E. STAT MRI	**Answer: D** (see p. 164)
Several days later, the patient develops hypokalemia and an ileus. After several IV KCl supplements, the potassium level goes down.	This refractory hypokalemia can be caused by all of the following EXCEPT: A. Hypomagnesemia B. Acidosis C. Renal failure D. Excessive NGT drainage E. Severe diarrhea	**Answer: B** (see p. 72)

A 44-year-old male with multiple episodes of gastric and duodenal ulcers develops recent weight loss.

He has also developed a perforated ulcer in his proximal Ileum.	Due to the refractory nature of his PUD and the unusual ulcer in the Ileum, which diagnosis first comes to mind? A. Insulinoma B. Glucagonoma C. Zollinger–Ellison syndrome D. Carcinoid syndrome E. Somatostatinoma	**Answer: C** (see p. 74)

The physician orders a secretin challenge test.

This test will result in an elevated lab value for which hormone if the diagnosis is correct?

A. Insulin
B. Glucagon
C. Serotonin
D. Somatostatin
E. Gastrin

Answer: E
(see p. 132)

To rule out MEN-I, a test must be screened.

What is the best initial screen for MEN-I?

A. Glucose
B. Gallstones
C. Calcium level
D. Somatostatin
E. Glucagon

Answer: C
(see p. 306)

The physical orders a test to localize the tumor.

What is a special scan that can help localize a gastrinoma?

A. Secretin scan
B. Gastrin-131 scan
C. Octreotide scan
D. Glucagon-131 scan
E. Insulin-130 scan

Answer: C
(see p. 307)

The scan reveals a tumor.

Looking at percentages, where is the most likely location of a gastrinoma tumor in Z-E syndrome?

A. Duodenum
B. Jejunum
C. Appendix
D. Pancreas
E. Spleen
F. Liver

Answer: A
(see p. 307)

A newborn develops vomiting. The vomitus is bilious (green).

An abdominal x-ray is taken, revealing a "double bubble" sign.

The double bubble sign reveals gas in the:

A. Colon and rectum
B. Stomach and rectum
C. Colon and small bowel
D. Duodenum and stomach
E. Rectum and small bowel

Answer: D
(see p. 384)

The patient is otherwise in no acute distress with normal vital signs. Further review of the abdominal x-ray reveals no gas in the small intestine or colon.	All the following are in the differential diagnosis EXCEPT: A. Annular pancreas B. Malrotation C. Duodenal atresia D. Hirschsprung's disease E. Intestinal atresia	Answer: D (see p. 386)
One diagnosis has a high mortality if it is missed.	The most likely life-threatening diagnosis is: A. Malrotation B. Renal cell carcinoma C. Medulloblastoma D. Ewing's syndrome E. Annular pancreas	Answer: A (see p. 388)
A quick diagnosis or "rule-out diagnosis" of this pathology is paramount.	The best and quickest study is: A. MRI B. PET scan C. Gastrografin enema D. RUQ ultrasound	Answer: C (see p. 223)
The contrast enema is normal, and an upper GI contrast study is undertaken that reveals duodenal atresia. The genotype returns as trisomy 21.	The next diagnostic test to get is: A. Vascular duplex of upper extremities B. HIDA scan C. Cardiac echocardiogram D. Brain CT E. Angiogram	Answer: C (see p. 470)

A 56-year-old male presents to his PCP with a chief complaint of headaches and "massive sweating" at times. He is adopted, so does not know his family history. He takes no medications. The headaches are getting progressively worse and now he thinks he is also having "panic attacks with racing of his heart."

His blood pressure in the office is checked twice and is 223/134.	What is the first diagnostic test to get from the lab? A. Cannabinoids screen B. Caffeine level C. Metanephrine level D. Serotonin level	Answer: C (see p. 300)
The lab test comes back very high.	What is the most likely diagnosis? A. Substance abuse B. Pheochromocytoma C. Renal artery stenosis D. Cushing's disease	Answer: B (see p. 299)

| The patient feels very hot and anxious and says his head is pounding with each heartbeat. | What is the immediate treatment for this patient?

A. Diuretic Lasix
B. ACE inhibitor
C. Benzodiazepines and antiserotonin blocker
D. β-Blocker and an α-blocker | **Answer: D**
(see p. 301) |

A 43-year-old obese female with three children undergoes an MRI for chronic back pain. Gallstones are found incidentally.

She has no family history of gallstones.	All of the following are risk factors for gallstones EXCEPT: A. Obesity B. Multiparous C. Hemolysis D. Female E. Weight loss F. High-fat diet	**Answer: F** (see p. 259)
Her PCP gives her the diagnosis of "asymptomatic gallstones."	The best treatment for her new diagnosis is: A. Percutaneous transhepatic cholangiography (PTC) B. Percutaneous cholecystostomy tube C. Laparoscopic cholecystectomy D. Weight loss E. Observation	**Answer: E** (see p. 260)
A year later she develops intermittent RUQ pain that radiates to her back after eating a fatty meal.	The best treatment option is: A. Percutaneous transhepatic cholangiography (PTC) B. Percutaneous cholecystostomy tube C. Laparoscopic cholecystectomy D. Weight loss E. Observation	**Answer: C** (see p. 273)
Her planned procedure is canceled, and a month later she develops constant, unrelenting RUQ pain, emesis, and a fever.	The best diagnostic test is: A. MRI B. CT C. Ultrasound D. PTC	**Answer: C** (see p. 247)
The diagnostic test reveals gallstones, a thickened gallbladder wall, and pericholecystic fluid.	The most likely diagnosis is: A. Choledocholithiasis B. Cholangitis C. Gallbladder cancer D. Acute cholecystitis E. Cholangiocarcinoma	**Answer: D** (see p. 261)

The diagnosis is confirmed.	The best treatment of her condition is: A. PTC B. ERCP C. Percutaneous cholecystostomy tube D. Laparoscopic cholecystectomy E. Open common bile duct exploration F. Liver resection	**Answer: D** (see p. 273)
Post procedure, she develops elevated bilirubin, and an MRCP reveals a gallstone in the distal common bile duct.	This condition is called: A. Choledocholithiasis B. Cholangitis C. Gallbladder cancer D. Acute cholecystitis E. Cholangiocarcinoma	**Answer: A** (see p. 260)
She requires another procedure to prevent obstruction of the duct.	The best procedure to remove this gallstone is: A. PTC B. ERCP C. Percutaneous cholecystostomy tube D. Laparoscopic cholecystectomy E. Open common bile duct exploration F. Liver resection	**Answer: B** (see p. 260)
On the study, a leak from the cystic duct (cystic duct leak) is found.	The treatment for this is: A. PTC (across sphincter) B. ERCP with stent placement across sphincter C. Percutaneous cholecystostomy tube D. Laparoscopic cholecystectomy with stent E. Open common bile duct exploration F. Liver resection	**Answer: B** (see p. 257)
Postprocedure CT scan reveals a large fluid collection in the RUQ (biloma).	The best treatment is: A. Emergent exploratory laparotomy B. Emergent laparoscopic drainage C. PTC D. ERCP with transduodenal drainage E. Percutaneous drain placement	**Answer: E** (see p. 274)

A 43-year-old female undergoes a gastric bypass for morbid obesity. Postoperatively, she develops tachycardia, severe abdominal pain, and hypotension.

A blood gas (ABG) is obtained: pH is 7.21, PaO_2 is 134 mm Hg, $PaCO_2$ is 37 mm Hg, and base deficit (BD) is −9 mEq/L.	This is most consistent with: A. Metabolic alkalosis B. Metabolic acidosis C. Respiratory alkalosis D. Respiratory acidosis	**Answer: B** (see p. 343)

She is taken to the O.R. for ex lap revealing a leak in an anastomosis. She awakens postoperatively with agitation and tachypnea. ABG reveals pH 7.56, PaO$_2$ of 156 mm Hg, PCO$_2$ of 20 mm Hg, and BD of 1 mEq/L.	This is most likely: A. Metabolic alkalosis B. Metabolic acidosis C. Respiratory alkalosis D. Respiratory acidosis	**Answer: C** (see p. 343)
She is heavily sedated and placed on pressure support to wean the ventilator. ABG reveals pH of 7.25, PaO$_2$ of 167 mm Hg, PaCO$_2$ of 67 mm Hg, and BD −1 mEq/L.	This is most consistent with: A. Metabolic alkalosis B. Metabolic acidosis C. Respiratory alkalosis D. Respiratory acidosis	**Answer: D** (see p. 343)
Postoperatively, she has massive NGT output. ABG reveals pH of 7.54, PaO$_2$ of 178 mm Hg, PaCO$_2$ of 41 mm Hg, and BD of +6 mEq/L.	This is most consistent with: A. Metabolic alkalosis B. Metabolic acidosis C. Respiratory alkalosis D. Respiratory acidosis	**Answer: A** (see p. 343)
One week postoperatively, she develops acute SOB and a swollen left leg. ABG reveals pH of 7.56, PaO$_2$ of 54 mm Hg, PCO$_2$ of 25 mm Hg, and BD of −2 mEq/L.	This is consistent with: A. Anastomotic leak B. Pneumonia C. Pulmonary embolism D. Myocardial infarction	**Answer: C** (see p. 90)
She develops hypoxia. FiO$_2$ is 100%, and PaO$_2$ is 66 mm Hg.	What might improve oxygenation? A. Increase tidal volume B. Increase respiratory rate (RR) C. Increase PEEP D. Add hypertonic saline E. Decrease tidal volume	**Answer: C** (see p. 517)
She remains sedated. ABG reveals pH of 7.21, PaO$_2$ of 178 mm Hg, and PCO$_2$ of 66 mm Hg.	What would normalize the pH? A. Increase PEEP B. Increase FiO$_2$ C. Increase RR D. Increase intravascular volume	**Answer: C** (see p. 347)

The patient continues to have acidosis. ABG reveals pH of 7.24, PaO$_2$ of 145 mm Hg, and PCO$_2$ of 55 mm Hg, and RR is 30 breaths/min.	What might help bring up the pH? A. Increase PEEP B. Increase FiO$_2$ C. Increase tidal volume D. Decrease RR	**Answer: C** (see p. 347)

A 23-year-old female snowboarding for the second time loses control and goes over a 40-feet cliff. When the ski patrol finds her, she is awake and talking, and she tells them she does not remember much except awaking covered by snow. She states, "I don't feel right," so the ski patrol brings her to the small full-service ER at the base of the mountain.

In the ER, she feels faint and then becomes completely unarousable.	A period of being awake after an initial loss of consciousness right after a TBI event, followed by a loss of consciousness after a period of time is termed: A. Rhythmic consciousness B. Lucid interval C. Episodic wakefulness D. Alternating GCS	**Answer: B** (see p. 518)
The patient is rapidly intubated to protect her airway.	Classic GCS indication for intubation is: A. GCS ≤12 B. GCS ≤10 C. GCS ≤9 D. GCS ≤8	**Answer: D** (see p. 155)
The patient is now intubated, sedated, and stable.	The best initial radiology test to evaluate brain injury is: A. X-ray for skull fx B. CT scan with contrast C. CT scan without IV contrast D. MRI	**Answer: C** (see p. 530)
CT scan shows a "lenticular" (lens-shaped) hematoma.	This is most likely a/an: A. Epidural hematoma B. Subdural hematoma C. DAI (diffuse axonal injury) D. IPH (intraparenchymal hemorrhage)	**Answer: A** (see p. 518)
CT also shows a crescent-shaped hematoma.	This is most likely a: A. DAI B. IPH C. Subdural hematoma D. IVH (intraventricular hematoma)	**Answer: C** (see p. 519)

On CT, there is a 12-mm midline shift, and the patient's GCS is now 3.	What is the definitive treatment? A. Ventriculostomy B. CSF drainage C. Craniectomy D. Lumbar puncture and ICP monitoring	**Answer: C** (see p. 518)

A 38-year-old male develops "brittle" diabetes, and he also has weight loss.

He then develops a lower extremity skin condition with redness and something almost like "psoriasis."	The first thing that comes to mind is: A. Somatostatinoma B. Pancreatic cancer C. Insulinoma D. Glucagonoma	**Answer: D** (see p. 305)
The patient really wants the skin condition to go away.	To treat this skin condition, the PCP recommends: A. Zinc and somatostatin B. Zinc and glucagon C. Zinc and cyproheptadine D. Zinc and ondansetron	**Answer: A** (see p. 305)
The PCP sends the patient to an endocrinologist.	The first localization study she orders is a/an: A. Gallbladder ultrasound B. HIDA scan C. CT scan of the abdomen D. CT scan of the pelvis E. Angiogram of the celiac vessels	**Answer: C** (see p. 305)
The tumor is localized.	The most likely anatomic location of this tumor is the: A. Head of the pancreas B. Tail of the pancreas C. Liver D. Spleen E. Gallbladder	**Answer: B** (see p. 305)
Treatment is needed.	The treatment of this tumor is: A. Chemotherapy B. Radiation therapy C. Both chemo and radiation therapy D. Whipple procedure E. Resection of the tail of the pancreas	**Answer: E** (see p. 277)
The pathology comes back.	The most likely tissue diagnosis is: A. Insulinoma B. Somatostatinoma C. Glucagonoma D. Gastrinoma E. Carcinoid	**Answer: C** (see p. 305)

A 27-year-old male was helping offload pallets from a forklift when the driver inadvertently pushed the gas pedal and pinned the patient's left lower leg against the wall, creating a severe closed crush injury. X-ray reveals a fibular fracture. On examination, his skin is intact, and his DP and PT pulses are palpable and 2/2.

Over time, the pain in the left lower leg is getting worse, but the pulses are still 2/2.	The presence of the distal pulses makes compartment syndrome an impossibility: A. True B. False	**Answer: B** (see p. 358)
On physical examination, the left lower leg feels "tight."	What is the classic physical finding associated with this compartment syndrome? A. Drop Tine test B. Numbness with active extension C. Pain on passive foot flexion D. Pain with knee flexion	**Answer: C** (see p. 358)
The orthopedic surgeon asks for an objective evaluation for compartment syndrome.	The best objective test for compartment syndrome is: A. Needle compartment pressures B. Check venous O_2 sats C. Muscle biopsy D. Ankle–brachial pressure index	**Answer: A** (see p. 358)
The pain persists, and the objective and clinical findings are c/w compartment syndrome.	The definitive treatment for lower extremity compartment syndrome is: A. Lasix diuresis B. Fibulectomy C. Percutaneous drain placement D. Four-compartment fasciotomy	**Answer: D** (see p. 358)

A 25-year-old male with a GSW to RUQ is admitted to the ER with a SBP of 70/palp. He is taken straight to the O.R. for an ex lap.

His next blood pressure is 60/palp.	The best IV resuscitation fluids include: A. Albumin B. Normal saline C. PRBCs and FFP D. Hypertonic saline	**Answer: C** (see p. 79)
Labs return with a fibrinogen of 50.	The best way to replace fibrinogen is: A. FFP B. Platelets C. Saline D. Cryoprecipitate	**Answer: D** (see p. 79)

His platelets are 20,000 postop.	The best way to improve platelets is with: A. FFP B. Platelets C. Saline D. Cryoprecipitate	**Answer: B** (see p. 79)
He has now received multiple blood and blood products.	What electrolyte need to be checked? A. Phosphorus B. Magnesium C. Ionized calcium D. Sodium	**Answer: C** (see p. 79)
Upon further information, the patient was on Coumadin for a DVT preinjury.	The best treatment option is: A. FFP B. Calcium C. Vitamin K D. PCC (Kcentra)	**Answer: D** (see p. 87)
Postoperatively, his HGB is 5.8.	What is the best treatment option? A. FFP B. DDAVP C. PRBCs D. Platelets	**Answer: C** (see p. 79)
It also now known that he was on hemodialysis three times a week.	The option to make his platelets work is: A. Glucagon B. DDAVP C. Calcium D. Methylprednisolone E. Somatostatin	**Answer: B** (see p. 80)
End points of resuscitation include pH and base deficit.	What other end point of resuscitation is needed? A. Lactic acid B. Procalcitonin C. WBC D. Somatostatin E. Glucagon	**Answer: A** (see p. 68)
He continues to ooze.	To increase von Willebrand's factor, what must be transfused? A. FFP B. Somatostatin C. PRBCs D. Cryoprecipitate E. Methylprednisolone	**Answer: D** (see p. 79)

A 30-year-old female breaks her finger in a car door. On x-ray in the local ER, the radiologist comments "subperiosteal bone resorption."

The patient relates a history of pancreatitis and kidney stones.	What is her most likely diagnosis? A. Hyperthyroidism B. Glucagonoma C. Addison's disease D. Hyperparathyroidism	Answer: D (see p. 132)
She also has a history of duodenal ulcers refractory to high-dose PPIs.	What diagnosis does this history prompt? A. Insulinoma B. Somatostatinoma C. Glucagonoma D. Hyperparathyroidism E. Gastrinoma	Answer: E (see p. 133)
She develops loss of peripheral vision and intermittent lactation.	This brings to mind: A. Carotid vascular atherosclerosis B. Diabetes C. Prolactinoma D. Somatostatinoma E. Glucagonoma	Answer: C (see p. 295)
The clinician steps back and sees all three of these diagnoses together.	The most likely endocrine disorder is: A. Pancreatic cancer B. Multiple endocrine neoplasia I C. Conn's syndrome D. Addison's disease E. Somatostatinoma	Answer: B (see p. 306)
Her calcium and parathyroid hormone levels are very elevated.	What is the most likely cause of her hyperparathyroidism? A. Parathyroid cancer B. Parathyroid hyperplasia C. Dialysis-dependent renal failure D. Parathyroid adenoma E. Familial hypocalciuric hypercalcemia	Answer: B (see p. 311)
For the hyperplasia, she underwent four-gland resection.	What else must be done? A. Place 30 mg of parathyroid tissue into forearm B. Iodine-131 nuclear ablation C. Thiazide diuretic D. Neck radiation	Answer: A (see p. 326)

A 25-year-old male is involved in a baseball bat and knife attack. He used his right hand and forearm for protection. He has lacerations in his forearm and multiple lacerations over the fingers.

He cannot feel any sensation in his fifth finger (pinky).	Which nerve is most likely injured? A. Radial B. Ulnar C. Medial D. Musculocutaneous E. Digital	**Answer: B** (see p. 439)
On further examination, he cannot flex his middle (third) finger at the DIP joint.	This most likely represents an injury to which ligament? A. Extensor digitorum B. Flexor digitorum superficialis C. Profundis flexorum D. Flexor digitorum profundus E. Collateral ligament	**Answer: D** (see p. 411)
His second digit "drops" and cannot be extended at the MP joint.	This most likely represents injury to which ligament? A. Extensor ligament B. Flexor digitorum superficialis C. Profundis flexorum D. Flexor digitorum profundus E. Collateral ligament	**Answer: A** (see p. 413)
On further examination, he cannot feel any sensation on the tip of his thumb.	This represents injury to what nerve? A. Radial B. Ulnar C. Median D. Musculocutaneous E. Digital	**Answer: C** (see p. 415)
The index finger of his left hand has flexion at the PIP joint and extension at his DIP joint. He cannot straighten this finger.	This most likely represents a: A. Gamekeeper's finger deformity B. Jersey finger deformity C. Boutonnière deformity D. Mallet finger deformity E. Dupuytren's deformity	**Answer: C** (see p. 413)
This diagnosis is confirmed.	It is most likely due to laceration of the: A. PIP extensor ligament B. Flexor digitorum superficialis C. Profundis flexorum D. Flexor digitorum profundus E. Collateral ligament F. DIP extensor ligament	**Answer: A** (see p. 410)

A 28-year-old male involved in a MCC presents with HR 120 and SBP of 110.

On examination, his right leg is shorter than the left leg and is internally rotated. A stat pelvis x-ray is taken.	The x-ray will most likely show: A. Anterior hip dislocation B. Posterior hip dislocation C. Femoral neck fx D. Proximal femur fx E. Pubic rami fractures	**Answer: B** (see p. 159)
The patient is in terrible pain.	The next step after the primary survey is: A. Reposition the hip on the ER table B. Buck's traction C. Lidocaine into lumbar roots D. Valium IV	**Answer: A** (see p. 368)
The patient then develops an HR of 140, and his SBP is 82/palp. Further review of the pelvis x-ray reveals a widened symphysis pubis.	The best action is starting blood transfusions and also: A. Manual compression of the abdominal aorta B. High proximal tourniquet C. Placement of a pelvic binder D. Buck's traction	**Answer: C** (see p. 161)
His blood pressure is now 130/83, HR 110, and FAST negative. He receives chest and pelvic x-rays.	The next diagnostic test is: A. Angiogram of the leg B. Doppler of the leg C. ABIs D. CT scans E. HIDA scan	**Answer: D** (see p. 97)
The patient is now hemodynamically normal. On extremity examination, he has an open right tib/fib fracture with exposed bone.	The next step in treatment is: A. NS bolus B. Dakin's irrigation C. IV antibiotics D. Betadine irrigation	**Answer: C** (see p. 115)
No other injuries are identified, and the patient has normal vital signs.	The next step in this patient's care involves: A. IV steroids B. O.R. for irrigation and débridement C. Kyphoplasty D. IV vasopressin	**Answer: B** (see p. 48)

A 44-year-old male develops painless hematuria.

He reports smoking 2 packs of cigarettes a day.	Due to the smoking, what is the first diagnosis that comes to mind? A. AV malformation B. Urethral neoplasm C. Bladder cancer D. Renal cell carcinoma	**Answer: C** (see p. 533)
The diagnosis needs to be confirmed or ruled out.	What is the best test to rule out this diagnosis? A. Ultrasound B. PET scan C. MRI D. Cystoscopy	**Answer: D** (see p. 546)
More testing is needed.	The first radiology test to workup painless hematuria is: A. MRI B. CT scan with IV contrast C. Ultrasound D. HIDA scan E. PET scan	**Answer: B** (see p. 245)
A CT scan reveals a right kidney mass with tumor extension into the IVC.	These findings are classic for which tumor? A. Renal cell carcinoma B. Transitional cell carcinoma C. Ureter neoplasm D. Ewing's carcinoma E. Sarcoma	**Answer: A** (see p. 532)
During resection in the O.R. the patient gets severely hypoxic. This hypoxia is refractory to 100% oxygen and high PEEP.	This is most likely due to: A. DVT B. Tumor embolus C. Urine embolus D. Air embolus	**Answer: B** (see p. 258)

Two college roommates go camping in a national forest. They both complain of spider bites. The first patient c/o severe abdominal pain, nausea, vomiting, and chills.

This patient killed the spider and placed it into a ziplock bag.	It most likely will have which of the following characteristics? A. Red hourglass shape on the abdomen B. Violin shape on the thorax C. Yellow egg sac on the abdomen D. Furry legs E. Purple dot on the head	**Answer: A** (see p. 166)

The second patient has a 3-cm very painful red area with a blister in the middle. He also killed the spider.	This spider will most likely have which of the following characteristics? A. Red hourglass shape on the abdomen B. Violin shape on the thorax C. Yellow egg sac on the abdomen D. Furry legs E. Purple dot on the head	**Answer: B** (see p. 165)
The spider in the first patient was identified by its markings.	It is identified as a: A. Brown recluse B. Tarantula C. Black widow D. Wolf spider E. Hobo spider	**Answer: C** (see p. 166)
Due to the patient's severe symptoms of abdominal pain and muscle cramps, the physician decides to treat him aggressively.	This treatment would include: A. Clonidine B. Antivenom C. Dexamethasone D. Calcium channel blocker	**Answer: B** (see p. 166)
The spider that bit the second patient with the painful red blister is also identified by its markings.	The most like identification is: A. Brown recluse B. Tarantula C. Black widow D. Wolf spider E. Hobo spider	**Answer: A** (see p. 165)
Due to the progressing erythema and blister in the second patient, the physician elects to treat this bite aggressively.	Treatment includes diphenhydramine and: A. Dexamethasone B. Dantrolene C. Dapsone D. Demerol	**Answer: C** (see p. 165)

A 42-year-old female presents to her PCP with c/o new onset of weight gain, acne, a fat bump on her upper back, and purple streaks on her lower abdomen. Her random glucose is 355, and her BP is 178/98.

She has been on no medications for years.	This clinical presentation is most c/w which of the following? A. Addison's disease B. Carcinoid syndrome C. Zollinger–Ellison syndrome D. Cushing's syndrome	**Answer: D** (see p. 297)

The PCP orders a screening test.	The most appropriate initial test is: A. Gastrin level B. Serotonin level C. Urine 17-OHCS D. Insulin	**Answer: C** (see p. 298)
The test comes back elevated.	The next test to differentiate normal versus abnormal cortisol production is the: A. Low-dose insulin B. Low-dose vasopressin C. Low-dose secretin D. Low-dose dexamethasone	**Answer: D** (see p. 298)
The study comes back with an elevated cortisol.	The next study to differentiate a pituitary versus ectopic ACTH source is: A. High-dose dexamethasone B. High-dose secretin C. High-dose insulin D. High-dose vasopressin stimulation test	**Answer: A** (see p. 298)
The high-dose test results in a much lower cortisol level.	This result is c/w: A. Small oat cell lung tumor B. Carcinoid tumor C. Pituitary source D. Ectopic source	**Answer: C** (see p. 298)
The patient cannot see in her peripheral vision.	A brain CT and MRI most likely reveals a: A. Pituitary gland mass B. Pituitary AVM C. Cerebellum mass D. Middle cerebellar artery aneurysm	**Answer: A** (see p. 298)
The patient is referred to a neurosurgeon.	The surgeon recommends what procedure? A. Craniotomy and cerebellum resection B. Interventional neuroradiology aneurysm coiling C. Craniotomy and aneurysm clipping D. Coiling of AVM E. Transsphenoidal adenomectomy	**Answer: E** (see p. 311)

Index

Note: Page locators followed by f indicates figure.